THE CIRCULATION

Fetus and Neonate: Physiology and Clinical Applications

Volume 1: The Circulation

THE CIRCULATION

Edited by
MARK A. HANSON
JOHN A. D. SPENCER
CHARLES H. RODECK

Department of Obstetrics and Gynaecology, University College and Middlesex School of Medicine, London

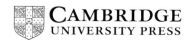

CAMBRIDGE
UNIVERSITY PRESS

Published by the Press Syndicate of the University of Cambridge
The Pitt Building, Trumpington Street, Cambridge CB2 1RP
40 West 20th Street, New York, NY 10011-4211, USA
10 Stamford Road, Oakleigh, Melbourne 3166, Australia

First published 1993

Printed in Great Britain at the University Press, Cambridge

A catalogue record for this book is available from the British Library

Library of Congress cataloguing in publication data

Fetus and neonate : physiology and clinical applications/edited by Mark A. Hanson,
John A. D. Spencer, Charles H. Rodeck.
p. cm.
Includes index.
Contents: v. 1. Circulation.
ISBN 0 521 41187 4 (hc : v. 1). – ISBN 0 521 42327 9 (pb : v. 1)
1. Fetus – Physiology.   2. Fetus – Diseases – Pathophysiology.
3. Infants (Newborn) – Physiology.   4. Infants (Newborn) – diseases –
Pathophysiology.   I. Hanson, Mark A.   II. Spencer, John A. D.
III. Rodeck, Charles. H.
[DNLM: 1. Fetus – physiology.   2. Infant, Newborn – physiology.
WD210.5 F4217]
RG610.F48 1993
618.3'2 – dc20
DNLM/DLC
for library of congress   92-13559   CIP

ISBN 0 521 41187 4 hardback
ISBN 0 521 42327 9 paperback

Contents

Preface to the series

The factual burden of a science varies inversely with its degree of maturity
P. Medawar 'Two Conceptions of Science': 'Anglo-Saxon Attitudes',
Henry Tizard Memorial Lecture, Encounter 143, August 1965

The idea for a series on the applications of Fetal and Neonatal Physiology to Clinical Medicine came from the need of our students for something intermediate between a textbook and review articles. Textbooks provide breadth of coverage but tend to lack critical discussion. Reviews can provide such discussion but represent the view of one authority and may need a balance. For the student, such reviews are not a substitute for original papers and are better taken after consumption of a full course of such papers rather than as an hors d'oeuvres to them.

We envisage the readership of the series as 'students' of the subject in the widest sense, from undergraduates learning about fetal and neonatal physiology as part of a basic science degree or preclinical medical students, to postgraduate and postdoctoral scientists and clinicians specializing in obstetrics, neonatology or paediatrics. We decided that all needs would best be met by producing a series of multiauthored volumes. This will allow rapid production of short texts that will keep the material focused whilst still allowing the subject to be reviewed from several points of view. None the less, we have decided to adopt a 'systems' approach because it has the advantages of simplicity and conformity to textbooks of physiology.

The chapters in each volume of the series are arranged in sections: Physiology, Pathophysiology and Clinical Applications. They are not intended to be all-inclusive but rather to demonstrate the applications of basic scientific research to clinical medicine via improved understanding of pathophysiological processes.

The series concentrates on late fetal and neonatal life (the perinatal period). In late gestation the fetus must have established the mechanisms which will permit it to make the transition to becoming a neonate, whilst still being highly adapted to the peculiar intrauterine environment in which it remains. The importance of making the transition successfully is underlined by the fact that this is one of the most dangerous periods of human life. In the course of it, some physiological processes continue, whilst others cease to function, undergo drastic change, or are initiated. The understanding of the underlying controlling processes constitutes one of the greatest challenges in physiology.

Our feeling that such a series is necessary has been reinforced by the increasing number of students who are keen to learn more about this fascinating area. They are aware of the possibility of obtaining biological information from the human fetus using non-invasive methods, but as they see the difficulties of interpreting such information in clinical practice, they perceive the need for a greater understanding of fundamental physiological processes. We hope that this series will stimulate some of them to take up research in this field.

Finally, the series stands for two things which seem temporarily out of fashion. First, by illustrating the clinical applications of basic research, it demonstrates how advances in modern medicine are based on animal research. We cannot, in setting out to improve the care of the human fetus or neonate, have one without the other. Secondly, we believe and teach that the knowledge gained using techniques from a range of disciplines (biochemistry, molecular biology, physics etc.) must ultimately be integrated into concepts of how the body works as a whole. Such integration is precisely the realm of physiology; nowhere is the power of the method more clearly evident than in the fetus and neonate. This synthesis into a whole is not to generalize, but to push our understanding to greater depths.

Mark Hanson
John Spencer
Charles Rodeck

University College London

Acknowledgements

MAH is indebted to the Wellcome Trust who have supported his research in fetal and neonatal physiology through some lean years for science in the UK. Dr Richard Barling encouraged us to develop the series and both he and Isla Fraser at Cambridge University Press have been extremely helpful and considerate. Finally we are indebted to Jinette Newns who undertook the painstaking work of preparing the manuscript of Volume One of the series in a cheerful and efficient manner.

Contributors

L. D. Allan
Department of Perinatal Cardiology, 15th Floor, Guy's Tower, St Thomas's Street, London SE1 9RT, UK.

D. J. P. Barker
Medical Research Council, Environmental Epidemiology Unit, Southampton General Hospital, Southampton SO9 4XY, UK.

R. Berger
R. Klinikum der Justus Liebig, Universität Giessen, Klinikstraße 32, 6300 Giessen, Germany.

A. D. Bocking
Department of Obstetrics and Gynecology, St Joseph's Hospital, 268 Grosvenor Street, London, Ontario N6A 4V2, Canada.

R. A. Brace
Department of Reproductive Medicine H-813, University of California, San Diego, California 92103, USA.

A. M. Carter
The Lawson Research Institute, The University of Western Ontario, 268 Grosvenor Street, London, Ontario N6A 4V2, Canada.

J. M. Dunn
Pediatric Heart Institute, St Christopher's Hospital for Children, Philadelphia, Pennsylvania 18134-1095, USA.

A. D. Edwards
Department of Paediatrics, University College and Middlesex School of Medicine, University College London, The Rayne Institute, University Street, London WC1E 6JJ, UK.

M. A. Hanson
Departments of Obstetrics & Gynaecology and Physiology, University College and Middlesex School of Medicine, University College London, 86–96 Chenies Mews, London WC1X 6HE, UK.

S. G. Haworth
Department of Paediatric Cardiology, Institute of Child Health, University of London, 30 Guilford Street, London WC1N 1EH.

M. A. Heymann
Department of Pediatrics, Cardiovascular Research Institute, School of Medicine, University of California, San Fransisco, California, USA.

H. S. Iwamoto
Department of Pediatrics, University of Cincinnati Medical Center, 231 Bethesda Avenue ML 541, Cincinnati, Ohio 45267-0541, USA.

A. Jensen
Klinikum der Justus Liebig, Universität Giessen, Klinikstraße 32, 6300 Giessen, Germany.

C. M. Law
Medical Research Council, Environmental Epidemiology Unit, Southampton General Hospital, Southampton, SO9 4XY, UK.

K. Maršál
Department of Obstetrics and Gynecology, General Hospital, S-214 01 Malmö, Sweden.

M. J. Morton
Department of Physiology, School of Medicine, Oregon Health Sciences University, 3181 SW Sam Jackson Park Road, Portland, Oregon 97201-3098, USA.

E. O. R. Reynolds
Department of Paediatrics, University College and Middlesex School of Medicine, University College London, The Rayne Institute, University Street, London WC1E 6JJ, UK.

P. Russo
Pediatric Heart Institute, St Christopher's Hospital for Children, Philadelphia, Pennsylvania 18134-1095, USA.

S. J. Soifer
Department of Pediatrics, Cardiovascular Research Institute, School of Medicine, University of California, San Fransisco, California, USA.

J. A. D. Spencer
Department of Obstetrics and Gynaecology, University College and Middlesex School of Medicine, University College London, 86–96 Chenies Mews, London WC1X 6HE, UK.

K. L. Thornburg
Department of Physiology, School of Medicine, Oregon Health Sciences University, 3181 SW Sam Jackson Park Road, Portland, Oregon 97201-3098, USA.

B. J. Trudinger
Department of Obstetrics and Gynaecology, Westmead Hospital, Westmead, NSW 2145, Australia.

A. M. Walker
Centre for Early Human Development, Monash Medical Centre, 24 Clayton Road, Clayton, Melbourne, Victoria 3168, Australia.

S. R. Weil
Pediatric Heart Institute, St Christopher's Hospital for Children, Philadelphia, Pennsylvania 18134-1095, USA.

T. Wheeler
Department of Human Reproduction and Obstetrics, Princess Anne Hospital, Coxford Road, Southampton SO9 4HA, UK.

J. S. Wyatt
Department of Paediatrics, University College and Middlesex School of Medicine, University College London, The Rayne Institute, University Street, London WC1E 6JJ, UK.

C. E. Wood
Department of Physiology, University of Florida College of Medicine, Gainseville, Florida 32610-0274, USA.

Physiology

1

The control of heart rate and blood pressure in the fetus: theoretical considerations

MARK A. HANSON

Introduction

The well-known interaction between arterial blood pressure and heart rate (via the baroreflex) in the adult provides the rationale for considering these two components of the fetal circulation together. In fact, much understanding of the control of the fetal circulation has come from attempts to extrapolate knowledge of circulatory control in the adult back to the fetus. Circulatory reflexes are more fully reviewed elsewhere (Hanson, 1989). The aim of this chapter is to review briefly the processes which determine fetal heart rate and arterial pressure, and to discuss the interaction between the two variables and the underlying physiological processes which determine it. Newer methods for measuring these variables are discussed, with particular reference to the clinical importance of understanding disturbances in them under pathophysiological conditions.

Determinants of heart rate

As in the adult, a plethora of factors act on the fetal heart to maintain its rate above the intrinsic rate of the sino-atrial node. Neural factors act directly on the sino-atrial node via the vagus and sympathetic nerves in the late gestation sheep fetus (Mott & Walker, 1983; Martin, 1985; Hanson, 1989) and indirectly via the release of catecholamines from the adrenal medulla (Jones & Robinson, 1975). These neural effects, which can form the efferent limb of reflex control of heart rate, appear to play a relatively small role in mid-gestation (see Chapter 8). In late gestation, hypoxia or asphyxia (whether produced by maternal inhalation of a hypoxic gas, cord occlusion, or restriction of uterine blood flow) produces an initial bradycardia followed by a slow increase in heart rate

1

which returns to or exceeds its control value over the next few minutes (Fig. 1.1). The early bradycardia under these circumstances is chemoreflex in origin as it is abolished by cutting the carotid sinus nerves bilaterally (Giussani et al., 1990) or by giving atropine (Caldeyro-Barcia et al., 1966; Martin, 1985) or vagotomy (Barcroft, 1946). This bradycardia is not baroreflex as it occurs before a rise in arterial pressure has time to develop, e.g. during brief uterine artery occlusions or when the rise is

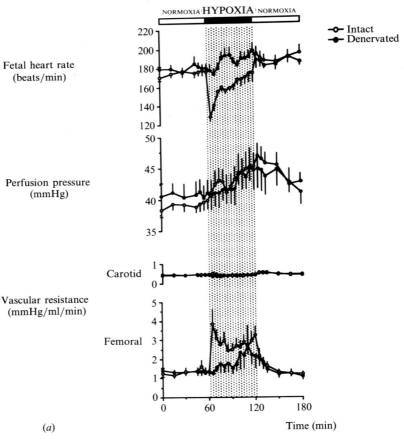

(a)

Fig. 1.1. Effect on fetal heart rate, mean arterial blood pressure and carotid and femoral vascular resistance in sheep of reducing arterial PO_2 to 12–15 mm Hg by lowering the PO_2 of the gas breathed by the ewe for one hour. (a) Intact animals vs. those with bilateral division of the carotid sinus nerves; (b) after pretreatment with atropine or saline vehicle; (c) after pretreatment with phentolamine or saline vehicle. (From Giussani et al., 1990, 1991.)

prevented by α- adrenergic blockade (Giussani et al., 1991), or transection of the spinal cord at L1–2 (Blanco, Dawes & Walker, 1983) which interrupts descending sympathetic outflow. The delayed increase in fetal heart rate is due to a β-adrenergic stimulation from the rise in plasma catecholamines (Cohn, Piasecki & Jackson, 1982; Jensen, Kunzel & Kastendieck, 1987; Martin, Kapoor & Scroop, 1987; Jones et al., 1988; Perez et al., 1989). Other humoral agents released in hypoxia or asphyxia may also be involved, but their precise role has yet to be determined. The most well known of these is arginine vasopressin (AVP) which is secreted

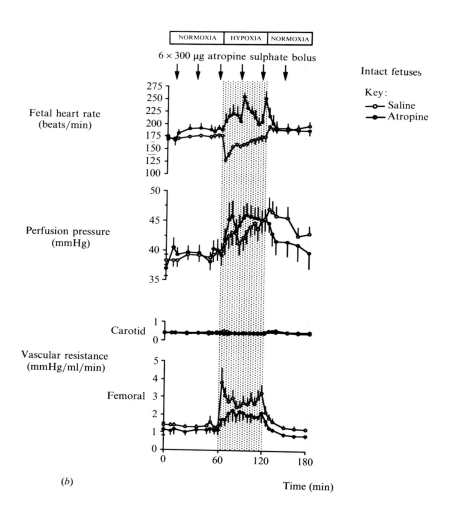

(b)

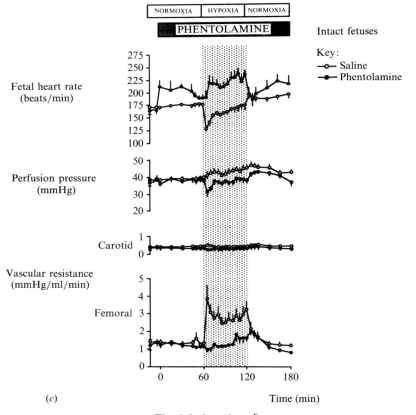

| NORMOXIA | HYPOXIA | NORMOXIA |

Fig. 1.1. (*continued*)

(*c*)   Time (min)

in large amounts in hypoxia, acidaemia, asphyxia or hypotension (Wood, 1989; Wood & Chen, 1989) and has been reported to reduce fetal heart rate (Iwamoto et al., 1979; Courtice et al., 1984; Dunlap & Valego, 1989; Irion, Mack & Clark, 1990; Piacquadio, Brace & Cheung, 1990).

Hence the so-called 'early decelerations' associated with contractions during normal labour (Martin, 1985) are thought to be via a rapidly acting reflex with the vagus as the efferent limb. The mechanisms involved in producing 'late decelerations' are not obviously reflex in origin as they are not blocked by atropine (Caldeyro-Barcia et al., 1966). Such decelerations in fetal heart rate are likely to be due to the direct effects of hypoxia on the sino-atrial node or conducting tissue, or possibly to the release of humoral agents which depress the heart.

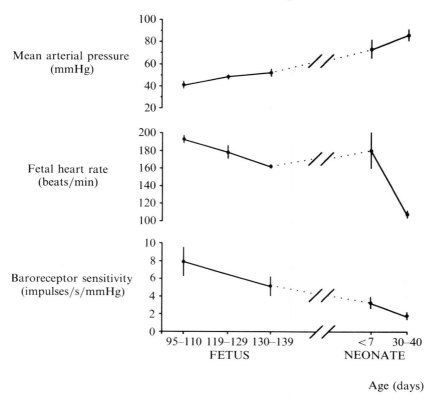

Fig. 1.2. Mean arterial blood pressure, fetal heart rate and sensitivity of baro-receptor afferents in late gestation and postnatally in the sheep. (Data from Kitanaka et al., 1989; Blanco et al., 1988; Dawes, 1985; Dawes et al., 1980.)

It is possible to produce prolonged *increases* in mean fetal heart rate by reflex and non-reflex means, e.g. in pyrexia from fever or from maternal exposure to high environmental temperatures (Walker, 1988). Haemor-rhage also elevates fetal heart rate (Brace, 1987). However, the presence of an elevated fetal heart rate does not itself imply hypoxaemia or acidaemia (see Dawes, 1991).

Fetal heart rate declines steadily throughout later gestation in the sheep (Kitanaka et al., 1989) (Fig. 1.2) and human fetus, accompanied by a rise in stroke volume as the heart grows and a rise in mean arterial pressure. The fall in heart rate cannot simply be explained in terms of a baroreflex (see below). Nor is the fall in heart rate due solely to increasing vagal tone, as vagotomy in late gestation does not produce an increase in heart rate to values seen in mid-gestation. The decline in fetal heart rate may depend on changes at the level of the sino-atrial node, but the mechanisms are not known.

Determinants of arterial blood pressure

In the simplest terms, mean arterial pressure is determined by cardiac output (i.e. combined ventricular output in the fetus) and total peripheral resistance. These two components are under both extrinsic and intrinsic control, as is the case for heart rate alone. Indeed, the major determinant of combined ventricular output in late gestation is fetal heart rate, as the mechanical constraints on the heart permit only small changes in stroke volume (see Chapter 6). Extrinsic mechanisms affecting the peripheral arterioles form the efferent limb of reflex control, predominantly by α-adrenergic means. Thus the rise in mean arterial pressure occurring during hypoxia can be reduced by cutting the carotid sinus nerves (Giussani et al., 1990, Fig. 1.1(a)) or by α-adrenergic blockade with phentolamine (Giussani et al., 1991, Fig. 1.1(c)). Again, such reflexes have an indirect component via the release of catecholamines from the adrenal medulla. Many other humoral agents may also play a role and these are reviewed in Chapter 4.

Mean arterial pressure increases steadily during late gestation in the sheep fetus (Dawes, 1985; Kitanaka et al., 1989). This is partly accounted for by the increase in cardiac output during this period but more importantly to the fact that vascularity does not increase at the same rate as body size, hence peripheral vascular resistance rises. Changes in compliance have a pronounced effect on the pressure and flow velocity waveforms (see Fig. 1.3). One example is the changing 'Windkessel' capacitance in moving more distally in the circulation. Another is that arterial pressure at any point will be affected if the distribution of flow to vascular beds of varying compliance changes. Blood volume and pressure is sometimes related to the concept of mean systemic filling pressure (Guyton, 1986) although this method has not been applied to the fetal circulation. Finally, the effects of changes in viscosity cannot be ignored, especially under conditions of chronic hypoxaemia when the haematocrit increases owing to enhanced erythropoiesis.

The shape of the pressure waveform changes in moving from the central to the peripheral circulation. The amplitude of the pressure oscillation increases, and that of the velocity oscillation decreases, with (*a*) Linear pressure–volume relationship

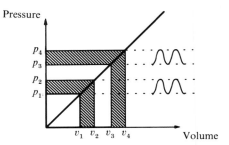

(*b*) Effect of compliance on pressure–volume relationship

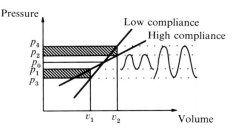

(*c*) Curvilinear pressure–volume relationship

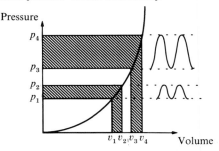

Fig. 1.3. Effect of resistance and compliance on pressure/flow relationship for a slow sine wave. (*a*) At constant stroke volume ($V_2-V_1 = V_4-V_3$) an increase in resistance increases the level of the pressure oscillation from P_2-P_1 to P_4-P_3 at constant compliance. (*b*) Reducing compliance amplifies the pressure oscillation from P_2-P_1 to P_4-P_3 even though mean pressure (P_0) and stroke volume (V_2-V_1) remain constant. (*c*) In fact, the pressure/volume plot is alinear, as compliance falls at greater distension. Both amplitude of the oscillation and mean pressure increase at greater volume, even though stroke volume remains constant ($V_2-V_1 = V_4-V_3$).

8   *Mark A. Hanson*

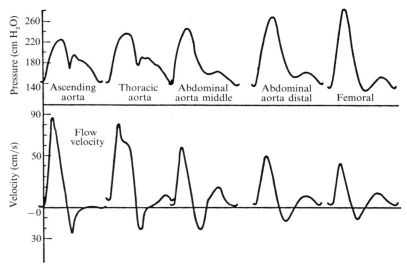

Fig. 1.4. Changes in the pressure and velocity waveforms in moving distally in the circulation. Note increase in amplitude of pressure oscillation, decline in amplitude of velocity waveform and appearance of dicrotic wave. (From McDonald, 1974.)

distance from the heart (see Fig. 1.4). Several components are involved in this change. First, there is the loss of a detectable incisura in moving further from the aortic semi-lunar valves. A pronounced dicrotic wave now appears due to reflections from the periphery. These reflections are due to collision of the blood with vessel walls at points of branching, and also to the increased rigidity of more peripheral vessels. The reflected pressure component adds to the forward-going pressure, whereas the reflected flow component subtracts from the forward-going flow (Fig. 1.5). This produces a temporary reduction or even cessation of flow, so that the flow waveform has a clearly biphasic pattern. The effects on blood velocity are even more pronounced, sometimes producing a period of reversed velocity before the dicrotic wave. These effects will be greater during peripheral vasoconstriction (Fig. 1.6).

For pulsatile changes, characterization of pressure and flow waveforms is often performed in the frequency domain and restriction of flow is described by impedance. Impedance to flow is considered in terms of the modulus of impedance: for a sinusoidal oscillation this is given by the amplitude of the pressure sine wave/ amplitude of the flow sine wave. The pressure and flow waveforms are usually not in phase and both the extent

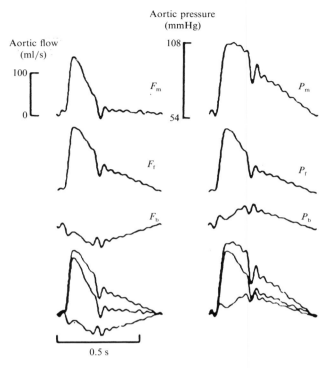

Fig. 1.5. Relation between measured (F_m, P_m), forward (F_f, P_f) and reflected (F_b, P_b) flow (F) and pressure (P). The lower part of each panel shows how a summation of forward and reflected waves gives the measured flow or pressure. (From Van Den Bos et al., 1976.)

of this phase difference (the phase angle) and the modulus of impedance depend on the frequency of the sinusoidal oscillation (Fig. 1.7). This type of analysis shows the relative contributions of the components of impedance. If the pressure and flow oscillations are in phase (phase angle = 0°), the impedance is a pure resistance. Its value, which is high, will be altered by vasoconstriction or dilatation. If the flow oscillation leads the pressure oscillation (phase angle tending to −90°), then capacitance plays the major role in impedance. If on the other hand the pressure leads the flow (phase angle tending to +90°), then the major component is inductance (due to the inertia of the blood).

When the waveform is not a sine wave, as in the arterial system, Fourier analysis must be used to characterize it by a collection of sine waves of various frequencies, the fundamental or first harmonic being the

10   *Mark A. Hanson*

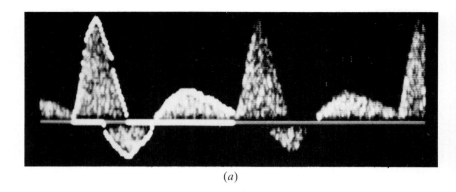

(a)

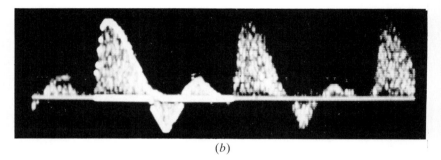

(b)

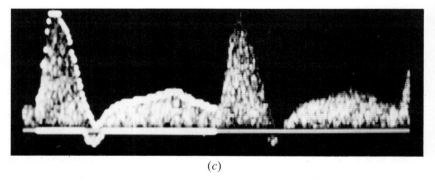

(c)

Fig. 1.6. Doppler flow–velocity waveforms derived using continuous wave instrument applied to femoral artery of anaesthetized newborn lamb. (a) Is control (PI = 5.78). (b) Shows vasoconstriction produced by close intraarterial injection of phenylephrine (PI = 5.80); note that PI hardly changes as both systolic and diastolic components change in proportion. (c) Shows vasodilatation by similar injection of hydralazine (PI = 3.16); both systolic and diastolic components have increased but there is a small fall in PI. Route of injection ensured that no changes occurred in central arterial or venous blood pressure or in heart rate.

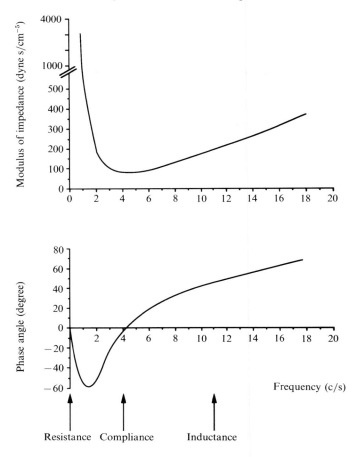

Fig. 1.7. Effect of frequency of oscillation on modulus of impedance and phase angle. See text for discussion.

frequency of the heart beat. The modulus of impedance and the phase angle would then be plotted against the frequency for each sine wave. Whilst the method is valuable for understanding the dynamics of the circulation, changes in vascular tone due to vasoconstriction or vasodilatation in fact only affect the modulus of impedance to any degree at low frequencies, i.e. at the point where it is determined by resistance. In the physiological range, the magnitude of impedance is low compared to peripheral resistance.

It is also possible to consider the function of the arterial system in the time domain. This was done in a way in Fig. 1.5. A more detailed

theoretical analysis employs the 'unit impulse' method, in which it is
envisaged that the heart is replaced by a device connected to the root of
the aorta which suddenly imposes a large step increase in flow (Laxminarayan, Sipkema & Westerhof, 1977). With a simple Windkessel, pressure
and flow would decline exponentially. For a system in which there is
reflection from the periphery (e.g. an elastic tube closed at one end), the
pressure should have a second peak. As this is not prominent in vivo, it
stresses the diffuse nature of the wave reflected from the periphery in the
physiological range (Fig. 1.5).

Interaction of heart rate and arterial blood pressure in the fetus

The inverse relation between fetal arterial pressure and heart rate
described above is well established for the sheep fetus. Unfortunately, no
comparable data exists for the human fetus or indeed for any primate
fetus, although the fall in fetal heart rate over this period in the human is
well established. The inverse relation suggests the operation of a baroreflex, although cause and effect cannot be established merely from a
correlation of this kind. The baroreflex has been shown to operate in the
sheep fetus in late gestation (Itskovitz, Lagamma & Rudolph, 1983) as a
transient rise in arterial pressure, produced by intravenous injection of
phenylephrine, produces a fall in fetal heart rate which is abolished by
chemodenervation or by atropine. The developmental process is however complicated by the fact that the sensitivity of the baroreceptors (in
terms of the change in their rate of discharge per mm Hg increase in
arterial pressure) falls over this period of gestation (Blanco et al., 1988)
(see Fig. 1.2). It may be that a reduction in baroreflex 'gain' occurs as a
consequence of the rise in mean arterial pressure, as during hypertension
in postnatal life, but, if this is the case, it is surprising that the relation
between arterial pressure and heart rate over late gestation is linear.
Further work is needed in this area.

The interaction between peripheral resistance and heart rate has been
much studied in the adult, and this would repay study in the fetus. During
exercise in the adult, for example, a balance is struck between the
vasodilator mechanisms in the exercising muscles and the vasoconstriction necessary to redistribute cardiac output away from non-essential
tissues and to increase arterial pressure to provide improved perfusion.
To permit such a rise in pressure to occur, the baroreflex gain is reduced
(Persson, Ehmke & Kirchhelm, 1989). Whilst muscular exercise of this

intensity is not a feature of fetal life, the redistribution of cardiac output has similarities with that seen in the fetus during a period of hypoxaemia. It will be important to investigate this further as under such circumstances the fetus depends upon its circulation for survival.

Changes in venous return may also affect heart rate in the adult, this being the basis for the Bainbridge reflex (Guyton, 1986). It is therefore conceivable that changes in umbilical venous blood flow might produce changes in fetal heart rate, although this has not been investigated directly.

Under conditions of hypoxaemia or asphyxia where the changes in blood gases and the rise in arterial pressure will stimulate not only arterial chemoreceptors but also arterial baroreceptors, interaction between chemoreflexes and baroreflexes must be considered. Such interaction has been described in the adult (Rowell & O'Leary, 1990) although whether such interaction occurs in the fetus is not known.

The variation of fetal heart rate

Interest in fetal heart rate variation has increased enormously over the last 15–20 years, and some form of continuous fetal heart rate monitoring is now very common during labour. A computerized acquisition and analysis system has been developed (for review see Dawes, 1991) in order that the variation can be measured. The system reduces interobserver error and makes judgements more objective (Dawes, 1991). Prolonged loss of fetal heart rate variation and absence of accelerations is commonly held to be a cause for concern either antenatally or intrapartum. However, the possibility that the low variation is simply due to behavioural state has to be taken into account (Nijhuis, 1991) and healthy babies can be born vaginally despite records being taken which did not show accelerations (especially before 34 weeks).

Fetal heart rate variation is reduced in intrauterine growth retardation associated with maternal hypertension or proteinuric preeclampsia but reduced variation does not correlate with the presence of acidosis at delivery (Henson et al., 1983, 1984). Smith et al. (1988), reported that reduced variation was associated with chronic hypoxaemia (deduced from lower than normal umbilical artery PaO_2 at delivery). It is also associated with a rise in liquor erythropoietin, hypoglycaemia and a rise in plasma alanine. Cordocentesis has also been used to correlate reduced fetal heart rate variation with hypoxaemia in utero (Visser et al., 1990).

The degree of the reduction in fetal heart rate variation, and whether both short- and long-term variation are reduced, may indicate the severity of the hypoxaemia/presence of acidaemia (see Dawes, 1991).

However, the physiological processes underlying heart rate variation have not been established. The key studies of Dalton, Dawes and Patrick (1977) on the sheep fetus showed that the majority of the variation could be accounted for by fetal body and breathing movements and that variation was greater in the low voltage electrocortical state. Administering neuromuscular blockade to the fetus therefore reduced fetal heart rate variation. However, hypoxia is known to inhibit fetal breathing and body movements, so it would be expected to reduce heart rate variation.

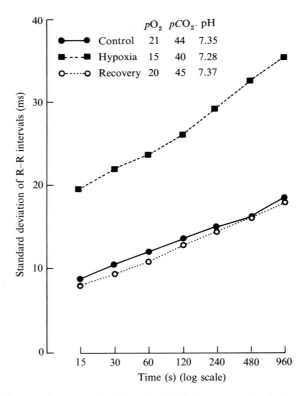

Fig. 1.8. Observations on a fetal lamb of 135 days gestation before (solid line) during (interrupted line), and after (dotted line) hypoxia induced by giving the ewe a low O_2 mixture to breath for one hour. The standard deviations of heart periods (R–R intervals) rose during hypoxia at all observational epochs from 15 s to 16 min and rapidly returned to the initial values on recovery. (From Dalton et al., 1977.)

But in fact in the sheep heart rate variation increases during acute hypoxia (Dalton et al., 1977, Fig. 1.8) and in man variation increases during labour in association with the mild hypoxaemia produced by contractions. A distinction needs therefore to be drawn between the effect of acute hypoxia, which appears to increase variation in both man and animals, and that of chronic hypoxaemia (as in intrauterine growth retardation, rhesus incompatibility) which appears to reduce variation. More work is urgently needed if the physiology underlying the difference, which is essential for assessing its clinical significance, is to be understood. For example, it is necessary to know whether the variation normally present is a manifestation of the mechanisms which control fetal heart rate, e.g. baro- and chemoreflexes. Evidence for this in the sheep comes from the work of Itskovitz et al. (1983) who showed that chemodenervated fetuses had a more variable fetal heart rate than did intact fetuses. By extrapolation, one could argue that the greater the afferent input the more tightly controlled fetal heart rate would be, so that its variation would be reduced under conditions of hypoxia/acidaemia when chemoreceptor discharge increases. But this argument ignores the plethora of other factors which are changing simultaneously and which will greatly affect the control system. For example, if the 'gain' of one component of the system, which provides an error signal to the controller, increases, one would predict the variability to increase.

Other methods for studying heart rate have been used in the adult. One is to use a fractal analysis technique to examine how rigidly fetal heart rate is determined under various circumstances, based on the assumption that heart rate is more chaotically, rather than randomly, determined (for review see Goldberger, 1991). A plot of the power spectrum of the heart rate derived from Fourier analysis would therefore be expected to show major differences between normoxic and hypoxic fetuses. This technique is useful if determination of the power of certain frequency components aids identification of their likely origin. For example, postnatally the establishment of a major component of heart rate variation with a frequency at the concurrent frequency of breathing is the standard method for demonstrating the presence of respiratory sinus arrhythmia. The phase plot technique (where heart rate at time t is plotted against rate at time $t + x$), or indeed a plot of successive R–R intervals (see Chapter 13) might reveal whether the underlying control mechanisms change in gain under various conditions (Fig. 1.9). It must be borne in mind that the method only provides a *description* of the heart rate pattern, giving by itself no insight into the underlying mechanisms which influence this

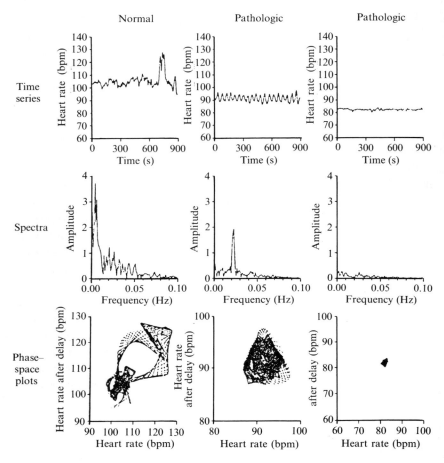

Fig. 1.9. Simulation of plots of heart rate dynamics under normal and two pathological conditions. At the top, heart rate is plotted as a time series, showing an acceleration in the normal trace (left), a sinusoidal pattern in one pathological trace (centre) and a loss of variation in the other pathological trace (right). In the middle, Fourier transformation is used to derive a spectral, frequency–amplitude plot. The normal trace shows a broad spectrum, the sinusoidal pattern now shows a clear peak at its characteristic frequency and the 'flat trace' reveals low power at all frequencies. At the bottom, the data is shown as a phase–space plot. The normal trace shows a plot consistent with a strange (chaotic) attractor, the sinusoidal pattern suggests a periodic attractor and the flat trace resolves into a fixed point attractor. (Adapted from Goldberger, 1991.)

pattern. A major problem is the choice of the time interval to be used for the phase plot. For example, if the heart rate pattern has a major component which is a sine wave of period 3 min, then a phase plot using 3 min as the interval will appear very different from one in which a different interval is chosen.

Disturbances of fetal arterial blood pressure

The work reviewed in Chapter 12 makes it clear that birth weight to placental weight ratio is an important determinant of arterial blood pressure and the risk of cardiovascular disease in later life. The recent data on young children suggests that the differences in systolic pressure may be evident even at age 4, suggesting that subjects statistically more likely to develop hypertension in later life are already on a different trajectory for increasing blood pressure. This raises the possibility that the disturbance in blood pressure regulation has occurred prenatally, and that it is somehow related to fetal growth. Barker has focused attention on the balance between fetal and placental weight. The placenta receives about 40% of the combined ventricular output at term, and hence as a single organ it must determine to a large degree the level of fetal arterial pressure. A working hypothesis is therefore that fetuses with a relatively larger placental to body weight ratio may have to exert a greater degree of peripheral vasoconstriction to maintain arterial blood pressure within normal limits. This may produce greater muscularization of the walls of the peripheral arterioles, favouring increased resistance and reduced compliance; it may also cause resetting of baroreflex sensitivity downwards, permitting further rises in arterial blood pressure to occur postnatally (as occurs in hypertension later in life). The causes of such a mismatch between fetal and placental weight are not known, although as the processes which control placental growth, and indeed those which control fetal growth, are unknown, one can only speculate. Animal studies do not at present give a clear lead, although mean arterial pressure is reported to be lower in growth retarded fetal guinea pigs (Detmer, Gu & Carter, 1991) and sheep (Robinson, Jones & Kingston, 1983). Recent evidence from Barker's group suggests that maternal nutritional status during pregnancy may be all-important. The physiological mechanisms involved here are open to investigation, and preliminary evidence suggests (Jansson & Persson, 1991) that guinea pigs experimentally growth retarded in utero show a greater mean blood pressure at 3–4 months of age postnatally than do those which are appropriately grown.

Effects of long-term hypoxaemia/asphyxia in utero

In view of the interaction between chemo- and baroreflexes discussed above, the effects of chronic hypoxaemia/asphyxia on cardiovascular control in utero will be worth investigating. The initial effects of hypoxia for about 1 h on the sheep fetus near term are well established, i.e. a transient bradycardia, rise in mean arterial pressure, redistribution of combined ventricular output, cessation of fetal breathing and body movements and switching of the electrocortical state (ECoG) to a high voltage pattern. However, if the hypoxia is maintained for several hours to a day or more, these changes are reversed and fetal behaviour becomes normal. Chronic hypoxia for up to 3 wk in sheep fetuses does not produce long-term changes in fetal heart rate, occurrence of heart rate acceler-ations and decelerations, mean arterial pressure, fetal breathing or in ECoG (Bocking et al., 1988a,b; Kitanaka et al., 1989). The mechanisms underlying this 'adaptation' are unknown. Are they due to adaptation of the chemo- or baroreceptors themselves? Or do they represent changes in CNS control mechanisms in the face of continually increased afferent input from these receptors? Or does the secretion of some endocrine factor (e.g. from the placenta) bias the formation of the system in favour of a reduced response? The adaptive processes occur over a timescale which is too short to permit increased haemopoiesis to raise the O_2-carrying capacity of the blood, but changes in CNS blood flow or in metabolism (and hence in tissue PO_2) may be involved.

Conclusion

The application to the fetus of ideas about the interaction between blood pressure and heart rate, derived from the adult, has produced useful insights but there are still huge gaps in understanding. It will be very important to understand the processes which control fetal heart rate for effective use of fetal heart rate monitoring in the future. The new observations which suggest that cardiovascular disease in adult life may have intrauterine origins will have far-reaching consequences, and, unless the underlying physiology of this phenomenon is clear, it will not be possible to develop treatment strategies. Animal research has paved the way in this field of research, but there remain crucial differences between animals and man which must be resolved. This may not be possible until similar techniques can be applied in parallel in man and animals. One crucial development will be a technique for measuring human fetal arterial blood pressure repeatedly in utero. Such a method has been developed for measuring pulmonary arterial pressure in the neonate (Muswer et al., 1990) using vessel wall compliance, but to date the only measurements of fetal intravascular pressure in the human have been made acutely before termination of pregnancy by ultrasound-guided needling.

References

Barcroft, J. (1946). *Researches on Pre-natal Life*. Oxford: Blackwell Scientific Publications.

Blanco, C. E., Dawes, G. S., Hanson, M. A. & McCooke, H. B. (1988). Carotid baroreceptors in fetal and newborn sheep. *Pediatric Research, 24*, 342–46.

Blanco, C. E., Dawes, G. S. & Walker, D. W. (1983). Effect of hypoxia on polysynaptic hind-limb reflexes of unanaesthetized fetal and newborn lambs. *Journal of Physiology, 339*, 453–66.

Bocking, A. D., Gagnon, R., Milne, K. M. & White, S. E. (1988a). Behavioral activity during prolonged hypoxemia in fetal sheep. *Journal of Applied Physiology, 65*, 2420–6.

Bocking, A. D., Gagnon, R., White, S. E., Homan, J., Milne, K. M. & Richardson, B. S. (1988b). Circulatory responses to prolonged hypoxemia in fetal sheep. *American Journal of Obstetrics & Gynecology, 159*, 1418–24.

Bocking, A. D., White, S., Gagnon, R. & Hansford, H. (1989). Effect of prolonged hypoxemia on fetal heart rate accelerations and decelerations in sheep. *American Journal of Obstetrics & Gynecology, 161*, 722–7.

Brace, R. A. (1987). Fetal blood volume responses to fetal haemorrhage: autonomic nervous system contribution. *Journal of Developmental Physiology, 9*, 97–103.

Caldeyro-Barcia, R., Mendez-Bauer, C., Poseiro, J. J., Escarcena, L. A., Pose, S. V., Bieniarz, J., Arnt, I., Gulin, L. & Althabe, O. (1966). Control of human fetal heart rate during labor. In *The Heart and Circulation in the Newborn and Infant*, ed. D. E. Cassels. pp. 7–36. Grune and Stratton. New York and London.

Cohn, H. E., Piasecki, G. J. & Jackson, B. T. (1982). The effect of ß-adrenergic stimulation on fetal cardiovascular function during hypoxemia. *American Journal of Obstetrics & Gynecology, 144*, 810.

Courtice, G. P., Kwong, T. E., Lumbers, E. R. & Potter, E. K. (1984). Excitation of the cardiac vagus nerve by vasopressin in mammals. *Journal of Physiology, 354*, 547–56.

Dalton, K. J., Dawes, G. S. & Patrick, J. E. (1977). Diurnal, respiratory and other rhythms of fetal lambs. *American Journal of Obstetrics & Gynecology, 127*, 414–24.

Dawes, G. S. (1985). The control of fetal heart rate and its variability in lambs. In *Fetal heart rate monitoring*, ed. W. Kunzel. pp. 184–190. Springer-Verlag. Berlin.

Dawes, G. S., Johnston, B. M. & Walker, D. W. (1980). Relationship of arterial pressure and heart rate in fetal, new-born and adult sheep. *Journal of Physiology*, **309**, 405–17.

Dawes, G. S. (1991). Computerized measurement of fetal heart-rate variation antenatally and in labour. *Recent Advances in Obstetrics and Gynaecology*. pp. 57–68. Longman.

Detmer, A., Gu, W. & Carter, A. M. (1991). The blood supply to the heart and brain in the growth retarded guinea pig fetus. *Growth and Developmental Physiology*, **15**, 153–60.

Dunlap, C. E., III & Valego, N. K. (1989). Cardiovascular effects of dynorphin A-(1—13) and arginine vasopressin in fetal lambs. *American Journal of Physiology*, **256**, R1318–24.

Giussani, D. A., Spencer, J. A. D., Moore, P. J. & Hanson, M. A. (1990). The effect of carotid sinus nerve section on the initial cardiovascular response to acute isocapnic hypoxia in fetal sheep in utero. *Journal of Physiology*, **432**, 33P.

Giussani, D. A., Spencer, J. A. D., Moore, P. J. & Hanson, M. A. (1991). Effect of phentolamine on initial cardiovascular response to isocapnic hypoxia in intact and carotid sinus denervated fetal sheep. *Journal of Physiology*, **438**, 56P.

Goldberger, A. L. (1991). Is the normal heartbeat chaotic or homeostatic? *NIPS*, **6**, 87–91.

Guyton, A. C. (1986). *Textbook of Maternal Physiology*. Saunders, P.A., (ed.), Chapter 23.

Hanson, M. A. (1989). The importance of baro- and chemoreflexes in the control of the fetal cardiovascular system. *Journal of Developmental Physiology*, **10**, 491–511.

Hanson, G. L., Dawes, G. S. & Redman, C. W. G. (1983). Antenatal fetal heart rate variability in relation to fetal acid–base status at caesarean section. *British Journal of Obstetrics and Gynaecology*, **90**, 516–21.

Henson, G. L., Dawes, G. S. & Redman, C. W. G. (1984). Characterisation of the reduced heart rate variation in growth-retarded fetuses. *British Journal of Obstetrics and Gynaecology*, **91**, 751–5.

Irion, G. L., Mack, C. E. & Clark, K. E. (1990). Fetal hemodynamic and fetoplacental vascular response to exogenous arginine vasopressin. *American Journal of Obstetrics & Gynecology*, **162**, 1115–20.

Itskovitz, J., Lagamma, E. F. & Rudolph, A. M. (1983). Baroreflex control of the circulation in chronically instrumented fetal lambs. *Circulation Research*, **52**, 589–96.

Iwamoto, H. S., Rudolph, A. M., Keil, L. C. & Heymann, M. A. (1979). Hemodynamic responses of the sheep fetus to vasopressin infusion. *Circulation Research*, **44**, 430.

Jansson, T. & Persson, E. (1991). Intrauterine growth retarded guinea pigs with more than 45% reduction in birthweight have elevated blood pressure at 3.4 months of age. Society for Gynecological Investigation. 38th Annual Meeting, San Antonio, Texas, March 1991 (abstract no 327).

Jensen, A., Kunzel, W. & Kastendieck, E. (1987). Fetal sympathetic activity, transcutaneous PO_2, and skin blood flow during repeated asphyxia in sheep. *Journal of Developmental Physiology*, **9(4)**, 337–46.

Jones, C. T. & Robinson, R. O. (1975). Plasma catecholamines in fetal and adult sheep. *Journal of Physiology,* **248**, 15–33.

Jones, C. T., Roebuck, M. M., Walker, D. W. & Johnston, B. M. (1988). The role of the adrenal medulla and peripheral sympathetic nerves in the physiological responses of the fetal sheep to hypoxia. *Journal of Developmental Physiology,* **10**, 17–36.

Kitanaka, T., Alonso, J. G., Gilbert, R. D., Siu, B. L., Clemons, G. K. & Longo, L. D. (1989). Fetal responses to long-term hypoxemia in sheep. *American Journal of Physiology,* **256**, R1348–54.

Laxminarayan, S., Sipkema, P. & Westerhof, N. (1977). Characterization of the arterial system in the time domain. *IEEE Transactions, Bio-medical Engineering.*

McDonald, D. A. (1974). *Blood Flow in Arteries.* 2nd Edition. Edward Arnold, London.

Martin, C. B. (1985). Pharmocological aspects of fetal heart rate regulation during hypoxia. In *Fetal Heart Rate Monitoring,* ed. Kunzel, W., pp. 170–84. Springer-Verlag, Berlin.

Martin, A. A., Kapoor, R. & Scroop, G. C. (1987). Hormonal factors in the control of heart rate in the normoxaemic and hypoxaemic fetal, neonatal and adult sheep. *Journal of Developmental Physiology,* **9**, 465–80.

Mott, J. C. & Walker, D. W. (1983). Neural and endocrine regulation of circulation in the fetus and newborn. In *Handbook of Physiology,* pp. 837–83. Bethseda, MD.: American Physiology Society. Cardiovascular System III.

Muswer, N. N., Poppe, D., Smallhorn, J. F., Hellman, J., Whyte, H., Smith, B. & Freedom, R. M. (1990). Doppler echocardiographic measurement of pulmonary artery pressure from ductal Doppler velocities in the newborn. *Journal of the American College of Cardiology,* **15**, 446–56.

Nijhuis, J. G. (1991). Fetal behavioural states. In *Fetal Monitoring,* ed. J. A. D. Spencer. pp. 24–27. Oxford University Press.

Perez, R., Espinoza, M., Riquelme, R., Parer, J. T. & Llanos, A. J. (1989). Arginine vasopressin mediates cardiovascular responses to hypoxemia in fetal sheep. *American Journal of Physiology,* **256**, R1011–18.

Persson, P. B., Ehmke, H. & Kirchhelm, H. R. (1989). Cardiopulmonary-arterial baroreceptor interaction in control of blood pressure. *News in Physiological Sciences,* **4**, 56–8.

Piacquadio, K. M., Brace, R. A. & Cheung, C. Y. (1990). Role of vasopressin in mediation of fetal cardiovascular responses to acute hypoxia. *American Journal of Obstetrics & Gynecology,* **163**, 1294–1300.

Robinson, J. S., Jones, C. T. & Kingston, E. J. (1983). Studies on experimental growth retardation in sheep. The effects of maternal hypoxaemia. *Journal of Developmental Physiology,* **5**, 89–100.

Rowell, L. B. & O'Leary, D. S. (1990). Reflex control of the circulation during exercise: chemoreflexes and mechanoreflexes. *Journal of Applied Physiology,* **69**, 407–18.

Smith, J. H., Anand, K. J. S., Cotes, P. M., Dawes, G. S., Harkness, R. A., Howlett, T. A., Rees, L. H. & Redman, C. W. G. (1988). Antenatal fetal heart rate variation in relation to the respiratory and metabolic status of the compromised human fetus. *British Journal of Obstetrics and Gynaecology,* **95**, 980–9.

Van Den Bos, G. C., Westerhof, N., Elzinga, G. & Sipkema, P. (1976).

Mark A. Hanson

Reflection in the systemic arterial system: effects of aortic and carotid occlusions. *Cardiovascular Research,* **10**, 565–73.

Visser, G. H. A., Sadovsky, G. & Nicolaides, K. H. (1990). Antepartum heart rate patterns in small-for-gestational-age third-trimester fetuses: Correlations with blood gas values obtained at cordocentesis. *American Journal of Obstetrics and Gynecology,* **162**, 698–703.

Walker, D. W. (1988). Effects of increased core temperature on breathing movements and electro-cortical activity in fetal sheep. *Journal of Developmental Physiology,* **10(6)**, 513–23.

Wood, C. E. (1989). Sinoaortic denervation attenuates the reflex responses to hypotension in fetal sheep. *American Journal of Physiology,* **256**, R1103–10.

Wood, C. E. & Chen, H.-G. (1989). Acidemia stimulates ACTH, vasopressin, and heart rate responses in fetal sheep. *American Journal of Physiology,* **257**, R344–9.

2

Regional distribution of cardiac output

ARNE JENSEN AND RICHARD BERGER

Introduction

In the first part of this chapter the distribution of combined ventricular output during normoxaemia will be described. Then the cardiovascular responses to hypoxaemia and asphyxia will be discussed with respect to the different methods by which the lack of oxygen is induced. These include maternal hypoxaemia, graded reduction in umbilical blood flow, graded reduction in uterine blood flow, repeated brief arrest of uterine blood flow, prolonged arrest of uterine blood flow, reduction in fetal blood volume, and chronic hypoxaemia induced by various methods. The following section of this chapter deals with circulatory responses of immature fetuses to hypoxaemia and asphyxia. The next two sections describe the interaction between O_2 delivery and tissue metabolism and cardiovascular mechanisms involved in fetal circulatory responses to oxygen lack. In the second part of this chapter, blood flow and oxygen delivery to the principal fetal organs during hypoxaemia and asphyxia are examined and discussed in relation to organ function.

The distribution of cardiac output in the fetus during normoxaemia

In chronically prepared fetal sheep at 0.85 of pregnancy (3–4 days after surgery) mean heart rate is ≈170 beats/min, arterial pressure is 44 mm Hg, ascending aortic pH is 7.40, PO_2 is 24 mm Hg, PCO_2 is 47 mm Hg, haemoglobin oxygen saturation is 67%, haemoglobin is 8.6 g/dl, and oxygen content is 7.8 ml/dl (Itskovitz, LaGamma & Rudolph, 1987; Jensen, Roman & Rudolph, 1991). The corresponding values of samples withdrawn simultaneously from various major fetal vessels, including descending aorta, umbilical vein, abdominal inferior vena cava, superior vena cava, and superior sagittal sinus, are presented in Table 2.1. The

Table 2.1. *Fetal heart rate, blood pressures, blood gases, pH, and oxygen content in nine normoxaemic fetal sheep at 0.9 gestation*

Heart rate (beats/min)	167 ± 19
Mean aortic pressure (torr)	44.2 ± 3.5
Umbilical venous pressure (torr)	11.1 ± 4.83
Vena cava pressure (torr)	3.3 ± 2

Ascending aortic values

PO_2 (torr)	24.1 ± 2.4
PCO_2 (torr)	47.3 ± 3.9
pH	7.40 ± 0.013
Base excess	4.60 ± 3.19
O_2 saturation (%)	67.3 ± 3.9
Haemoglobin (g/dl)	8.6 ± 1.3
O_2 content (ml/dl)	7.76 ± 1.1

Superior vena cava values

PO_2 (torr)	18.7 ± 1.9
PCO_2 (torr)	51.2 ± 4.6
pH	7.37 ± 0.03
Base excess	5.20 ± 3.08
O_2 saturation (%)	45.7 ± 6.4
Haemoglobin (g/dl)	8.9 ± 1.4
O_2 content (ml/dl)	5.44 ± 1.11

Descending aortic values

PO_2 (torr)	21.7 ± 2.3
PCO_2 (torr)	50.6 ± 4.5
pH	7.39 ± 0.026
Base excess	5.57 ± 3.57
O_2 saturation (%)	58.2 ± 5.8
Haemoglobin (g/dl)	8.8 ± 1.3
O_2 content (ml/dl)	6.83 ± 1.2

Abdominal inferior vena cava values

PO_2 (torr)	17.1 ± 2.0
PCO_2 (torr)	54.2 ± 3.3
pH	7.37 ± 0.03
Base excess	5.78 ± 3.15
O_2 saturation (%)	40.3 ± 6.4
Haemoglobin (g/dl)	8.9 ± 1.4
O_2 content (ml/dl)	4.85 ± 1.28

Umbilical vein values

PO_2 (torr)	32.8 ± 3.7
PCO_2 (torr)	43.9 ± 4.0
pH	7.42 ± 0.03
Base excess	5.24 ± 2.99
O_2 saturation (%)	86.1 ± 3.1
Haemoglobin (g/dl)	8.5 ± 1.3
O_2 content (ml/dl)	9.78 ± 1.5

Superior sagittal sinus values

PO_2 (torr)	17.4 ± 0.9
PCO_2 (torr)	52.9 ± 5.0
pH	7.38 ± 0.03
Base excess	5.80 ± 3.61
O_2 saturation (%)	41.0 ± 1.9
Haemoglobin (g/dl)	9.7 ± 1.0
O_2 content (ml/dl)	5.3 ± 0.4

Source: Jensen, Roman & Rudolph, 1991.

values of umbilical venous, ascending and descending aortic oxygen saturation given in this table are in remarkable agreement with those from acutely instrumented fetal sheep published by Dawes, Mott & Widdicombe (1954).

Under physiological conditions, as reflected by these blood gas values (Table 2.1), the combined ventricular output (cardiac output) at 0.9 gestation is approximately 480 ml/min/kg fetal weight. Its distribution to the principal fetal organs, the resulting blood flow and O_2 delivery, and the vascular resistances are presented in Table 2.2. About 55% and 45% of the cardiac output are distributed to the fetal body and to the placenta, respectively. About 30% are directed to the fetal carcass, including skeletal, muscle, bones, skin, and connective tissues and 11% to the lungs. During normoxaemia only small fractions of the cardiac output are distributed to the brain (3%), heart (2.6%), small gut (2.6%), kidneys (2.3%), and adrenals (0.006%) (Jensen et al., 1991). In the human fetus cerebral blood flow comprises a larger fraction of the cardiac output, because the brain/ body weight ratio is higher than in sheep.

This normal distribution of blood flow changes dramatically in late gestation during hypoxaemia and even more so during asphyxia. The following sections describe the general changes in the distribution of fetal organ blood flows when oxygen is in short supply. The effect of various experimental interventions that result in fetal hypoxaemia and a redistribution of blood flow and oxygen delivery will be emphasized. Table 2.3 summarizes the results of the most significant studies on changes in blood gas tensions and organ blood flows in relative terms.

Cardiovascular responses to oxygen lack induced by various methods
Effects of maternal hypoxaemia

Maternal hypoxaemia is usually produced by manipulating the inspired fraction of oxygen, to reduce maternal arterial PO_2 to about 40 mm Hg. This results in fetal arterial PO_2 values of about 10–12 mm Hg. Due to hyperventilation of the ewe, fetal blood PCO_2 falls too. To study the effects of isocapnic hypoxaemia on the fetal circulation, it is necessary to increase carbon dioxide concentrations in the inspired gas mixture ($FiCO_2 = 3$–4%).

The resulting moderate fetal hypoxaemia (arterial $PO_2 = 10$–12 mm Hg) causes a fall in heart rate and an increase in arterial blood pressure (Cohn et al., 1974), but combined ventricular output does not fall as long

Table 2.2. *Fetal combined ventricular output and organ blood flow, distribution of cardiac output, O_2 delivery, and vascular resistance in nine chronically prepared fetal sheep at 0.9 gestation*

	Blood flow (ml/min per 100 g)	% Cardiac output	O_2 delivery (ml/min per 100 g)	Vascular resistance (mm Hg/ml per min per 100 g)
Combined ventricular output	478 ± 94[a]	100	—	
Umbilical blood flow	213 ± 55[a]	44.0 ± 9.3	—	0.16 ± 0.03[c]
Total body blood flow	315 ± 63[a]	56.0 ± 9.3	21.34 ± 6.75[a]	0.13 ± 0.02[c]
Upper body organs				
Brain	87.4 ± 20.6	3.00 ± 1.11	6.71 ± 1.45	0.49 ± 0.11
Cerebrum	79.5 ± 18.3	2.00 ± 0.70	6.11 ± 1.34	0.54 ± 0.13
Cerebellum	119.5 ± 24.1	0.32 ± 0.11	9.16 ± 1.58	0.35 ± 0.06
Diencephalon	105.7 ± 32.2	0.25 ± 0.12	7.94 ± 1.66	0.42 ± 0.13
Midbrain	134.5 ± 42.5	0.19 ± 0.10	10.05 ± 2.01	0.33 ± 0.11
Medulla	144.5 ± 46.0	0.15 ± 0.07	10.83 ± 2.44	0.31 ± 0.11
Hypophysis	67.8 ± 36.7	0.01 ± 0.01	5.05 ± 2.25	0.76 ± 0.37
Choroid plexus	458.1 ± 265.9	0.04 ± 0.02	34.3 ± 18.70	0.13 ± 0.09
Heart	163.1 ± 46.5	2.55 ± 0.62	12.29 ± 2.19	0.27 ± 0.08
Upper carcass	21.6 ± 4.7	15.91 ± 4.48	1.66 ± 0.34	1.99 ± 0.53
Scalp	33.7 ± 10.4	0.21 ± 0.07	2.65 ± 9.80	1.34 ± 0.48
Body skin	23.0 ± 6.3	0.17 ± 0.09	1.84 ± 0.74	1.90 ± 0.54
Upper body, total	113 ± 24[a]	23.0 ± 5.4	8.58 ± 1.42[a]	0.38 ± 0.11[c]

Lower body organs

Adrenals	174.3 ± 118.6	0.06 ± 0.04	10.83 ± 6.75	0.84 ± 1.57
Kidneys	154.8 ± 40.2	2.34 ± 0.76	10.61 ± 3.95	0.28 ± 0.07
Spleen	345.1 ± 244.7	1.01 ± 0.71	21.64 ± 15.0	0.53 ± 0.92
Small gut	89.1 ± 29.8	2.65 ± 1.47	6.08 ± 2.23	0.50 ± 0.18
Large gut	41.3 ± 10.6	0.27 ± 0.12	2.78 ± 0.75	1.04 ± 0.25
Pancreas	35.3 ± 12.9	0.08 ± 0.04	2.33 ± 0.74	1.33 ± 0.54
Lower carcass	19.0 ± 5.0	13.82 ± 2.70	0.38 ± 0.14	2.32 ± 0.74
Body skin	26.1 ± 13.7	0.16 ± 0.06	1.81 ± 1.10	1.90 ± 0.79
Lower body, total	138 ± 35[a,b]	25.4 ± 4.3	9.24 ± 2.27[a,b]	0.31 ± 0.08[c,d]
Lungs	162.2 ± 74.4	11.81 ± 5.12	5.68 ± 2.52	0.35 ± 0.27

[a] (ml/min per kg). [b] Not including umbilical blood flow. [c] (mm Hg/ml per min per kg).
[d] Not including umbilical vascular resistance.
Source: Jensen, Roman & Rudolph, 1991.

Table 2.3. *Fetal changes during hypoxaemia and asphyxia*

(a)

	Cohn et al., 1974 Maternal hypoxaemia (FiO_2 = 6%)		Peeters et al., 1979 Maternal hypoxaemia (FiO_2 = 10%)	Yaffe et al., 1987 Reduction of uterine blood flow by 75%	Jensen et al., 1987b Arrest of uterine and ovarian blood flow
	without acidaemia	with acidaemia			
Heart rate (bpm)	−	no change	−	−	− −
Arterial blood pressure (mm Hg)	+	−	—	+	+
pH	no change	−	—	− −	− −
PO_2 (mm Hg)	−	no change	−	−	− −
PCO_2 (mm Hg)	no change	no change	—	+	—
Blood flow changes					
Umbilical cord (ml/min/100 g)	no change	no change	no change	no change	− −
Fetal body (ml/min/100 g)	no change	−	—	—	− − −
Brain	+	+	+	no change	no change
Heart	+ +	+ +	+ +	no change	no change
Adrenal	+ + +	+ + +	+ + +	+ + +	+ + +
Liver (arterial)	—	—	−	—	− −
Kidney	−	− −	− −	−	− − −
Lungs	− −	− −	—	—	− −
Gastrointestinal tract	no change	−	no change	−	− − − −
Carcass	no change	− −	−	−	− −

(b)

	Itskovitz et al., 1987 Reduction of umbilical blood flow by 50%[a]	Block et al., 1990 Arrest of uterine blood flow plus maternal hypoxaemia		Jensen et al., 1991 Graded reduction of uterine blood flow[a]	Toubas et al., 1981 Reduction in fetal blood volume by 15%
		hypoxaemia with severe acidaemia	agonal heart rate pattern		
Heart rate (bpm)	–	–	– –	–	–
Arterial blood pressure (mm Hg)	+	no change	– –	+	–
pH	no change	– – –	– – –	– –	
PO_2 (mm Hg)	–	– – –	– – –	–	no change
PCO_2 (mm Hg)	no change	+ + +	+ + + +	+	+
Blood flow changes					
Umbilical cord (ml/min/100 g)	– –	– – –	– – – –	no change	–
Fetal body (ml/min/100 g)	no change	– –	– – –	no change	no change
Brain	+	no change	– – –	+	no change
Heart	no change	+ +	– –	+ +	no change
Adrenal	+ +	+ + +	– –	+ + +	no change
Liver (arterial)	no change	——	——	——	no change
Kidney	no change	– –	– –	no change	
Lungs	– –	——	——	——	– –
Gastrointestinal tract	no change	– –	——	no change	–
Carcass	+	——	– –	–	–

[a] To effect a reduction in fetal oxygen delivery by 50%.

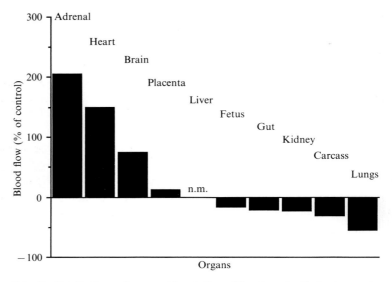

Fig. 2.1. Redistribution of organ blood flow (% of control) during maternal hypoxaemia ($FiO_2 = 6\%$) in chronically prepared fetal sheep near term. Fetal PO_2 in the carotid artery was reduced from 21 ± 1 mm Hg to 12 ± 1 mm Hg with no change in arterial pH. (From Cohn et al., 1974.)

as blood pH is maintained. When hypoxaemia is accompanied by acid-aemia cardiac output falls by about 20% (Cohn et al., 1974), umbilical blood flow is maintained, while blood flow to the fetal body is reduced by 40% (Cohn et al., 1974; Parer, 1980).

The distribution of the combined ventricular output changes in the fetus much the way it does in the adult. There is a circulatory centraliz-ation of blood flow in favour of the brain, heart, and adrenals, and at the expense of peripheral organs, including lungs, kidneys, gastrointestinal tract, and carcass (Fig. 2.1) (Cohn et al., 1974; Peeters et al., 1979). This holds true for normally grown and growth retarded fetuses.

Fetal hypoxaemia is also accompanied by a redistribution of umbilical venous blood flow. The fraction of blood bypassing the liver through the ductus venosus increases from 55% to 65% (Edelstone, Rudolph & Heymann, 1980; Reuss & Rudolph, 1980), thus contributing consider-ably to the maintenance of oxygen delivery to the fetus. In addition, there is a preferential streaming of umbilical venous blood across the foramen ovale via the left ventricle towards the upper body circulation to maintain oxygen delivery to the heart and brain (Reuss & Rudolph, 1980).

During fetal hypoxaemia the proportion of superior vena cava blood flow directed through the foramen ovale into the upper body segment is slightly increased (Cohn et al., 1974). The venous blood returning to the heart via the abdominal inferior vena cava is reduced by 50%. Thus, blood returning from the umbilical vein, superior vena cava and inferior vena cava contributes 32%, 30% and 44% respectively to venous return (Reuss & Rudolph, 1980).

In summary, during moderate hypoxaemia cardiac output is maintained (unlike hypoxaemia plus acidaemia) and the circulating blood is redistributed to the brain, heart, and adrenals at the expense of peripheral organs, including the lungs, i.e. circulatory centralization. These changes are accompanied by a changing pattern of venous return and by a preferential streaming of umbilical venous blood through the ductus venosus and the foramen ovale to the upper body segment.

Reduction in umbilical blood flow

Reduction in umbilical and placental blood flow can be achieved by compression of the umbilical vein (Künzel et al., 1977), compression of the fetal abdominal aorta (Edelstone et al., 1980), by snaring the umbilical cord (Itskovitz et al., 1987), and by an embolization of the placental vascular bed (Clapp et al., 1981).

A reduction of arterial and/or venous umbilical blood flow causes a decrease in oxygen delivered to the fetus. Unlike during maternal hypoxaemia, this does not decrease umbilical venous oxygen content (Künzel et al., 1977; Itskovitz et al., 1987). Therefore, a reduction in umbilical blood flow, e.g. by 50%, results in a similar reduction in oxygen delivery to the fetus.

Due to the favourable relationship between uterine and umbilical blood flow, umbilical venous PCO_2 does not change, and fetal arterial blood pH does not change even though umbilical blood flow and hence fetal oxygen delivery is reduced to 50% of normal.

A compression of the umbilical cord is accompanied by an increase in arterial blood pressure, a fall in heart rate, and a fall in combined ventricular output (Künzel et al., 1977; Itskovitz, Goetzman & Rudolph, 1982a; Itskovitz et al., 1987).

Reduced umbilical blood flow is accompanied by a redistribution of blood flow to the fetal organs that is different from that observed during maternal hypoxaemia (Fig. 2.2). Blood flows to the brain (+43%), heart

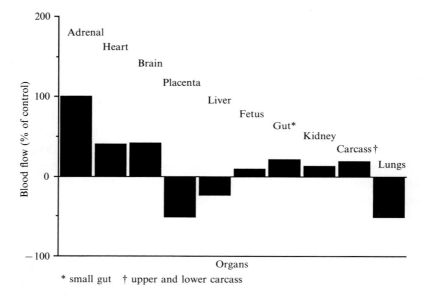

Fig. 2.2. Redistribution of organ blood flow (% of control) during reduction of umbilical blood flow and hence oxygen delivery by 50% in chronically prepared fetal sheep near term. Fetal oxygen content in the ascending aorta was reduced from 7.41 ± 0.90 ml/dl to 6.34 ± 0.87 ml/dl, pH did not change. (From Itskovitz et al., 1987.)

(+41%) and adrenals (+100%) increase. However, unlike during maternal hypoxaemia, blood flows to the peripheral organs, including those to the kidney, gastrointestinal tract, and spleen do not change, and that to the carcass increases (+20%). Only blood flow to the lungs falls (−50%).

The fraction of umbilical blood flow shunted through the ductus venosus increases by 30% when umbilical blood flow is reduced by 75% (Edelstone et al., 1980). However, the proportion of venous return from both inferior and superior venae cavae increases relative to that from the umbilical vein. Therefore, the oxygen content of the blood crossing the foramen ovale falls and oxygen delivery to the brain and heart is maintained by increasing blood flow (Itskovitz et al., 1987).

Reduction in uterine blood flow

Uterine blood flow can be reduced by various methods, including compression of the maternal aorta (Jensen, Künzel & Hohmann, 1985*b*;

Jensen, Hohmann & Künzel, 1987*a,b*; Jensen, Künzel & Kastendieck, 1987*c*; Jensen, Lang & Künzel, 1987*d*), the uterine arteries (Yaffe et al., 1987) or the uterine veins (Künzel et al., 1975) or by embolization of the uterine vascular bed (Creasy et al., 1973).

The haemodynamic effects of reduced uterine blood flow depend largely on the severity of the reduction. The most severe insult of course is arrest of uterine blood flow that interrupts both materno-fetal oxygen delivery and feto-maternal carbon dioxide clearance. Due to collateral blood supply to the sheep uterus including that provided by the ovarian arteries, arrest of uterine blood flow can only be achieved by complete compression of the abdominal maternal aorta below the renal arteries.

Graded reduction in uterine blood flow

Graded reduction in uterine blood flow to achieve a fall in fetal oxygen delivery by 50% and a final carotid arterial PO_2 of 16 mm Hg is associated with fetal bradycardia of mild degree and an increase in fetal aortic pressure (Skillman et al., 1985; Jensen et al., 1991). These changes are similar to those occurring during maternal hypoxaemia and with umbilical cord compression, but of different degree. Also, whereas combined ventricular output decreases during cord compression, it does not change significantly with graded uterine blood flow reduction (Jensen et al., 1991).

The redistribution of cardiac output and of blood flow to individual organs during graded reduction of uterine blood flow is qualitatively similar, but quantitatively different from that observed during arrest of uterine blood flow (Fig. 2.3). Blood flow to the brain, heart, and adrenals increases and that to the carcass and to the skin falls, while umbilical blood flow is maintained (Jensen et al., 1991). If arterial PO_2 falls below 14 mm Hg, umbilical blood flow falls (Cohn et al., 1985).

During graded reduction in uterine blood flow umbilical venous blood directed through the ductus increases, as does the fraction of umbilical venous blood crossing the foramen ovale. There is a significant increase in blood returning from both superior and abdominal inferior vena cava and from the umbilical vein via the ductus venosus that crosses the foramen ovale to the upper body segment. However, due to the oxygen content being higher in the umbilical venous and in the superior vena cava blood than in the abdominal inferior vena cava blood, the relative contribution to the oxygen delivered to the heart and brain by blood derived from the former is much higher than that contributed by the abdominal vena cava (Jensen et al., 1991).

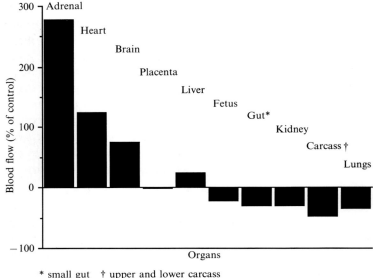

* small gut   † upper and lower carcass

Fig. 2.3. Redistribution of organ blood flow (% of control) during graded reduction of uterine blood flow to achieve a reduction in fetal oxygen delivery by 50% in chronically prepared fetal sheep near term. Fetal oxygen content in the ascending aorta was reduced from 7.76 ± 1.1 ml/dl to 4.78 ± 0.9 ml/dl; pH decreased from 7.40 to 7.25. (From Jensen et al., 1991.)

Repeated brief arrest of uterine blood flow

Repeated reductions in uterine blood flow occur quite frequently during the second stage of labour and expose the fetus to various degrees of hypoxaemia. In spite of its clinical relevance, there are only a few systematic studies devoted to this particular mode of repeated restriction of oxygen delivery to the fetus. One of these studies tried to mimic changes in the uterine vascular bed in the second stage of labour by repeatedly inflating a balloon catheter, which was advanced into the abdominal maternal aorta (Jensen et al., 1985a), in an acute fetal sheep model. Uterine blood flow was intermittently arrested 11 times within 33 min. Each single asphyxial episode lasted 30, 60 or 90 s. Depending on the duration of asphyxia there is a repeated fall in arterial oxygen saturation, heart rate, skin blood flow and transcutaneously measured PO_2 ($tcPO_2$), whereas arterial blood pressure and plasma catecholamine concentrations rise (Jensen et al., 1985a) (Fig. 2.4). With increasing duration of repeated arrest of uterine blood flow fetal skin blood flow decreases to such an extent that the transcutaneous PO_2-signal is suppressed even though central oxygenation is restored. This suggests that in the presence of fetal bradycardia, low transcutaneous PO_2 readings may be used as an index of poor skin blood flow and hence of a circulatory redistribution (Fig. 2.5), as proposed previously (Jensen & Künzel, 1980). This view is supported by close correlations between fetal skin blood flow and plasma catecholamine concentrations (Jensen et al., 1987c).

The observation that reduced blood flow to the fetal skin during repeated reduction in uterine blood flow can be detected by transcutaneous PO_2-measurements has been confirmed by studies in which microspheres were injected into the fetal circulation (Jensen et al., 1987a). These studies showed that reduced skin blood flow is accompanied by both increased sympathetic activity, as assessed by plasma catecholamine concentrations, and a redistribution of systemic blood flow (Fig. 2.5). This may be of clinical significance, because early detection of fetal circulatory centralization through variables that depend on skin blood flow may improve fetal surveillance during complicated labour (Jensen & Künzel, 1980; Jensen et al., 1985a, 1987a,c).

The pattern of redistribution of fetal blood flow after repeated brief episodes of asphyxia, caused by arrest of uterine blood flow for 90 s, is different from that during prolonged asphyxia or maternal hypoxaemia. Myocardial blood flow, for instance, which increases during various interventions (Cohn et al., 1974; Peeters et al., 1979; Itskovitz et al., 1987; Jensen et al., 1991) was not increased significantly 4 min after the last asphyxial episode. This suggests that increased myocardial flows recover more rapidly after repeated than after prolonged asphyxia (Fig. 2.5).

Another difference is that blood flow to the lungs increases under these experimental conditions (Fig. 2.5). This may be related to either vasodilatation in the lungs or to increased arterial pressure in the pulmonary artery due to a transient constriction of the ductus arteriosus (Jensen et al., 1987a).

Prolonged arrest of uterine blood flow

Prolonged arrest of uterine blood flow for 4 min causes severe fetal asphyxia. Heart rate, arterial oxygen content, pH, and combined ventricular output fall, and arterial blood pressure, PCO_2, and lactate concentrations rise rapidly (Jensen et al., 1987b).

This acute severe asphyxia is accompanied by rapid changes in both the fetal and the umbilical circulation. To study the changes in organ blood

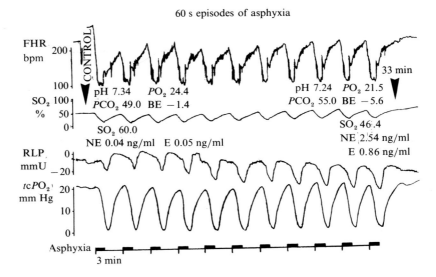

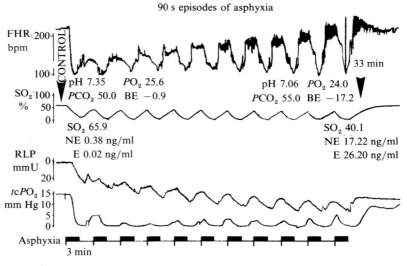

Fig. 2.4. Repeated brief arrest of uterine blood flow for 60 s and 90 s in acutely prepared fetal sheep near term. Original recordings of (from the top) fetal heart rate (FRH), oxygen saturation (SO_2), skin perfusion (mm units deflection) and transcutaneous PO_2 ($tcPO_2$). Note: In contrast to 60 seconds, arrest of uterine blood flow for 90 seconds suppresses the transcutaneous PO_2 signal, although O_2 saturation returns to normal. This is due to increasing catecholamine concentrations that reduce skin blood flow during repeated asphyxia. After asphyxia (bottom) oxygen saturation of haemoglobin is high and all variables recover. With decreasing catecholamine concentrations blood flow to the skin, transcutaneous PO_2, and heart rate return to normal. (From Jensen et al., 1985a.)

Recovery after episodes of 90 s of asphyxia

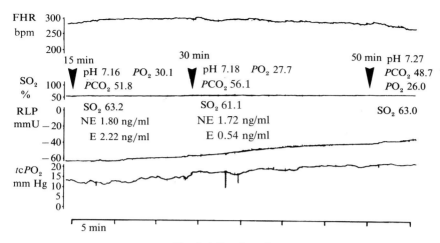

Fig. 2.4 *Continued.*

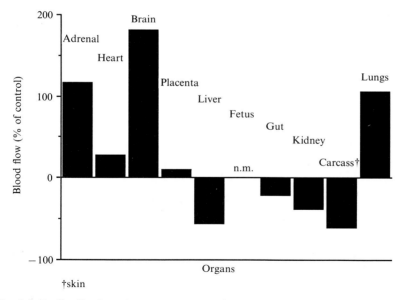

Fig. 2.5. Redistribution of organ blood flow (% of control) during repeated brief arrest of uterine blood flow in acutely prepared fetal sheep near term. Eleven asphyxial episodes were induced within 33 minutes by occlusion of the maternal aorta for 90 s. Fetal PO_2 in the femoral artery remained unchanged before and after asphyxia (23.9 ± 1 vs. 24.7 ± 1.6 mm Hg); pH fell from 7.26 to 7.02. (From Jensen et al., 1987a.)

flow distribution at short intervals a modification of the isotope labelled microphere method has been devised, in which microspheres are injected serially during continuous withdrawal of the reference blood samples (Jensen et al., 1987*b*). The redistribution of cardiac output is qualitatively similar to that observed during graded reduction in uterine blood flow and during maternal hypoxaemia, in that the fractions of cardiac output distributed to the brain, heart, and adrenals increase, while those to peripheral organs fall drastically (Fig. 2.6). However, there are distinct differences, for example, cardiac output falls markedly. Furthermore, there are differences in cerebral vascular resistance and in both blood flow and oxygen delivery to the brain, in that cerebral blood flow does not rise. Thus, oxygen delivery to the cerebrum falls whereas that to the brain stem is maintained, reflecting a redistribution of brain blood flow in favour of brain stem areas (Fig. 2.6) (Jensen et al., 1987*b*).

If severe asphyxia caused by arrest of uterine blood flow is prolonged, circulatory centralization cannot be maintained (Fig. 2.7). Rather, there is a decentralization with a decrease in vascular resistance in peripheral

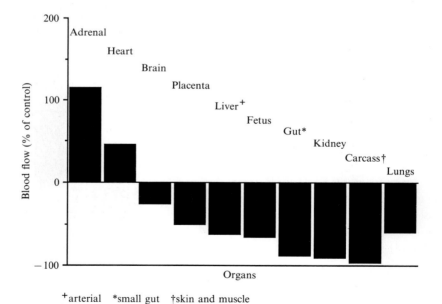

Fig. 2.6. Redistribution of organ blood flow (% of control) during arrest of uterine blood flow for 4 minutes, caused by occlusion of the maternal aorta in unanaesthetized fetal sheep near term. Oxygen saturation in the femoral artery fell from 43% to 4%, pH fell from 7.30 to 7.05. (From Jensen et al., 1987b.)

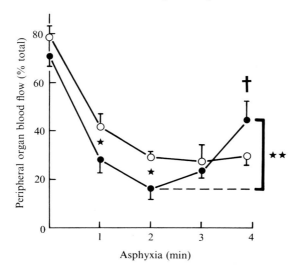

Fig. 2.7. Changes in blood flow to peripheral organs during acute asphyxia in four surviving (open circle) and five non-surviving (filled circle) fetal sheep near term. Note, that, unlike in surviving fetuses, at the nadir of asphyxia (at 4 min) in non-surviving fetuses, the proportion of blood flow directed to peripheral organs was significantly higher than at 2 min of asphyxia (**, $P = 0.01$; 2 min vs. 4 min). (From Jensen et al., 1987*b*.)

organs and an increase in resistance in central organs, including those in the brain and the heart. Also umbilical resistance rises and hence placental blood flow falls. These changes, which are associated with severe metabolic derangements and severe acidaemia below pH 7.0, will lead to fetal demise, unless immediate resuscitation occurs (Jensen et al., 1987*b*).

During decentralization at the nadir of asphyxia (Fig. 2.7), the loss of peripheral vascular resistance may be related to the severity of local acidosis causing the vascular smooth muscle in peripheral arteries to dilate (Jensen et al., 1988). The fate of the fetus during severe asphyxia is determined by the degree of hypoxic myocardial depression and by the depletion of cardiac glycogen stores. Agonal heart rate patterns, increasing degree of cardiac failure and the resulting increase in central venous pressures precede fetal death.

There is one report on fetal circulatory derangements during reduction of blood flow through common hypogastric artery by 75% leaving the ovarian anastomoses intact. In that study cardiac output and umbilical blood flow were maintained. However, an increase in vascular resistance in the brain and heart was observed. The fact that these changes occurred during moderate acidaemia (pH 7.14 ± 0.02) and the fact that they were accompanied by only minor reductions in peripheral blood flows renders these results difficult to interpret (Yaffe et al., 1987).

Fetal haemorrhage

A reduction in fetal oxygen delivery can also be produced by reduction in fetal blood volume, i.e. anaemic hypoxaemia (Itskovitz, Goetzman & Rudolph, 1982*b*). A fall in blood volume by 15–20% is accompanied by a reduction in heart rate (−20%), arterial blood pressure (−10%), and cardiac output (−25%).

The resulting redistribution of fetal organ blood flow is different from that observed during hypoxaemia and asphyxia (Fig. 2.8), in that blood flows to the heart, brain and adrenals are maintained, but not increased. Blood flows to almost all peripheral organs and that to the placenta fall (Itskovitz et al., 1982*b*).

The fraction of umbilical venous blood passing through the ductus venosus increases and contributes about 30% to the cardiac output. Hence, ductus venosus derived blood flow and oxygen delivery to the

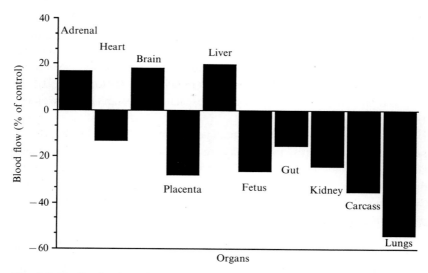

Fig. 2.8. Redistribution of organ blood flow (% of control) during reduction in fetal blood volume by 15% in chronically prepared fetal sheep near term. Fetal PO_2 in the descending aorta did not change (23.7 ± 3.4 vs. 23.5 ± 2.9 mm Hg), pH fell from 7.39 to 7.30. (From Toubas et al., 1981.)

upper and lower body segments also increase by 30% (Itskovitz et al., 1982*b*). Prolonged but quantitatively similar volume losses, e.g. 30% over a period of 2 h, cause less pronounced changes in cardiovascular variables (Brace & Cheung, 1986).

Chronic hypoxaemia

A number of experimental models have been devised in sheep, guinea pigs and rats to produce chronic fetal hypoxaemia with consequent intrauterine growth retardation. These include prolonged maternal hypoxaemia (Jacobs et al., 1988; Kitanaka et al., 1989), reduction of placental size by preconceptual removal of endometrial caruncles (Robinson et al., 1979), placental damage by embolization of the utero-placental bed (Clapp et al., 1981), embolization of the fetal placental vascular bed (Block et al., 1990), ligation of uterine (Lafeber, Rolph & Jones, 1984) or umbilical (Emmanoulides, Townsend & Bauer, 1968) vessels, and maternal heat stress (Alexander et al., 1987). However, fetal growth retardation can also be produced by substrate restriction without any apparent changes in fetal oxygen delivery (Mellor, 1983).

All of these perturbations are associated with a decrease in placental size and/or transfer function that is directly related to the magnitude of retardation in fetal growth (for review see Clapp, 1988). The actual mechanisms involved in reduction of fetal growth are not well under-stood. However, there is clear evidence for oxygen lack being one important factor. But there are also structurally unknown placental signals to consider that might initiate the cessation of fetal growth before hypoxaemia occurs (Jones, 1985). Placental membranes play an import-ant role in the production of prostaglandins, particularly prostacyclin (PGI_2), one of the most potent vasodilators (Lewis, Moncada & O'Grady, 1983). There is, for instance, a substantial reduction in prosta-cyclin production in placentae of fetuses that are chronically hypoxaemic and growth retarded (Jogee, Myatt & Elder, 1983). Whether this re-duction in prostacyclin concentrations is related to an elevated vascular resistance in the fetus is at present unclear.

Reduced fetal growth is associated with a number of metabolic and endocrine changes including hypoglycaemia, hypoinsulinaemia, in-creased concentrations of glucagon, lactate, alanine, triglycerides (for review see Robinson, Falconer & Owens, 1985), cortisol (Clapp et al., 1982), catecholamines, β-endorphins and decreased concentrations of growth-promoting factors, i.e. T_3, T_4, somatomedins and prolactin,

ACTH, insulin-like growth factor (IGF-2). Ovine placental lactogen and growth hormone are unchanged (Robinson et al., 1985; Clapp, 1988; Jones et al., 1988*a*).

The consumption of oxygen and glucose by the fetus is reduced in absolute terms, but are maintained in terms of fetal body mass (Owens et al., 1987). However, the utero-placental consumption of glucose per weight of placenta is reduced and a greater proportion of that glucose or other substrates is converted to lactate by the placenta. And there is also an increase in the fraction of lactate produced by utero-placental tissues that is secreted into the fetal circulation (Owens, Falconer & Robinson, 1987).

Growth retarded fetuses tend to have a lower arterial blood pressure and a higher heart rate under control conditions (Robinson, Jones & Kingston, 1983) (Fig. 2.9). The chronic reduction in fetal oxygen delivery

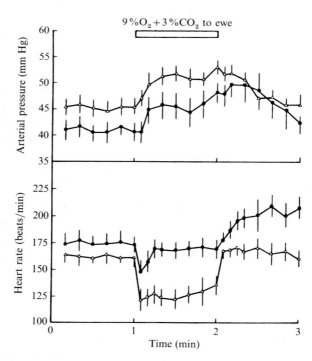

Fig. 2.9. The diagram shows the changes in blood pressure and heart rate in fetal sheep during maternal hypoxaemia (FiO_2 = 9%). Note that in the growth retarded fetuses (filled circle) blood pressure is lower and heart rate is higher than in the normal fetuses (open circle). (From Robinson et al., 1983.)

is compensated in part by an increased packed cell volume with an increased transport capacity for oxygen (Robinson et al., 1983; Jacobs et al., 1988).

Minor degrees of chronically reduced fetal oxygen delivery are not necessarily associated with major circulatory responses (Block et al., 1990). However, major changes in chronically reduced fetal oxygen delivery cause a circulatory centralization in favour of the brain and heart. This is reflected by a relative maintenance of the weight of central organs as compared to that of the fetal body in general and the fetal liver in particular. It has therefore been suggested that the brain/liver weight ratio can be used as an index of fetal growth retardation. The responses of growth-retarded fetuses to acute hypoxaemia or asphyxia are different from that observed in normal-sized fetuses, in that they develop acid-aemia more easily. Furthermore, bradycardia is brief and heart rate returns to control values quickly after the onset of acute hypoxaemia (Robinson et al., 1983), whereas tachycardia develops during recovery. This has been attributed to an increased sympathetic tone in growth-retarded fetuses (Jones & Robinson, 1975; Llanos et al., 1980), even though their adrenaline responses to hypoxaemia are not particularly high (Jones & Robinson, 1983).

During hypoxaemia in growth-retarded fetuses there is only a small increase in plasma glucose concentration that may be due to a failure to mobilize glycogen stores. This is accompanied by only a small decrease in insulin concentrations (Robinson et al., 1983), that may be explained by the fact that basal glucose concentrations in the fetal plasma are low and cannot be reduced further, because the reduction of peripheral glucose consumption is limited.

There is also evidence for an activation of the pituitary–adrenal axis in growth-retarded fetuses, because both plasma ACTH and cortisol concentrations are substantially higher during hypoxaemia than in normal-sized fetuses (Robinson et al., 1983). This may be related to the induction of preterm labour (Challis, Mitchell & Lye, 1984).

Circulatory changes during oxygen lack in immature fetuses

The knowledge of circulatory changes during oxygen lack in immature fetuses is scant. However, it is clear from the existing reports that there are distinct differences between immature and mature fetuses. In general, during normoxaemia, heart rate is higher and arterial blood pressure is lower in immature than in mature fetuses. Furthermore, as far as

Table 2.4. *Effect of acute hypoxaemia on heart rate, arterial blood pressure, and blood flow in young fetal sheep*

	88 days		98 days		135 days[a]	
Mean gestational age	Control	Hypoxaemia	Control	Hypoxaemia	Control	Hypoxaemia
Heart rate (b/min)	224 ± 27	237 ± 35	203 ± 16	226 ± 19[b]	160 ± 9	113 ± 27[b]
Arterial blood pressure (torr)	31 ± 6	30 ± 7	40 ± 3	39 ±	63 ± 7	76 ± 13[c]
Blood flow (ml/min per kg)						
Combined ventricular output	516 ± 95	445 ± 75	566 ± 65	497 ± 58	381 ± 38[b]	NA
Umbilical–placental	256 ± 81	163 ± 54[c]	300 ± 69	197 ± 65[d]	195 ± 54	NA
Fetal body	261 ± 34	282 ± 50	266 ± 36	228 ± 93	302 ± 42	NA
Vascular resistance (torr ml min per kg)						
Total	0.06 ± 0.02	0.07 ± 0.02	0.07 ± 0.01	0.10 ± 0.03	NA	NA
Umbilical–placental	0.13 ± 0.05	0.22 ± 0.13	0.14 ± 0.04	0.20 ± 0.07[b]	NA	NA
Fetal body	0.12 ± 0.03	0.11 ± 0.04	0.16 ± 0.03	0.19 ± 0.08	NA	NA

[a] Cohn et al., (1974).   [b] $P < 0.05$.   [c] $P < 0.01$.   [d] $P < 0.005$: significantly different from control value, paired t-test.
NA = not available.
Source: From Iwamoto et al., 1989.

the circulatory response to hypoxia or asphyxia during development is concerned, there appears to be a different balance of parasympathetic and sympathetic control of the fetal heart rate early in gestation, so that heart rate does not fall or even increases during maternal hypoxaemia (Walker et al., 1979).

There is only one systematic study available on the circulatory effects of maternal hypoxaemia on immature (i.e. 0.7 gestation) and very immature (i.e. 0.6 gestation) chronically prepared fetal sheep (Iwamoto et al., 1989). These authors examined in detail the changes of heart rate, arterial blood pressure, distribution of cardiac output, organ blood flows and vascular resistances during moderate hypoxaemia, i.e. 12–14 mm Hg PO_2 in the descending fetal aorta. Under these conditions, which were accompanied by slight fetal acidaemia, arterial blood pressure and heart rate did not change at 0.6 gestation, whereas heart rate increased significantly at 0.7 gestation (Table 2.4). As in mature fetuses, cerebral, myocardial, and adrenal blood flows increased and pulmonary blood flow decreased. The authors conclude that these responses mature early and are likely to be local vascular responses to decreases in oxygen content (Iwamoto et al., 1989). Furthermore, they found that combined ventricular output and umbilical–placental blood flow decreased in both groups (Table 2.4). Interestingly, in the fetuses at 0.6 gestation there was no change in blood flow to the carcass, i.e. musculo-skeletal and cutaneous circulations, gastrointestinal or renal circulations during hypoxaemia, whereas blood flow to the carcass fell in the fetuses at 0.7 gestation suggesting that peripheral vasomotor control starts to develop at approximately 0.7 gestation. This among other vasoactive substances may also involve arginine–vasopressin, which was increased at 0.7 gestation. But these differences in responses between 0.6 and 0.7 gestation may also indicate immaturity in chemoreceptor function, in the response of neurohormonal modulators, or in the response of regional receptor effector mechanisms (Iwamoto et al., 1989).

Only recently, comparative information on the effects of acute asphyxia, caused by arrest of uterine blood flow on chronically prepared fetal sheep at 0.6, 0.75 and 0.9 gestation have become available (Jensen, 1992). Under these conditions, heart rate fell during and recovered after asphyxia in all age groups (Fig. 2.10). However, there were major differences in the arterial blood pressure, which was significantly poorer at 0.6 than at 0.75 and 0.9 gestation. During 1 and 2 minute asphyxia, arterial blood pressure does not change significantly at 0.6, rises after a

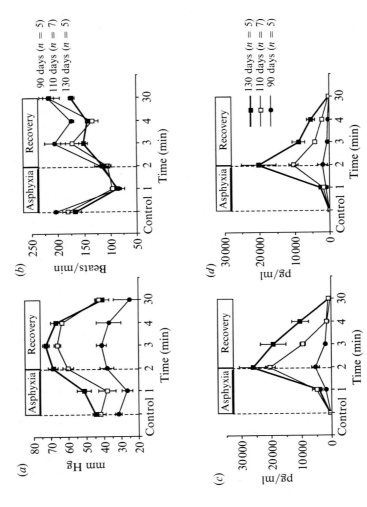

Fig. 2.10. Changes in (a) arterial blood pressure, (b) heart rate, (c) norepinephrine, and (d) epinephrine concentrations during arrest of uterine blood flow for 2 minutes in chronically prepared fetal sheep at 0.6, 0.75, 0.9 gestation. (From Jensen, 1992.)

transient decrease at 0.75 and progressively rises at 0.9 gestation (Fig. 2.10). These responses were accompanied by age-dependent changes in plasma concentrations of epinephrine and norepinephrine. Epinephrine concentrations did not change significantly and the increase in concentration of norepinephrine was blunted during asphyxia at 0.6 gestation, whereas high and extremely high plasma concentrations could be measured at 0.75 and 0.9 gestation, respectively.

There are also age-dependent differences in organ blood flow. For example, blood flow to the brain per 100 g is lowest, higher and highest at 0.6, 0.75 and 0.9 gestation, respectively (Jensen, 1992). Interestingly during recovery in the youngest group of fetuses, there was a steady increase in blood flow to all parts of the brain, including the germinal matrix. Whether this new finding may be related to the well-known fact that cerebral haemorrhage, in immature human fetuses originates from the germinal matrix in 80% of cases, remains to be established.

Blood flow to the myocardium increased progressively during asphyxia without differences between age groups and recovered thereafter in the fetuses at 0.75 and 0.9 gestation. In the youngest group of fetuses there was a tremendous increase in myocardial blood flow in the late recovery period, suggesting increased myocardial oxygen demands, e.g. by increased cardiac output.

The blood flow to the carcass is largely similar in fetuses of 0.75 and 0.9 gestation, in that it falls during asphyxia and recovers. However, at 0.6 gestation carcass blood flow at control is almost twice as high afterwards; it fell during asphyxia and rose above control after it. Taking these findings together it appears that in very immature fetuses a state of postasphyxial hyperperfusion of a number of organs develops, which may reflect a lack of control of vascular resistance. This view is supported by the fact that, at this point in gestation, in man and in sheep, asphyxia was followed by pronounced hypotension (Jensen, 1992). These observations during arrest of uterine blood flow as well as those from maternal hypoxaemia provide evidence that in the very immature fetal sheep at 0.6 gestation circulatory centralization is incomplete and may be ineffective in reducing oxygen delivery to and hence oxygen consumption of peripheral organs (Jensen et al., 1991). The fact that the age-dependence of fetal circulatory and metabolic centralization coincides with the maturation of the sympathetic nervous system as well as other neuro-hormonal systems, sheds light on the importance of these systems for intact survival of acute asphyxia.

Interaction between O_2 delivery and tissue metabolism

It has been recognized for a long time that hypoxaemia and asphyxia cause both a redistribution of blood flow (Cohn et al., 1974; Itskovitz et al., 1987; Jensen et al., 1987a,b, 1991) and a reduction in oxygen consumption (Jensen et al., 1987b, 1991). However, a direct relationship between blood flow changes during asphyxia and changes in oxygen consumption has been suggested only recently (Jensen et al., 1987b) (Fig. 2.11).

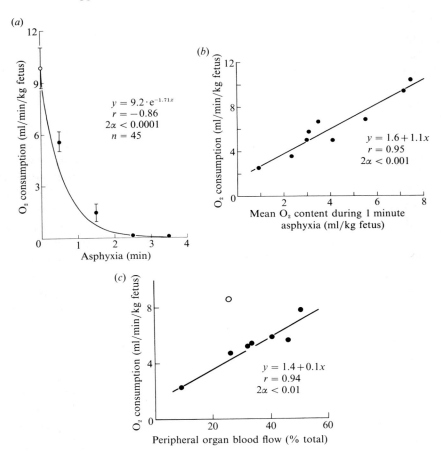

Fig. 2.11. Changes in fetal and placental oxygen consumption during arrest of uterine blood flow. Note, that O_2 consumption falls exponentially during asphyxia. Note also, that O_2 consumption correlates closely with both O_2 content in the descending aortic blood and blood flow to peripheral organs. This suggests that in the fetus O_2 delivery is a major determinant of oxygen consumption. (From Jensen et al., 1987b.)

The relationship between utero-placental oxygen delivery and fetal oxygen consumption is curvilinear, and fetal oxygen consumption only falls when utero-placental blood flow is reduced below 50% (Wilkening & Meschia, 1983). This, and the fact that it is known from adult physiology that mitochondrial oxygen consumption is maintained until oxygen partial pressure falls below a 'critical PO_2' of approximately 1 mm Hg, have precluded for a long time the possible conclusion that blood flow and oxygen delivery to fetal organs might determine the oxygen consumed in these organs.

Recently, it has been suggested that the relation between the availability of oxygen and the consumption of oxygen may be fundamentally different during fetal as compared with adult life (Jensen et al., 1987*b*) in that fetal oxygen consumption depends linearly on the delivery of oxygen, i.e. blood flow × O_2 content, to fetal organs (Fig. 2.11). It has been shown for whole cell preparations (Wilson, Owen & Erecinska, 1979), various individual fetal organs, e.g. the carotid body (Acker & Lübbers, 1977), the liver (Bristow et al., 1983), the kidney (Iwamoto & Rudolph, 1985), for organ parts (Jensen et al., 1991), and for the whole conceptus (Jensen et al., 1987*b*) that the amount of oxygen available determines the amount of oxygen consumed.

Furthermore, it has been concluded that, during asphyxia, changes in vasomotor activity, e.g. caused by the sympathetic nervous system, play an important part in regulating fetal oxygen consumption by changing blood flow and hence oxygen delivery to peripheral organs (Jensen et al., 1987*b*). Whether the fall of placental O_2 consumption parallels that of the fetus when maternal and/or fetal O_2 delivery to the placenta is decreased and how that fall in placental O_2 consumption might affect its endocrine functions is not known.

These findings, which have recently been confirmed by studies on the oxygen consumption of fetal sheep ventilated in utero after snaring the umbilical cord (Asakura, Ball & Power, 1990), are not at variance with studies showing a curvilinear relationship between utero-placental blood flow and fetal oxygen consumption. Depending on the oxygen delivered, the fetus can increase oxygen extraction across the utero-placental vascular bed, across the umbilical–placental vascular bed, and across the arterio-venous vascular bed of each individual organ. Therefore, oxygen consumption of the whole conceptus (i.e. fetus, placenta & membranes) of the fetus, and of the individual organs, will only decrease when oxygen extraction is maximal and oxygen delivery is further reduced beyond that point.

Additional support for this important mechanism has been provided by in vitro studies on fetal skeletal muscle cells (Braems & Jensen, 1991), and myocardial cells in monolayer culture (Braems, Dußler & Jensen, 1990). These showed that, unlike in the adult, in the fetus oxygen availability is a determinant of cellular oxygen consumption.

Evidence produced in vivo and in vitro suggests that, on transition from normoxia to hypoxia, the fetus is able to reduce oxygen consumption by decreasing oxygen delivery to peripheral organs (Jensen et al., 1987*b*; Braems & Jensen, 1991). This, along with increasing blood flow to central organs, helps to maintain oxygen consumption in central organs by maintaining oxygen delivery to the brain and to the heart, i.e. 'metabolic centralization'.

Conversely, on transition from hypoxia to normoxia the increase in oxygen delivery is paralleled by an increase in cellular oxygen consumption and in metabolic drive in most fetal organs. This mechanism, which may be of particular importance on transition from fetal to postnatal life when oxygen delivery and oxygen consumption rise (Dawes & Mott, 1959) provides optimal cell function at any given state of oxygenation.

In summary, circulatory centralization during hypoxia and asphyxia, caused by chemoreceptor mediated vascular reflexes, which involve, among others, the sympathetic nervous system, acts in concert with metabolic centralization, which maintains oxygen delivery to, oxygen consumption of and cell function in the brain and heart to ensure intact survival of the fetus (Jensen, 1991).

Cardiovascular mechanisms

Near term the common fetal cardiovascular response to acute oxygen lack is bradycardia, an increase in arterial blood pressure and an increase in heart rate variability (Dalton, Dawes & Patrick, 1977; Walker et al., 1979). These changes are in part mediated by peripheral arterial chemo-receptors (Giusssani et al., 1990; for review see Hanson, 1988), which co-activate parasympathetic (for review see Martin, 1985) and sympathetic pathways (Cohn, Piaseki & Jackson, 1978; Court et al., 1984; Jensen et al., 1987*a,b,c*). This was elegantly illustrated by Blanco, Dawes & Walker (1983), who transected the spinal cord at T12 and then were able to show that hypoxaemia no longer produced a rise in arterial blood pressure, due to ablation of sympathetic efferents, even though the fall in heart rate persisted, because the vagi were intact.

Because arterial blood pressure rises there is also an activation of baroreceptors (Blanco et al., 1985) which may result in a further decrease in fetal heart rate. During severe prolonged hypoxaemia myocardial suppression and, eventually, myocardial failure occurs. Unlike reflex bradycardia, bradycardia resulting from myocardial depression cannot be blocked by atropine (Itskovitz et al., 1982*a*).

There is a correlation between arterial oxygen content before the insult and the delay to the onset of bradycardia. The lower the PO_2 in the carotid arterial blood the shorter is the delay in the onset of bradycardia, the greater the decrease in heart rate and the more prolonged the duration of bradycardia (Itskovitz et al., 1982*a*). Conversely, during a reduction in umbilical blood flow the baroreceptor-mediated response precedes that of the carotid chemoreceptors, because arterial blood pressure rises before oxygen content falls.

During prolonged hypoxaemia, bradycardia tends to normalize. This is associated with an increased sympathetic activity of the neuro- and medullary sympathetic nervous system, which is accompanied by a release of catecholamines from the adrenal medulla and sympathetic nerves (Cohen et al., 1984; Jensen et al., 1985, 1987*a,c*; Jelinek & Jensen, 1991). The increased release of catecholamines results in a circulatory centralization in favour of the brain, heart and adrenals at the expense of peripheral organs (for review see Rudolph, 1984).

If during hypoxaemia the sympathetic effect on the heart is blocked by β-adrenoceptor antagonists the fall of fetal heart rate, cardiac output and umbilical blood flow is more pronounced. Furthermore, increased blood flow to the heart, brain and adrenals cannot be maintained (Parer, 1983; Court et al., 1984).

Blockade of α-adrenoceptors during hypoxaemia causes an increase in fetal heart rate and cardiac output, whereas arterial blood pressure and total vascular resistance fall. Then blood flow to the heart, adrenals, gut, spleen, and lungs are increased (Reuss et al., 1982). Blockade of α- and β-adrenoceptors results in fetal demise during hypoxaemia (Parer et al., 1978).

Ablation of peripheral sympathetic neurones by chemical sympathectomy, e.g. by 6-hydroxydopamine, leaves the adrenal medulla intact. Hence, circulating catecholamine concentrations do not change much (Iwamoto et al., 1983; Jensen & Lang, 1992). Changes of cardiac output during and after acute asphyxia are similar in intact as compared with sympathectomized fetuses (Fig. 2.12) (Jensen & Lang, 1992). However, during fetal hypoxaemia and asphyxia the increase in arterial blood

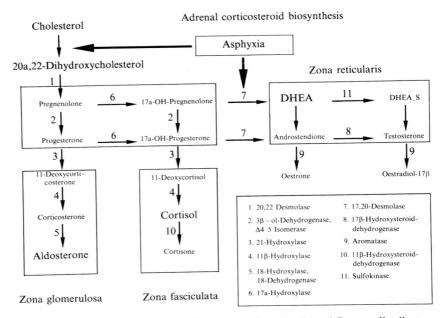

Fig. 2.12. Severe asphyxia, caused by arrest of uterine blood flow, redistributes corticosteroid biosynthesis in favour of the cortisol and aldosterone pathways and at the expense of the androgen pathway. This is related to the oxygen dependence of 17, 20 desmolase. (From Jensen et al., 1988.)

pressure is delayed (Iwamoto et al., 1983; Lewis & Sischo, 1985; Jensen & Lang, 1988). This may be associated with a slow initial rise in plasma catecholamine concentrations (Jones et al., 1988*b*). In sympathectomized fetuses the redistribution of organ blood flow during hypoxaemia and asphyxia is different from that in intact fetuses (Fig. 2.12), in that blood flows to the gastro-intestinal tract and to the kidneys do not change (Iwamoto et al., 1983; Jensen & Lang, 1988). The effect of chemical sympathectomy on the carcass, skeletal muscle and skin blood flows depends on the severity of asphyxia (Iwamoto et al., 1983; Jensen & Lang, 1988). The increase in vascular resistance, which usually occurs during arrest of uterine blood flow, is completely blunted in the gastrointestinal tract and markedly delayed in the carcass (Jensen & Lang, 1988, 1992). During maternal hypoxaemia, the increase in blood flow to the heart, brain and adrenals is not significantly affected in sympathectomized fetuses (Iwamoto et al., 1983). However, during arrest of uterine blood

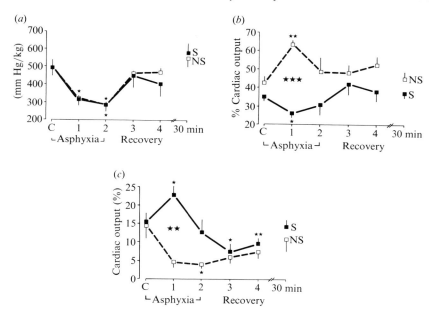

Fig. 2.13. (*a*) Cardiac output and its distribution to the placenta, (*b*), and carcass, (*c*), of intact (NS) and sympathectomized (S) chronically prepared fetal sheep near term during arrest of uterine blood flow. (From Jensen & Lang, 1988.)

flow, the initial increase in blood flow to the brainstem is blunted (Jensen & Lang, 1988; 1992). Furthermore, the percentage of the cardiac output directed to the placenta is reduced, while that to the carcass is increased as compared with intact fetuses (Fig. 2.13). Therefore, in sympathectomized fetuses circulatory centralization is less effective in protecting the fetus against adverse effects of asphyxia (Jensen & Lang, 1988, 1992).

But there are also other mechanisms to consider that are involved in the regulation of blood flow during oxygen lack. Fetal hypoxaemia is accompanied by an increase in plasma renin activity (Robillard et al., 1981), which converts angiotensin I to angiotensin II, a potent vasoconstrictive hormone (Scroop et al., 1986; Martin, Kapoor & Scroop, 1987*b*). Furthermore, there is a rise in vasopressin (AVP) during hypoxaemia (Rurak, 1978). Infusion of vasopressin causes bradycardia and a circulatory centralization (Rurak, 1978).

Acute hypoxia is associated with a reduction in fetal blood volume. In the regulation of these changes atrial natriuretic factor (ANF) may be involved (Cheung & Brace, 1988). Whether the rise in ANF concentrations observed during acute hypoxia is a direct or an indirect effect of hypoxia has yet to be determined (Cheung & Brace, 1988).

Circulatory changes during volume loss, e.g. through fetal haemorrhage, are in part governed by the autonomic nervous system (Brace, 1987). Furthermore, there are a number of hormones released, including AVP (Rurak, 1978; Robillard et al., 1979; Drummond et al., 1980), renin (Robillard et al., 1982; Iwamoto & Rudolph, 1981), catecholamines (Jones et al., 1985; Lewis & Sischo, 1985), ACTH, and cortisol (Rose, Morris & Meis, 1981). Prolonged but quantitatively similar volume losses, e.g. 30% over a period of 2 h, cause less pronounced hormone changes (Brace & Cheung, 1986).

Furthermore, during hypoxia there is clear evidence for the activation of the pituitary adreno-cortical axis, resulting in increased ACTH and cortisol concentrations (see Jones et al., 1988*b*; Challis et al., 1989). Among other responses these two hormones allegedly help to maintain the arterial blood pressure during hypoxaemia (Jones et al., 1988*b*).

Another group of substances related to changes in cardiovascular variables during hypoxaemia are β-endorphins (Skillman & Clark, 1987). Blocking endogenous opiate receptors by naloxone results in a pronounced fall in heart rate, and a decrease in cardiac output and placental blood flow, while peripheral vascular resistance rises. This suggests that endogenous opioids may modulate the cardiovascular response to hypoxia (LaGamma et al., 1982). Other peptides, e.g. neuropeptide Y (NPY) have been reported to cause vasoconstriction, but the actual mechanism has not yet been determined (Emson & Quidt, 1984).

Changes in blood flow to fetal organs during hypoxaemia and asphyxia

Brain

Blood flow to the fetal brain increases during various interventions that result in a fall in arterial oxygen content. These include maternal hypoxaemia (Cohn et al., 1974; Peeters et al., 1979), graded reduction in umbilical blood flow (Itskovitz et al., 1987) and graded reduction in uterine blood flow (Jensen et al., 1991). However, during arrest of uterine blood flow, blood flow to the brain does not increase in spite of an increase in arterial blood pressure, suggesting an increase in cerebral vascular resistance (Jensen et al., 1987*b*). This cerebral reflex vasoconstriction during acute severe asphyxia is accompanied by a steep rise in plasma catecholamine concentrations, suggesting that an activation of the sympathetic nervous system through arterial chemoreceptors is involved (Jensen et al., 1985*b*).

Thus, during acute asphyxia caused by arrest of uterine blood flow (Jensen et al., 1987*b*) oxygen delivery to the brain falls, whereas it is maintained during moderate hypoxaemia (Jones et al., 1977; Peeters et al., 1979; Richardson et al., 1989; Jensen et al., 1991).

A recent study on the effect of mild chronic hypoxaemia (of approximately 17 mm Hg PO_2 in the fetal ascending aorta) caused by embolization of the umbilical circulation, revealed that there may be threshold arterial oxygen contents, above which cerebral blood flow does not change (Block et al., 1990). This may be explained, in part, by an increased oxygen extraction across the cerebral vascular bed, but there are other mechanisms to consider including reduced cerebral oxygen consumption.

During hypoxaemia, the increase in blood flow to the brainstem is greater than that seen in other regions despite the fact that this area has the highest resting blood flow in the fetal brain (Jensen et al., 1987*b*, 1991; Itskovitz et al., 1987; Richardson et al., 1989). This may have survival value for the fetus because neuronal activity in important autonomic centres in the brainstem is maintained.

Autoregulation of fetal cerebral blood flow is operative in the fetal lamb near term during normoxia (Tweed et al., 1983). However, it has been demonstrated that during hypoxaemia autoregulation of cerebral blood flow is lost. Then cerebral blood flow varies with arterial blood pressure. But this is not always true. For instance, during acute asphyxia caused by arrest of uterine blood flow, cerebral vascular resistance increases and hence cerebral blood flow does not increase in spite of a steep increase in arterial blood pressure. Thus, under these very acute conditions, autoregulation of cerebral blood flow is intact, even though arterial oxygen content is poor (Jensen et al., 1987*b*). Whether this is related to the rapidity of the change in carotid arterial oxygen content over time, and hence to the intensity of carotid arterial chemoreceptor stimulation, is at present unknown. Interestingly, during repeated occlusion of the umbilical cord, blood flow to the grey matter increased, whereas that to the white matter decreased, a pattern of redistribution that was consistent with brain lesions (Clapp et al., 1988).

A fall in oxygen delivery to the cerebrum can be compensated, within limits, by an increase in cerebral oxygen extraction. If oxygen delivery continues to fall, cerebral oxygen consumption falls (Richardson et al.,

1989). Then, due to increasing cerebral oxygen deficiency, glucose, the main fuel of the brain (Makowski et al., 1972), is metabolized anaerobically, lactate concentration rises, and concentrations of high-energy phosphates fall in the cerebrum (Myers, 1977; Wagner et al., 1986). Finally, cerebral metabolism may collapse when synthesis of high-energy phosphates through aerobic or anaerobic glycolysis fails. Then neuronal membranes depolarize and voltage-gated Ca^{2+} channels open and Ca^{2+} flux into the cytoplasm increases. There is also an enhanced release of excitatory neurotransmitters (such as glutamate), and hence an increased N-methyl-D-aspartate (NMDA) receptor stimulation which further increases the flux of Ca^{2+} into the neurones, resulting in neuronal death.

There are also other adverse effects of asphyxia on the brain, e.g. the generation of oxygen radicals, which destroy multiple unsaturated fatty acids of the cell membranes. These membrane defects lead to a further increase in Ca^{2+} influx, which enhances energy-consuming cellular processes. Then both membranes and organelles of the neurones will be destroyed by lipases, proteases and endonucleases. Thus, a vicious circle is maintained that eventually results in neuronal death.

Functionally, there are a number of effects elicited by hypoxaemia and asphyxia on the brain, e.g. on the electrocortical activity and on fetal breathing. In normoxaemic fetal sheep there are episodic changes in electrocortical activity, characteristic of the sleep states seen postnatally, before 3 weeks term (Dawes et al., 1972). Then, fetal breathing movements (which are almost continuous before 115 days) are confined to episodes of low voltage activity. In this electrocortical state rapid eye movements occur, whereas gross fetal body movements are associated with high voltage electrocortical activity. These obvious functional changes between high and low voltage activity are accompanied by changes in arterial blood pressure, heart rate, blood flow to the brain and to the brainstem and in plasma catecholamine concentrations, suggesting changing sympathetic tone during high and low voltage activity (Jensen et al., 1986; Reid et al., 1990).

During hypoxia there is an increase in the relative incidence of episodes of high voltage activity (Martin, Voersmans & Jongsma, 1987a), whereas severe asphyxia is associated with an increased proportion of episodes of low voltage activity. Eventually, fetal electrocortical activity becomes isoelectric (Mann, Prichard & Symmes, 1970).

During hypoxaemia, fetal breathing movements and REM are reduced (Boddy et al., 1974; Bocking & Harding, 1986). This is due to central inhibition (Dawes et al., 1983). During prolonged hypoxaemia the incidence of breathing movements returns to normal values within 14 h (Koos et al., 1988).

Heart

During normoxaemia in the unanaesthesized fetal sheep near term, heart rate varies between 140 and 180 beats/min and the combined ventricular output is 450 ml/min/kg fetal body weight. There is only a small rise in cardiac output (10–15%) during tachycardia and only a small increase in stroke volume when end-diastolic filling pressures rises (Thornburg & Morton, 1983; Rudolph, 1985). Furthermore, cardiac output is very sensitive to changes in afterload (Gilbert, 1982). These findings suggest that the fetal heart operates at the upper limit of its function curve under physiological conditions (Rudolph, 1985). This may be related to structural differences between the adult and the fetal heart in which myofibril content is less (Maylie, 1982) and the sarcoplasmic reticulum and the T-tubule-system is poorly developed (Hoerter, Mazet & Vassort, 1982).

Hypoxaemia and asphyxia cause a fall in heart rate and combined ventricular output (Rudolph & Heymann, 1976). Although arterial blood pressure, and hence afterload, rise there is a small increase in stroke volume. In this situation coronary and myocardial blood flows are increased to meet cardiac oxygen demands by increasing oxygen delivery (Cohn et al., 1974; Peeters et al., 1979; Itskovitz et al., 1987; Jensen et al., 1991). The reduction in preductal aortic oxygen content by 50% does not affect cardiac consumption of either oxygen or that of glucose or lactate (Fisher, Heymann & Rudolph, 1982).

Unlike hypoxaemia, acidaemia reduces cardiac performance (Fisher, 1986). This may be related to depletion of cardiac glycogen stores which, in turn, may cause ECG changes (Hökegard et al., 1979).

Liver

The fetal hepatic vascular bed is different from that of the adult in that the ductus venosus connects the umbilical vein with the abdominal inferior vena cava. There are also branches of the umbilical vein to the left and right lobe of the liver, the latter communicating with the portal vein (Rudolph, 1983). About 55% of umbilical venous blood bypasses the liver through the ductus venosus. The remainder is distributed to the lobes of the liver. The left lobe of the liver is almost exclusively supplied by umbilical venous blood, whereas the right liver lobe is supplied by both umbilical and portal venous blood. The contribution of hepatic arterial blood is small (3–4%) (see Rudolph, 1985).

During maternal hypoxaemia sufficient to cause a fall in fetal oxygen tension to about 12 mm Hg in the carotid artery, umbilical blood flow is largely maintained, whereas blood flow to the fetal body tends to fall (Cohn et al., 1974). The fraction of umbilical blood passing through the ductus venosus increases from 55 to 65 %, whereas that going to the liver falls by a similar amount (Reuss & Rudolph, 1980; Bristow et al., 1983). Due to a reduction of O_2 content in the umbilical venous and portal venous blood, O_2 delivery to the liver falls drastically.

During a reduction in umbilical blood flow O_2 content does not change. However, hepatic and fetal O_2 delivery falls. This is accompanied by an increased fraction of blood distributed to the ductus venosus at the expense of that to the liver. Within the liver, umbilical venous blood flow to the right lobe is more reduced than that to the left. Portal venous blood is maintained (Edelstone et al., 1980; Itskovitz et al., 1987).

During reduction in uterine blood flow there is also a redistribution of umbilical venous blood towards the ductus venosus (10%). However, the mechanisms involved are poorly understood. There may be changes in vascular resistance in the ductus venosus related to transmural pressures (Edelstone et al., 1978). But there are also direct hypoxaemic effects and neurohormonal mechanisms to consider (Coceani et al., 1984).

During hypoxaemia, fetal hepatic oxygen consumption falls linearly in relation to the fall in O_2 delivery, but the fall in O_2 consumption is smaller in the left than in the right lobe of the liver suggesting functional differences (Bristow et al., 1983). During reduction in umbilical blood flow, O_2 delivery to the liver decreases, whereas hepatic O_2 consumption is maintained due to an increased O_2 extraction (Rudolph et al., 1989).

During maternal hypoxaemia, or during reduction in uterine blood flow, liver glycolysis is enhanced and glucose is released into the inferior vena cava blood. This covers approximately 30–40% of the fetal consumption of glucose when oxygen is in short supply (Bristow et al., 1983, Rudolph et al., 1989). There is no firm evidence for a significant gluconeogenesis in the sheep fetus (Gleason & Rudolph, 1986). The fall in net uptake of lactate by the liver may contribute to the rise in fetal blood lactate concentration.

Placenta

Umbilical blood flow falls during arrest of uterine blood flow (Jensen et al., 1987*b,d*) However, umbilical and hence placental blood flow is largely maintained during maternal hypoxaemia and during graded reduction in uterine blood flow, whereas blood flow to the fetus, particularly to the lower body segment, tends to fall (Cohn et al., 1974; Itskovitz et al., 1987; Jensen et al., 1991). At any rate, oxygen delivery from the placenta to the fetus falls. Studies of transplacental oxygen diffusion in sheep have demonstrated that umbilical and uterine blood form an exchange system that tends to produce equilibration in the venous concentrations of the two blood streams (Rankin et al., 1971).

The overall efficiency of this exchange system, however, is less than that of an ideal venous equilibration as shown by the observations that the uterine–umbilical venous PO_2 difference is consistently positive and ranges among animals between 12 and 20 mm Hg, and that the uterine-umbilical venous PCO_2 difference is consistently negative and averages approximately −3 mm Hg (Wilkening & Meschia, 1983). This limitation may result from several factors, e.g., configuration of maternal and fetal vessels, uneven placental perfusion, low O_2 diffusion capacity, or the high O_2 affinity of fetal blood (Wilkening & Meschia, 1983).

During oxygen lack there is no obvious improvement in the efficiency of the placenta to supply the fetus with oxygen, i.e. to reduce the uterine–umbilical venous O_2 difference. The reduced oxygen delivery to the fetus is compensated initially by an increased O_2 extraction to maintain O_2 consumption. However, below an O_2 delivery of 0.5 mmol/min/kg, fetal O_2 consumption starts to fall (Künzel et al., 1977; Wilkening & Meschia, 1983). During reduction in uterine blood flow, net placental consumption of glucose falls and there is evidence for substantial provision of glucose and lactate to the fetus. Fetal production of lactate increases sharply and much of this appears to be consumed by the placenta at a rate sufficient to account for the deficit in net glucose consumption (Gu, Jones & Parer, 1985).

Kidney

During a graded moderate reduction of uterine or umbilical blood flow there are no significant changes in renal blood flow (Itskovitz et al., 1987; Jensen et al., 1991). Maternal hypoxaemia causes an increase in renal vascular resistance and a fall in renal blood flow by 20% (Cohn et al., 1974; Weismann & Robillard, 1988). However, glomerular filtration rate is maintained, suggesting that renal vasoconstriction is likely to occur at the efferent rather than the afferent arteriolar level (Robillard et al., 1981). When renal blood flow falls there is an increase in plasma renin and vasopressin concentrations and an increased reabsorption of water (Robillard et al., 1981). There is only a transient fall in glomerular filtration rate if fetal hypoxaemia is prolonged. During recovery from hypoxaemia filtration rate and urine production increase above control values (Wlodeck et al., 1989).

A decrease in renal blood flow during fetal hypoxaemia causes a marked reduction in renal oxygen delivery and oxygen extraction increases. Eventually, renal oxygen consumption falls if hypoxaemia persists (Iwamoto & Rudolph, 1985).

In normoxia the kidneys metabolize lactate and release glucose, whereas during hypoxaemia they metabolize glucose and release lactate (Iwamoto & Rudolph, 1985). Obviously, renal gluconeogenesis prevails during normoxaemia, whereas glycolysis prevails during hypoxia.

Lungs

During fetal life gas exchange occurs in the placenta. Pulmonary blood flow is low, supplying only nutritional requirements for lung growth and perhaps serving some metabolic or para-endocrine functions (see Heymann, 1984). About 8–10% of the cardiac output is directed to the lungs (Rudolph & Heymann, 1970). The high pulmonary vascular resistance is in part due to the thickness of the vascular smooth muscle (Reid, 1979). Furthermore, low PO_2 during fetal life may contribute to an increased pulmonary vascular resistance.

From studies in sheep it has emerged that autonomic control of pulmonary vascular resistance is poor. Bilateral section of cervical or thoracic sympathetic nerves does not significantly change pulmonary vascular resistance (Colebatch et al., 1965). Similarly, bilateral cervical vagotomy had no effect. Also, selective pharmacologic blockade using phentolamine and atropine did not change resting pulmonary vascular tone (Rudolph, Heymann & Lewis, 1977). Interestingly, a combination of α- and β-adrenergic and parasympathetic blockade could prevent pulmonary vasoconstriction (Lewis, Heymann & Rudolph, 1976), suggesting that pulmonary vascular responses to hypoxia are not mediated directly by these autonomic pathways (Heymann, 1984). On the other hand, electrical (Colebatch et al., 1965), and hormonal stimulation (Smith, Morris & Assali, 1964) can alter pulmonary vascular resistance. Whether these mechanisms are invoked during fetal hypoxaemia is not clear (Heymann, 1984).

Prostaglandins have been reported to be involved in the regulation of pulmonary blood flow. At present, it appears that they have a modulatory effect on pulmonary vasoconstriction during hypoxaemia, which is blunted by indomethacin (Cassin, 1982). Recently, further evidence for a major role of leucotrienes, lipooxygenase-dependent derivatives of arachidonic acid metabolism, in regulating pulmonary blood flow has been produced. Maternal hypoxaemia, graded reduction of umbilical and uterine blood flow increase pulmonary vascular resistance and decrease pulmonary blood flow (Itskovitz et al., 1987; Jensen et al., 1991). In immature and mature human newborns there is evidence that reduced pulmonary blood flow during asphyxia might be related to patent ductus arteriosus and to respiratory distress syndrome (see Chapter 11).

Adrenals

Adrenal blood flow increases during maternal hypoxaemia, and during graded reduction in uterine and/or umbilical blood flow (Cohn et al., 1974; Itskovitz et al., 1987; Jensen et al., 1991), suggesting that this organ is important when oxygen is at short supply. The adrenals are therefore considered to be 'central' organs along with the brain and the heart. During normoxaemia adrenal medullary blood flow is twice as high as adrenal cortical blood flow. During isocapnic hypoxaemia the increase in blood flow ($+145\%$) is similar in the two areas (Jensen et al., 1985b). These changes in blood flow may be related to adrenal function in that catecholamines, e.g. norepinephrine and epinephrine, are released during hypoxaemia in large quantities from the adrenal medulla (Comline & Silver, 1961; Jelinek & Jensen, 1991). There is also a significant release of cortisol (Jones et al., 1977), which is related to an increased release of ACTH from the pituitary (Jones et al., 1988b), and of aldosterone (Robillard et al., 1984).

During severe asphyxia caused by arrest of uterine blood flow, the release of medullary and cortical hormones is different in that concentrations of norepinephrine, epinephrine, and aldosterone increase and those of cortisol and dehydroepiandrosterone decrease. Furthermore, there appears to be a redistribution of adrenal corticosteroid biosynthesis during asphyxia, in favour of the cortisol pathway and at the expense of the androgen pathway (Jensen et al., 1988) (Fig. 2.12).

Intestines

Blood flow to the intestinal tract is maintained during maternal hypoxaemia and during graded reduction in uterine and umbilical blood flow (Cohn et al., 1974; Itskovitz et al., 1987; Jensen et al., 1991) and intestinal oxygen consumption does not change, because oxygen extraction rises (Edelstone & Holzman, 1984). Only severe reduction in fetal arterial oxygen content resulted in a marked fall in intestinal blood flow (Jensen et al., 1987b; Yaffe et al., 1987). Then, in spite of an increased oxygen extraction, intestinal oxygen consumption falls and a mesentery acidosis develops (Edelstone & Holzman, 1984). In human newborns this might be related to necrotizing enterocolitis.

Spleen

Splenic blood flow is reduced during maternal hypoxaemia and severe asphyxia caused by arrest of uterine blood flow. During the latter insult, splenic blood flow is virtually arrested (Jensen et al., 1987b; Jensen & Lang, 1988). This may be related to the fact that the spleen is almost exclusively innervated by the sympathetic nervous system (Fillenz, 1966).

Carcass

The fetal carcass largely consists of skin, muscle, bones and connective tissues. Blood flow to the carcass falls during more severe maternal hypoxaemia or a reduction in uterine blood flow (Cohn et al., 1974; Jensen et al., 1991). It rises, however, during graded reduction in umbilical blood flow (Itskovitz et al., 1987). Interestingly, oxygen consumption of the carcass decreases twice as much during uterine blood flow reduction (Jensen et al., 1991) than during umbilical blood flow reduction (Itskovitz et al., 1987), even though in both studies total fetal oxygen delivery is reduced by similar amounts, i.e. by 50% (Fig. 2.15). This suggests that the delivery of oxygen to the carcass, which is considerably lower in the former study, may determine the consumption of oxygen in the carcass (Fig. 2.11; Fig. 2.14). This view is supported by studies in which uterine blood flow was arrested (Jensen et al., 1987b) (Fig. 2.11) which provided the first evidence that the amount of oxygen

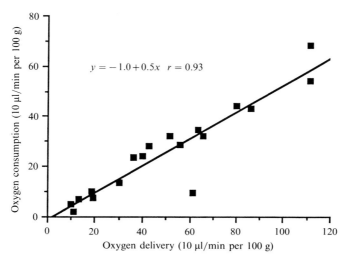

Fig. 2.14. Close correlation between O_2 delivery and O_2 consumption in the lower carcass of chronically prepared fetal sheep near term during graded reduction in uterine blood flow. Note, that O_2 delivery determines O_2 consumption. (From Jensen et al., 1991.)

delivered to peripheral organs determines the amount of oxygen consumed by these organs. This important mechanism enables the fetus to conserve oxygen in peripheral organs, e.g. the carcass, to maintain oxidative metabolism in central organs when oxygen is at short supply.

Skin and scalp

For a long time, reduced blood flow to the skin of the neonate has been recognized as an index of asphyxia and hence of circulatory redistribution (Apgar, 1953). However, blood flow to the skin of the fetus has only recently been studied systematically, to establish whether changes in cutaneous blood flow reflect a centralization of the fetal circulation (Jensen & Künzel, 1980; Jensen et al., 1985, 1987a,b,c,d).

In normoxaemic fetal sheep near term blood flow to the skin of the hips and shoulders is about 22–26 ml/min/100 g and that to the scalp is significantly higher and ranges between 29 and 34 ml/min/100 g (Jensen et al., 1986). During isocapnic hypoxaemia with a carotid arterial PO_2 of 12 mm Hg, blood flow to the skin and scalp falls by 18% and 23% respectively, as does blood flow to most of the peripheral organs, including the lungs (Jensen, 1989).

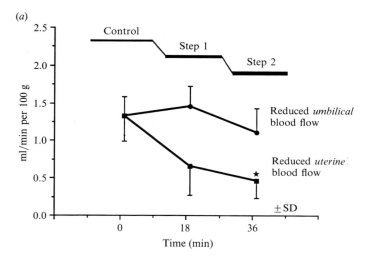

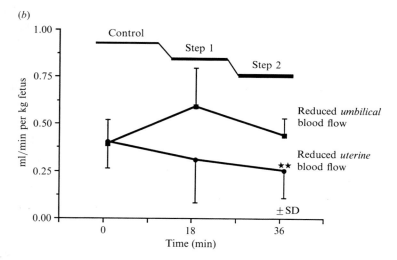

Fig. 2.15. Comparison between changes of (*a*) O_2 delivery and (*b*) O_2 consumption during graded reduction of umbilical (Itskovitz et al., 1987) and uterine blood flow (Jensen et al., 1991) to achieve a reduction in total fetal O_2 delivery by 50% in chronically prepared fetal sheep near term.

Graded reduction in uterine blood flow reduces blood flow to the skin and scalp by about 50–60% (Jensen et al., 1991), whereas arrest of uterine blood flow reduces blood flow to the skin by 95% and that to the scalp by 85% (Jensen et al., 1987*b*). At control and during acute asphyxia blood flows to the two cutaneous areas correlate linearly. However, throughout acute asphyxia blood flow to the scalp was five to ten times higher than that to the body skin, indicating a different responsiveness of the skin vasculature in certain areas (Jensen et al., 1985, 1987*a*). The fact that during acute asphyxia the time course of the fall in blood flow to peripheral organs is largely similar to that in the skin and scalp, suggests that decreased cutaneous blood flow reflects redistribution of the fetal circulation (Jensen et al., 1985, 1987*a,b,c,d*). This is related to the fact that asphyxia increases sympathetic nervous activity through arterial chemoreflex mechanisms and hence causes an almost generalized peripheral vasoconstriction.

Skin blood flow is quite a sensitive index of circulatory centralization, because blood flow to the skin decreases more than that to any other peripheral organ. Furthermore, skin blood flow depends largely on sympathetic activity, which is known to increase rapidly during asphyxia through chemoreceptor-mediated mechanisms (Hanson, 1988).

Acknowledgements

The authors acknowledge the invaluable help of Yves Garnier in designing the artwork and typing the manuscript. We are also endebted to James F. Clapp III, MetroHealth Medical Center, Cleveland, Ohio, USA, for revising the manuscript.

References

Acker, H. & Lübbers, D.W. (1977). The kinetics of local tissue PO_2 decrease after perfusion stop within the carotid body of the cat in vivo and in vitro. *Pflügers Archives,* **369**, 135–40.

Alexander, G., Hales, J. R. S., Stevens, D. & Donnelly, J. B. (1987). Effects of acute and prolonged exposure to heat on regional blood flows in pregnant sheep. *Journal of Developmental Physiology,* **9**, 1–15.

Apgar, V. A. (1953). A proposal for a new method of evaluation of the newborn infant. *Current Research in Anaesthesia and Analgesia,* **32**, 260–7.

Asakura, H., Ball, K. & Power, G. G. (1990). Interdependence of arterial PO_2 and O_2 consumption in the fetal sheep. *Journal of Developmental Physiology,* **13**, 205–13.

Blanco, C. E., Dawes, G. S. & Walker, D. W. (1983). Effect of hypoxia on polysynaptic hindlimb reflexes of unanesthetized fetal and newborn lambs. *Journal of Physiology,* **339**, 453–66.

Blanco, C. E., Dawes, G. S., Hanson, M. A. & McCooke, H. B. (1985). Studies of carotid baroreceptor afferents in fetal and newborn lambs. In *Physiological Development of the Fetus and Newborn*, ed. C. T. Jones & P. W. Nathanielsz. pp. 595–598. Academic Press, London.

Block, B. S., Schlafer, D. H., Wentworth, R. A., Kreitzer, L. A. & Nathanielsz, P. W. (1990). Regional blood flow distribution in fetal sheep with intrauterine growth retardation produced by decreased umbilical placental perfusion. *Journal of Developmental Physiology,* **13**, 81–5.

Bocking, A. D. & Harding, R. (1986). Effects of reduced uterine blood flow on electrocortical activity, breathing, and skeletal muscle activity in fetal sheep. *American Journal of Obstetrics and Gynecology,* **154**, 655–62.

Boddy, K., Dawes, G. S., Fisher, R. L., Pinter, J. & Robinson, J. S. (1974). Foetal respiratory movements, electrocortical and cardiovascular responses to hypoxaemia and hypercapnia in sheep. *Journal of Physiology*, **243**, 599–618.

Brace, R. A. (1987). Fetal blood volume responses to fetal haemorrhage: autonomic nervous contribution. *Journal of Developmental Physiology,* **9**, 97–103.

Brace, R. A. & Cheung, C. Y. (1986). Fetal cardiovascular and endocrine responses to prolonged fetal hemorrhage. *American Journal of Physiology,*, **251**, R417–24.

Braems, G. & Jensen, A. (1991). Hypoxia reduces oxygen consumption of fetal skeletal muscle cells in monolayer culture. *Journal of Developmental Physiology,* **16**, 209–15.

Braems, G., Dußler, I. & Jensen, A. (1990). Oxygen availability determines oxygen consumption of fetal myocardial cells in monolayer culture. Scientific Program and Abstracts, 36th Annual Meeting of Society for Gynecologic Investigation, p. 243.

Bristow, J., Rudolph, A. M., Itskovitz, J. & Barnes, R. (1983). Hepatic oxygen and glucose metabolism in the fetal lamb. *Journal of Clinical Investigation,* **71**, 1047–61.

Cassin, S. (1982). Humoral factors affecting pulmonary blood flow in the fetus and newborn infant. In *Cardiovascular Sequelae of Asphyxia in the Newborn*. Report of the 83rd Ross Conference on Pediatric Research, ed. G. J. Peckham & M. A. Heymann. pp. 10–18. Ross Laboratories, Columbus, Ohio.

Challis, J. R. G., Mitchell, B. F. & Lye, S. J. (1984). Activation of fetal adrenal function. *Journal of Developmental Physiology,* **6**, 93–105.

Challis, J. R. G., Fraher, L., Oosterhuis, J., White, S. E. & Bocking, A. D. (1989). Fetal and maternal endocrine responses to prolonged reductions in uterine blood flow in pregnant sheep. *American Journal of Obstetrics and Gynecology,* **160**, 926–32.

Cheung, C. Y. & Brace, R. A. (1988). Fetal hypoxia elevates plasma atrial natriuretic factor concentration. *American Journal of Obstetrics and Gynecology,* **159**, 1263–8.

Clapp, J. F., Peress, N. S., Wesley, M. & Mann, L. I. (1988). Brain damage after intermittent partial cord occlusion in the chronically instrumented fetal lamb. *American Journal of Obstetrics and Gynecology,* **159**, 504–9.

Clapp, J. F., Szeto, H. H., Larrow, R., Hewitt, J. & Mann, L. I. (1981). Fetal metabolic response to experimental placental vascular damage. *American Journal of Obstetrics and Gynecology,* **140**, 446–51.

Clapp, J. F., Thabault, N. C., Hubel, C. A., McLaughlin, M. K. & Auletta, F. J. (1982). Ovine placental cortisol production. *Endocrinology,* **111**, 1728–30.

Clapp, J. F. (1988). Fetal endocrine and metabolic response to placental insufficiency. In *The Endocrine Control of the Fetus,* ed. W. Künzel & A. Jensen. pp 246–253, Springer-Verlag, Heidelberg.

Coceani, F., Adeagbo, E., Cutz, E. & Olley, P. M. (1984). Autonomic mechanisms in the ductus venosus of the lamb. *American Journal of Physiology,* **247**, H17–24.

Cohen, W. R., Piasecki, G. J., Cohn, H. E., Young, J. B. & Jackson, B. T. (1984). Adrenal secretion of catecholamines during hypoxemia in fetal lambs. *Endocrinology,* **114**, 383–90.

Cohn, H. E., Sacks, E. J., Heymann, M. A. & Rudolph, A. M. (1974). Cardiovascular responses to hypoxemia and acidemia in fetal lambs. *American Journal of Gynaecology and Obstetrics,* **120**, 817–24.

Cohn, H. E., Piaseki, G. J. & Jackson, B. T. (1978). The role of autonomic nervous control in the fetal cardiovascular response to hypoxemia. In *Fetal and Newborn Cardiovascular Physiology*, vol 2. ed. L. D. Longo & D. D. Reneau. pp 249, Garland, New York.

Cohn, H. E., Piaseki, G. J. & Jackson, B. T. (1982). The effect of beta-adrenergic stimulation on fetal cardiovascular function during hypoxaemia. *American Journal of Obstetrics and Gynecology,* **144**, 810–16.

Cohn, H. E., Jackson, B. T., Piasecki, G. J., Couen, W. R. & Novy, M. J. (1985). Fetal cardiovascular responses to asphyxia induced by decreased uterine perfusion. *Journal of Developmental Physiology,* **7**, 289–98.

Colebatch, H. J. H., Dawes, G. S., Goodwin, J. W. & Nadeau, R. A. (1965). The nervous control of the circulation in the foetal and newly expanded lungs of the lamb. *Journal of Physiology,* **178**, 544–62.

Comline, R. S. & Silver, M. (1961). The release of adrenaline and noradrenaline from the adrenal glands of the foetal sheep. *Journal of Physiology*, **156**, 424–44.

Court, D. J., Parer, J. T., Block, B. S. B. & Llanos, A. J. (1984). Effects of beta-adrenergic blockade on blood flow distribution during hypoxaemia in fetal sheep. *Journal of Developmental Physiology*, **6**, 349–58.

Creasy, R. K., DeSwiet, M., Kahanpaa, K. V., Young, W. P. & Rudolph, A. M. (1973). Pathophysiological changes in the foetal lamb with growth retardation. In *Foetal and Neonatal Physiology,* eds. R. S. Comline, K. W. Cross, G. S. Dawes & P. W. Nathanielsz, pp. 395–402, University Press, Cambridge.

Dalton, K.J., Dawes, G.S. & Patrick, J.E. (1977). Diurnal, respiratory and other rhythms of fetal lambs. *American Journal of Obstetrics and Gynecology*, **127**, 414.

Dawes, G. S., Mott, J. C. & Widdicombe, J. G. (1954). The foetal circulation in the lamb. *Journal of Physiology*, **126**, 563–87.

Dawes, G. S. & Mott, J. C. (1959). The increase in oxygen consumption of the fetal lamb after birth. *Journal of Physiology*, **146**, 295–315.

Dawes, G. S., Fox, H. E., Leduc, B. M., Liggins, G. C. & Richards, R. T. (1972). Respiratory movements and rapid-eye-movement sleep in the foetal lamb. *Journal of Physiology*, **220**, 119–43.

Dawes, G. S., Gardner, W. N., Johnston, B. M. & Walker, D. W. (1983).

Breathing in fetal lambs: the effect of brain stem and mid-brain transection. *Journal of Physiology*, **335**, 535–53.

Drummond, W. H., Rudolph, A. M., Keil, L. C., Gluckman, P. D., MacDonald, A. A. & Heymann, M. A. (1980). Arginine vasopressin and prolactin after hemorrhage in the fetal lamb. *American Journal of Physiology*, **238**, E214–19.

Edelstone, D. I., Rudolph, A. M. & Heymann, M. A. (1978). Liver and ductus venosus blood flows in fetal lambs in utero. *Circulation Research*, **42**, 426–33.

Edelstone, D. I., Rudolph, A. M. & Heymann M. A. (1980). Effects of hypoxaemia and decreasing umbilical blood flow on liver and ductus venosus blood flows in fetal lambs. *American Journal of Physiology*, **238**, H656–63.

Edelstone, D. I. & Holzman, I. R. (1984). Regulation of perinatal intestinal oxygenation. *Seminars in Perinatology*, **8**, 226–33.

Emmanoulides, G. C., Townsend, D. E. & Bauer R. A. (1968). Effects of single umbilical artery ligation in the lamb. *Pediatrics*, **42**, 919–27.

Emson, P. C. & Quidt, M. E. (1984). NPY – a new member of the pancreatic polypeptide family. *Trends in Neurosciences*, **7**, 31–5.

Fillenz, M. (1966). Innervation of the cat spleen. *Journal of Physiology*, **185**, 2–3.

Fisher, D. J., Heymann, M. A. & Rudolph, A. M. (1982). Fetal myocardial oxygen and carbohydrate metabolism in sustained hypoxemia in utero. *American Journal of Physiology*, **243**, H959–63.

Fisher, D. J. (1986). Acidemia reduces cardiac output and left ventricular contractility in conscious lambs. *Journal of Developmental Physiology*, **8**, 23–31.

Gilbert, R. D. (1982). Effects of afterload and baroreceptors on cardiac function in fetal sheep. *Journal of Developmental Physiology*, **4**, 299.

Giussani, D. A., Spencer, J. A. D., Moore, P. J. & Hanson, M. A. (1990). The effect of carotid sinus nerve section on the initial cardiovascular response to acute isocapnic hypoxia in fetal sheep in utero. *Journal of Physiology,* **432**, 33P.

Gleason, C. A. & Rudolph, A. M. (1986). Oxygenation does not stimulate hepatic gluconeogenesis in fetal lamb. *Pediatric Research*, **20**, 532–5.

Gu, W., Jones, C. T. & Parer, J. T. (1985). Metabolic and cardiovascular effects on fetal sheep of sustained reduction of uterine blood flow. *Journal of Physiology*, **368**, 109–29.

Hanson, M. A. (1988). The importance of baro- and chemoreflexes in the control of the cardiovascular system. *Journal of Developmental Physiology*, **10**, 491–511.

Heymann, M. A. (1984). Control of the pulmonary circulation in the perinatal period. *Journal of Developmental Physiology*, **6**, 281–90.

Hökegard, K. H., Karlson, K., Kjellmer, I. & Rosén, K. G. (1979). ECG-changes in the fetal lamb during asphyxia in relation to beta-adrenoceptor stimulation and blockade. *Acta Physiologica Scandinavica*, **105**, 195–203.

Hoerter, J., Mazet, F. & Vassort, G. (1982). Perinatal growth of the rabbit cardiac cell: Possible implications for the mechanism of relaxation. *Journal of Molecular and Cellular Cardiology*, **13**, 725–40.

Itskovitz, J., Goetzman, B. W. & Rudolph, A. M. (1982a). The mechanism of late deceleration of the heart rate and its relationship to oxygenation in normoxemic and chronically hypoxemic fetal lambs. *American Journal of Obstetrics and Gynecology*, **142**, 66–73.

Itskovitz, J., Goetzman, B. W. & Rudolph, A. M. (1982*b*). Effects of hemorrhage on umbilical venous return and oxygen delivery in fetal lambs. *American Journal of Physiology*, **242**, H543–8.

Itskovitz, J., LaGamma, E. F. & Rudolph, A. (1987). Effects of cord compression on fetal blood flow distribution and O_2 delivery. *American Journal of Physiology*, **252**, H100–9.

Iwamoto, H. S., Kaufman, T., Keil, L. C. & Rudolph, A. M. (1989). Responses to acute hypoxemia in the fetal sheep at 0.6–0.7 gestation. *American Journal of Physiology*, **256**, H613–20.

Iwamoto, H. S. & Rudolph, A. M. (1981). Role of renin-angiotensin system in response to hemorrhage in fetal sheep. *American Journal of Physiology*, **240**, H848–54.

Iwamoto, H. S., Rudolph, A. M., Mirkin, B. L. & Keil, L. C. (1983). Circulatory and humoral responses of sympathectomized fetal sheep to hypoxemia. *American Journal of Physiology*, **245**, H767–72.

Iwamoto, H. S. & Rudolph, A. M. (1985). Metabolic responses of the kidney in fetal sheep: effect of acute and spontaneous hypoxemia. *American Journal of Physiology*, **249**, F836–41.

Jacobs, R., Robinson, J. S., Owens, J. A., Falconer, J. & Webster, M. E. D. (1988). The effect of prolonged hypobaric hypoxia on growth of fetal sheep. *Journal of Developmental Physiology*, **10**, 97–112.

Jelinek, J. & Jensen, A. (1991). Catecholamine concentrations in plasma and organs of the fetal guinea pig during normoxaemia, hypoxaemia and asphyxia. *Journal of Developmental Physiology*, **15**, 145–52.

Jensen, A. & Künzel, W. (1980). The difference between fetal transcutaneous PO_2 and arterial PO_2 during labour. *Gynecologic and Obstetric Investigation*, **11**, 249–64.

Jensen, A., Künzel, W. & Kastendieck, E. (1985*a*). Repetitive reduction of uterine blood flow and its influence on fetal transcutaneous PO_2 and cardiovascular variables. *Journal of Developmental Physiology*, **7**, 75–87.

Jensen, A., Künzel, W. & Hohmann, M. (1985*b*). Dynamics of fetal organ blood flow redistribution and catecholamine release during acute asphyxia. In *The Physiological Development of the Fetus and Newborn*, ed. C. T. Jones & P. W. Nathanielsz. pp 405–410, Academic Press, London and Orlando.

Jensen, A., Bamford, O. S., Dawes, G. S., Hofmeyr, G. & Parkes, M. J. (1986). Changes in organ blood flow between high and low voltage electrocortical activity in fetal sheep. *Journal of Developmental Physiology*, **8**, 187–94.

Jensen, A., Hohmann, M. & Künzel, W. (1987*a*). Redistribution of fetal circulation during repeated asphyxia in sheep: effects on skin blood flow, transcutaneous PO_2, and plasma catecholamines. *Journal of Developmental Physiology*, **9**, 41–55.

Jensen, A., Hohmann, M. & Künzel, W. (1987*b*). Dynamic changes in organ blood flow and oxygen consumption during acute asphyxia in fetal sheep. *Journal of Developmental Physiology*, **9**, 543–59.

Jensen, A., Künzel, W. & Kastendieck, E. (1987*c*) Fetal sympathetic activity, transcutaneous PO_2, and skin blood flow during repeated asphyxia in sheep. *Journal of Developmental Physiology*, **9**, 337–46.

Arne Jensen and Richard Berger

Jensen, A., Lang, U. & Künzel, W. (1987*d*). Microvascular dynamics during acute asphyxia in chronically prepared fetal sheep near term. *Advances in Experimental Medicine and Biology*, **220**, 127–31.

Jensen, A., Gips, H., Hohmann, M. & Künzel, W. (1988). Adrenal endocrine and circulatory responses to acute prolonged asphyxia in surviving and non-surviving fetal sheep near term. In *The Endocrine Control of the Fetus*, ed. W. Künzel & A. Jensen. pp 64–79, Springer-Verlag, Berlin, Heidelberg, New York, London, Paris, Tokyo.

Jensen, A. & Lang, U. (1988). Dynamics of circulatory centralization and release of vasoactive hormones during acute asphyxia in intact and chemically sympathectomized fetal sheep. In *The Endocrine Control of the Fetus*, ed. W. Künzel & A. Jensen. pp. 135–149. Springer-Verlag, Berlin, Heidelberg, New York, London, Paris, Tokyo.

Jensen, A. & Lang, U. (1992). Foetal circulatory responses to arrest of uterine blood flow in sheep: effects of chemical sympathectomy. *Journal of Developmental Physiology*, **17**, 75–86.

Jensen, A. (1989). Die Zentralisation des fetalen Kreislaufs. Thieme Verlag, Stuttgart, New York.

Jensen, A. (1992). The role of the sympathetic nervous system in preventing perinatal brain damage. In *Oxygen, Basis of the Regulation of Vital Functions in the Fetus*, ed. W. Künzel. pp. 77–107, Springer Verlag, Heidelberg, Berlin, New York.

Jensen, A., Roman, Ch., Rudolph, A. M. (1991). Effects of reducing uterine blood flow on fetal blood flow distribution and oxygen delivery. *Journal of Developmental Physiology*, **15**, 309–23.

Jogee, M., Myatt, L. & Elder, M. G. (1983). Decreased prostacyclin production by placental cells in culture from pregnancies complicated by fetal growth retardation. *British Journal of Obstetrics and Gynecology*, **90**, 247–50.

Jones, C. T. & Robinson, R. O. (1975). Plasma catecholamines in foetal and adult sheep. *Journal of Physiology*, **285**, 395–408.

Jones, C. T., Boddy, K., Robinson, J. S. & Ratcliffe, J. G. (1977). Developmental changes in the responses of the adrenal glands of the foetal sheep to endogenous adrenocorticotrophin as indicated by hormonal responses to hypoxaemia. *Journal of Endocrinology*, **72**, 279–92.

Jones, C. T. & Robinson, J. S. (1983). Studies on experimental growth retardation in sheep. Plasma catecholamines in fetuses with small placenta. *Journal of Developmental Physiology*, **5**, 77–87.

Jones, C. T. (1985). Reprogramming of metabolic development by restriction of fetal growth. *Biochemical Society Transactions*, **13**, 89–91.

Jones, C. T., Rose, J. C., Kelly, R. T. & Hardgrave, B. Y. (1985). Catecholamine responses in fetal lambs subjected to hemorrhage. *American Journal of Obstetrics and Gynecology*, **151**, 475–8.

Jones, C. T., Gu, W., Harding, J. E., Price, D. A., & Parer, J. T. (1988*a*). Studies on the growth of the fetal sheep. Effects of surgical reduction in placental size, or experimental manipulation of uterine blood flow on plasma sulphation promoting activity and on the concentration of insulin-like growth factors I and II. *Journal of Developmental Physiology*, 179–89.

Jones, C. T., Roebuck, M. M., Walker, D. W. & Johnston, B. M. (1988*b*). The role of the adrenal medulla and peripheral sympathetic nerves in the physiological responses of the fetal sheep to hypoxia. *Journal of Developmental Physiology*, **10**, 17–36.

Jones, M. D., Sheldon, R. E., Peeters, L. L., Meschia, G., Battaglia, F. C. & Makowski, E. L. (1977). Fetal cerebral oxygen consumption at different levels of oxygenation. *Journal of Applied Physiology*, **43**, 1080–4.

Kitanaka, T., Alonso, J. G., Gilbert, R. D., Siu, B. L., Clemons, G. K. & Longo, L. D. (1989). Fetal responses to long-term hypoxemia in sheep. *American Journal of Physiology*, R1348–54.

Koos, B. J., Kitanaka, T., Matsuda, K., Gilbert, R. D. & Longo, L. D. (1988). Fetal breathing adaption to prolonged hypoxaemia in sheep. *Journal of Developmental Physiology*, **10**, 161–6.

Künzel, W., Kastendieck, E., Böhme, U. & Feige, A. (1975). Uterine hemodynamics and fetal response to vena caval occlusion in sheep. *Journal of Perinatal Medicine*, **3**, 260–8.

Künzel, W., Mann, L. I., Bhakthavathsalan, A., Airomlooi, J. & Liu, M. (1977). The effect of umbilical vein occlusion on fetal oxygenation, cardiovascular parameters, and fetal electroencephalogram. *American Journal of Obstetrics and Gynecology*, **128**, 201–8.

Lafeber, H. N., Rolph, T. P. & Jones, C. T. (1984). Studies on the growth of the fetal guinea pig. The effects of ligation of the uterine artery on organ growth and development. *Journal of Developmental Physiology*, **6**, 441–59.

LaGamma, E. L., Itskovitz, J. & Rudolph A. M. (1982). Effects of naloxone on fetal circulatory responses to hypoxia. *American Journal of Obstetrics and Gynecology*, **143**, 933.

Lewis, A. B., Heymann, M. A. & Rudolph, A. M. (1976). Gestational changes in pulmonary vascular responses in fetal lambs in utero. *Circulation Research*, **39**, 536.

Lewis, A. B. & Sischo W. (1985). Cardiovascular and catecholamine responses to hypoxemia in chemically sympathectomized fetal lambs. *Developmental Pharmacology and Therapeutics*, **8**, 129–40.

Lewis, P. J., Moncada, S. & O'Grady, J. eds. (1983). *Prostacyclin in Pregnancy*. Raven, New York.

Llanos, A. J., Green, J. R., Creasy, R. K. & Rudolph, A. M. (1980). Increased heart rate response to parasympathetic and beta adrenergic blockade in growth retarded fetal lambs. *American Journal of Obstetrics and Gynecology*, **136**, 808–13.

Makowski, E. L., Schneider, J. M., Tsoulos, N. G., Colwill, J. R., Battaglia, F. C. & Meschia, G. (1972). Cerebral blood flow, oxygen consumption and glucose utilization of fetal lambs in utero. *American Journal of Obstetrics and Gynaecology*, **114**, 292–303.

Mann, L. I., Prichard, J. W. & Symmes, D. (1970). EEG, ECG, and acid–base observations during acute fetal hypoxia. *American Journal of Obsterics and Gynecology*, **106**, 39–51.

Martin, C. B. (1985). Pharmacological aspects of fetal heart rate regulation during hypoxia. In *Fetal Heart Rate Monitoring*, ed. W. Künzel. pp. 170–184. Springer Verlag, Berlin, Heidelberg, New York, Tokyo.

Martin, C. B., Voersmans, T. M. G. & Jongsma, H. W. (1987*a*). Effect of reducing uteroplacental blood flow on movements and on electrocortical activity of fetal sheep. *Gynecologic and Obstetric Investigation*, **23**, 34–9.

Martin, A. A., Kapoor, R. & Scroop, G. C. (1987*b*). Hormonal factors in the control of heart rate in normoxaemic and hypoxaemic fetal, neonatal and adult sheep. *Journal of Developmental Physiology*, **9**, 465–80.

Maylie, J. G. (1982). Excitation-contraction coupling in neonatal and adult myocardium of cat. *American Journal of Physiology*, **242**, H834–43.

Mellor, D. (1983). Nutritional and placental determinants of foetal growth rate in sheep and consequences for the newborn lamb. *British Veterinary Journal*, **139**, 307–24.

Myers, R. E. (1977). Experimental models of perinatal brain damage: Relevance to human pathology. In *Intrauterine Asphyxia and the Developing Fetal Brain*, ed. L. Gluck, pp. 37–97, Year Book Publication Co., New York.

Myers, R. E. (1979). Lactic acid accumulation as cause of brain edema and cerebral necrosis resulting from oxygen deprivation. In *Advances in Perinatal Neurology,* ed. R. Korobkin & C. Guilleminault. pp 85–114. Spectrum Publishers, New York.

Owens, J. A., Falconer, J. & Robinson, J. S. (1987). Effect of restriction of placental growth on fetal and utero-placental metabolism. *Journal of Developmental Physiology*, **9**, 225–38.

Parer, J. T., Krueger, T. R., Harris, J. L. & Reuss, L. (1978). Autonomic influences in umbilical circulation during hypoxia in fetal sheep. *Abstracts of Scientific Papers, E.J. Quilligan Symposium*. San Diego, CA.

Parer, J. T. (1980). The effect of acute maternal hypoxia on fetal oxygenation and the umbilical circulation in the sheep. *European Journal of Obstetrics and Gynecology and Reproductive Biology*, **10**, 125–36.

Parer, J. T. (1983) The influence of beta-adrenergic activity on fetal heart rate and the umbilical circulation during hypoxia in fetal sheep. *American Journal of Obstetrics and Gynecology*, **147**, 592–7.

Peeters, L. L. H., Sheldon, R. E., Jones, Jr, M. D., Makowski, E. L. & Meschia, G. (1979). Blood flow to fetal organs as a function of arterial oxygen content. *American Journal of Gynecology and Obsterics*, **135**, 637–46.

Rankin, J. H. G., Meschia, G., Makowski, E. L. & Battaglia, F. C. (1971). Relationship between uterine and umbilical venous PO_2 in sheep. *American Journal of Physiology*, **220**, 1688–92.

Reid, L. (1979). The pulmonary circulation: Remodelling in growth and disease. *American Review of Respiratory Disease*, **119**, 531–46.

Reid, D. L., Jensen, A., Phernetton, T. M. & Rankin, J. H. G. (1990). Relationship between plasma catecholamine levels and electrocortical state in the mature fetal lamb. *Journal of Developmental Physiology*, **13**, 75–9.

Reuss, M. L. & Rudolph, A. M. (1980). Distribution and recirculation of umbilical and systemic venous blood flow in fetal lambs during hypoxia. *American Journal of Obstetrics and Gynecology*, **141**, 427–32.

Reuss, M. L., Parer, J. T., Harris, J. L. & Krueger, T. R. (1982). Hemodynamic effects of alpha-adrenergic blockade during hypoxia in fetal sheep. *American Journal of Obstetrics and Gynecology*, **142**, 410–15.

Richardson, B. S., Rurak, D., Patrick, J. E., Homan, J. & Carmichael, L. (1989). Cerebral oxidative metabolism during sustained hypoxemia in fetal sheep. *Journal of Developmental Physiology*, **11**, 37–43.

Robillard, J. E., Weitzman, R. E., Fisher, D. A. & Smith Jr, F. G. (1979). The dynamics of vasopressin release and blood volume regulation during fetal hemorrhage in the lamb fetus. *Pediatric Research*, **13**, 606–10.

Robillard, J. E., Weitzman, R. E., Burmeister, L. & Smith F. G. (1981). Developmental aspects of the renal response to hypoxaemia in the lamb fetus. *Circulation Research*, **48**, 128–38.

Robillard, J. E., Gomez, R. A., Meernik, J. G., Kuehl, W. D. & Vanorden, D. (1982). Role of angiotensin II on the adrenal and vascular responses to hemorrhage during development in fetal lambs. *Circulation Research*, **50**, 645–50.

Robillard, J. E., Ayres, N. A., Gomez, R. A., Nakamura, K. T. & Smith Jr, F.G. (1984). Factors controlling aldosterone secretion during hypoxemia in fetal lambs. *Pediatric Research*, **18**, 607–11.

Robinson, J. S., Kingston, E. J., Jones, C. T. & Thornburn, G. D. (1979). The effect of removal of endometrial caruncles on fetal size and metabolism. *Journal of Developmental Physiology*, **1**, 379–98.

Robinson, J. S., Jones, C. T. & Kingston, E. J. (1983). Studies on experimental growth retardation in sheep. The effects of maternal hypoxaemia. *Journal of Developmental Physiology*, **5**, 89–100.

Robinson, J. S., Falconer, J., Owens, J. A. (1985). Intrauterine growth retardation: clinical and experimental. *Acta Paediatrica Scandinavica* (supplement), **319**, 135–42.

Rose, J. C., Morris, M. & Meis, P. J. (1981). Hemorrhage in newborn lambs: effects on arterial blood pressure, ACTH, cortisol, and vasopressin. *American Journal of Physiology*, **240**, E585–90.

Rudolph, A. M. & Heymann, M. A. (1970). Circulatory changes during growth in the fetal lamb. *Circulation Research*, **26**, 289–99.

Rudolph, A. M. & Heymann, M. A. (1976). Cardiac output in the fetal lamb: The effects of spontaneous and induced changes of heart rate on right and left ventricular output. *American Journal of Obstetrics and Gynecology*, **124**, 183–92.

Rudolph, A. M., Heymann, M. A. & Lewis, A. B. (1977). Physiology and pharmacology of the pulmonary circulation in fetus and newborn. In *Lung Biology in Health and Disease. Development of the Lung*, ed. W. A. Hodson. pp. 497–523. Marcel Dekker, New York.

Rudolph, A. M. (1983). Hepatic and ductus venosus blood flows during fetal life. *Hepatology*, **3**, 254.

Rudolph, A. M. (1984). The fetal circulation and its response to stress. *Journal of Developmental Physiology*, **6**, 11–19.

Rudolph, A. M. (1985). Distribution and regulation of blood flow in the fetal and neonatal lamb. *Circulation Research*, **57**, 811–21.

Rudolph, C., Roman, C. & Rudolph, A. M. (1989). Effect of acute umbilical cord compression on hepatic carbohydrate metabolism in the fetal lamb. *Pediatric Research*, **25**, 228–33.

Rurak, D. W. (1978). Plasma vasopressin levels during hypoxaemia and the cardiovascular effects of exogenous vasopressin in foetal and adult sheep. *Journal of Physiology*, **277**, 341–57.

Scroop, G. C., Marker, J. D., Stankewytsch-Janusch, B. & Seamark, R. F. (1986). Angiotensin I and II and the assessment of baroreceptor function in fetal and neonatal sheep. *Journal of Developmental Physiology*, **8**, 123–38.

Skillman, C. A., Plessinger, M. A., Woods, J. R. & Clark, K. E. (1985). Effect of graded reductions in uteroplacental blood flow on the fetal lamb. *American Journal of Physiology*, **249**, H1098–105.

Skillman, C. A. & Clark, K. E. (1987). Fetal beta-endorphin levels in response to reductions in uterine blood flow. *Biology of the Neonate*, **51**, 217–23.

Smith, R. W., Morris, J. A. & Assali, N. S. (1964). Effects of chemical mediators on the pulmonary and ductus arteriosus circulation in the fetal lamb. *American Journal of Obstetrics and Gynecology*, **89**, 252–60.

Thornburg, K. L. & Morton, M. J. (1983). Filling and arterial pressures as determinants of RV stroke volume in fetal sheep. *American Journal of Physiology*, **244**, H656–63.

Toubas, P. L., Silverman, N. H., Heymann, M. A. & Rudolph, A. M. (1981). Cardiovascular effects of acute hemorrhage in fetal lambs. *American Journal of Physiology*, **240**, H45–8.

Tweed, W. A., Cote, J., Pash, M. & Lou, H. (1983) Arterial oxygenation determines autoregulation of cerebral blood flow in the fetal lamb. *Pediatric Research*, **17**, 246–9.

Wagner, K. R., Ting, P., Westfall, M. V., Yamaguchi, S., Bacher, J. D. & Myers, R. E. (1986). Brain metabolic correlates of hypoxia-ischemic cerebral necrosis in mid-gestational sheep fetuses: significance of hypotension. *Journal of Cerebral Blood Flow and Metabolism*, **6**, 425–34.

Walker, A. M., Cannata, J. P., Dowling, M. H., Ritchie, B. C. & Maloney, J. E. (1979). Age-dependent pattern of autonomic heart rate control during hypoxia in fetal and newborn lambs. *Biology of the Neonate*, **35**, 198–208.

Weismann, D. N. & Robillard, J. E. (1988). Renal hemodynamic responses to hypoxemia during development: Relationships to circulating vasoactive substances. *Pediatric Research*, **23**, 155–61.

Wilkening, R. B. & Meschia, G. (1983). Fetal oxygen uptake, oxygenation, and acid-base balance as a function of uterine blood flow. *American Journal of Physiology*, **244**, H749–55.

Wilson, D. F., Owen, Ch. S. & Erecinska, M. (1979). Quantitative dependence of mitochondrial oxydative phosphorylation on oxygen concentration: A mathematical model. *Archives of Biochemistry and Biophysics*, **195**, 494–504.

Wlodek, M. E., Challis, J. R. G., Richardson, B. & Patrick, J. (1989). The effects of hypoxaemia with progressive acidaemia on fetal renal function in sheep. *Journal of Developmental Physiology*, **12**, 323–8.

Yaffe, H., Parer, J. T., Block, B. S. & Llanos, A. J. (1987). Cardiorespiratory responses to graded reductions of uterine blood flow in the sheep fetus. *Journal of Developmental Physiology*, **9**, 325–36.

3

Regulation of blood volume in utero

ROBERT A. BRACE

Introduction

Fetal blood circulates through the fetal body, umbilical cord, and fetal side of the placenta. Although often termed fetoplacental blood volume, the simpler phrase fetal blood volume will be used in this chapter to refer collectively to all blood which is pumped by the fetal heart. Recent studies suggest that the regulation of blood volume in the fetus is an order of magnitude more dynamic than in the adult. Two lines of evidence support this concept. First, rates of fluid movement into and out of the vascular space are several times greater in the fetus than in the adult. Secondly, the fetus restores its circulating blood volume to normal following experimentally induced volume disturbances in roughly one tenth of the time taken by the adult. The present chapter expands on these ideas and provides an overview of current knowledge of blood volume and its regulation in the fetus. Though a few studies of human fetuses provide a limited data base, the majority of information on the regulation of blood volume in utero has been derived from chronically catheterized ovine fetuses and very little is known about other species. Thus, this chapter attempts to synthesize, compare and integrate data from the human and sheep fetuses.

Fetal blood volume under normal conditions

Blood volume averages approximately 75 ml/kg of body weight in adult humans compared to 60 ml/kg in adult sheep. Early studies suggested that blood volume averaged over 150 ml/kg of body weight in both human and sheep fetuses (Barcroft & Kennedy, 1939; Morris, Morgan & Gobuty, 1974) but more recent studies indicate that fetal blood volume in humans and sheep averages approximately 110 ml/kg (Yao, Moinian & Lind,

1969; Brace, 1983*a*). As 30–33% of the fetal blood is within the umbilical cord and fetal side of the placenta (Barcroft, Barron & Windle, 1937; Yao et al., 1969), the volume of blood within the fetal body per unit body mass is only slightly higher than in the adult, averaging 80 ml/kg. This is the same as the blood volume in the newborn if placental transfusion is prevented (Yao et al., 1969). Once correction is made for body fat, there may be no difference in the volume of blood within the body of the fetus and adult relative to body weight.

In the human, fetal blood volume has been estimated using three different methods. (i) Using a plasma label and indicator dilution techniques, a volume of 168 ml/kg was found in previable fetuses undergoing termination of pregnancy (Morris et al., 1974). (ii) Using a red cell label for measurement, estimated blood volume in the term fetus was 105–115 ml/kg as determined from the sum of blood volume in the newborn plus the residual volume in the cord and placenta (Yao et al., 1969). (iii) In human fetuses undergoing intravascular packed cell transfusions, blood volume, as calculated from changes in haematocrit, averaged 101 ml/kg (Nicolaides, Clewell & Rodeck, 1987). In comparison, volume measurements in the fetal sheep using a plasma label, a red cell label, and haematocrit changes at transfusion have produced estimates for fetal blood volume of between 77 and 159 ml/kg (Creasy et al., 1970; Brace, 1983*a*). The different values in both humans and sheep are due to methodological differences and are discussed below.

Although the accuracy of measurement techniques in the human fetus has yet to be determined, there have been careful studies of measurement errors in the ovine fetus (Brace, 1983*a*). The primary problem which occurs when plasma labels are used for indicator dilution measurements is that the label is lost rapidly from the fetal vascular space, due in part to the fact that the capillaries of fetal sheep are 15 times more permeable to plasma proteins than adult capillaries (Gold & Brace, 1988). Thus, the Evans blue dye or radiolabelled albumin used for the volume measurement was lost rapidly from the fetal vascular space, resulting in the inclusion into the estimated blood volume of a significant portion of the fetal interstitial space. A problem with the red cell label is that plasma volume is slightly underestimated. However, the error in the ovine fetus is only 2–3 ml/kg and thus is very small compared to the error made with either a plasma label or double indicator dilution measurements (Brace, 1983*a*). Thus, measurement of fetal blood volume with a red cell label provides the most accurate estimate of true volume.

The calculation of fetal blood volume during intravascular transfusions is based on the assumption that the volume of blood in the fetal circulation at the end of transfusion equals the initial volume plus the volume transfused. However, several studies have shown that very rapid shifts of fluid from the plasma occur in the ovine fetus under a number of conditions including during transfusion (Brace, 1983*b*; Brace, 1989). This leads to an underestimate of fetal blood volume from transfusion data. In fetal sheep, which were slowly transfused, the error caused an underestimate of 33 ml/kg (Brace, 1989*a*). Human fetuses are usually transfused rapidly so it is likely that the measurement error would be less than 33 ml/ kg. However, the extent of the error has not been determined. In addition, the underestimate may be systematically less in younger (i.e., smaller) human fetuses because they require less volume to be transfused and hence less time is required.

Changes in blood volume during gestation

There is a large increase in fetal size during development, accompanied by a large increase in blood volume. In 1939, Barcroft and Kennedy reported that blood volume in the ovine fetus increased from 23 ml at 9–10 weeks gestation to 640 ml at 20 weeks (term = 21 weeks). More recently, Creasy et al. (1970) found values as high as 768 ml at 20 weeks. Near-term volumes as high as 988 ml can be calculated from the data of Caton et al. (1975). Fig. 3.1 is a composite of data from a number of published studies and illustrates the changes in ovine fetal blood volume during the last 60% of gestation. Note that the volume determined using labelled red cells is less than that determined using plasma or double indicator dilution techniques.

In the human fetus, Morris et al. (1974) found blood volume increased from approximately 18.5 ml at 16 weeks gestation to 81 ml at 22 weeks. Nicolaides et al. (1987) reported that the mean blood volume in anaemic fetuses increased from 26 ml at 18 weeks to 152 ml at 31 weeks gestation. Yao et al. (1969) estimated fetal blood volume at the time of delivery as the sum of neonatal volume plus the residual volume within the cord and placenta. By combining these and other data, Fig. 3.2 compares the developmental changes in human fetal blood volume from 16 weeks gestation to term.

By comparing maximal values in Figs. 3.1 and 3.2, it can be seen that blood volume in the ovine fetus is 50% greater than that of the human fetus at term. This difference is due to a difference in weight. That is, the term ovine fetus weighs on average 50% more than the term human fetus.

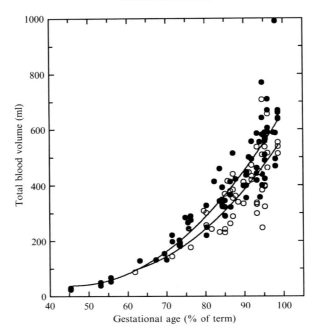

Fig. 3.1. Blood volume of the ovine fetus as a function of gestational age. Filled circles represent volumes determined with plasma label or double indicator dilution technique (upper regression line: $Y = 489.6 - 19.61X + .02133X^2$, $r = .913$, $P < .00001$). Open circles represent volumes determined with red cell label (lower regression line: $Y = 662.3 - 22.52X + .2158X^2$, $r = .783$, $P < .00001$).

Thus, relative to body weight, the human and ovine fetuses appear to have equal blood volumes.

The conclusion that human and ovine fetuses have similar blood volumes relative to body weight can be reached by a careful analysis of the published data in view of the methodological errors discussed above: in early studies in sheep using a plasma label for measurement, Barcroft and Kennedy (1939) found individual values for ovine fetal blood volume as high as 350 ml/kg prior to midgestation. They also found that the relative blood volume decreased to 140 ml/kg at term (Fig. 3.3). Thus, it has been widely accepted that weight normalized fetal blood volume was greater in early compared to late gestation. This concept was accepted in part because the placenta has a greater weight than the fetus in early gestation and it seemed logical that a larger placenta would contain a greater proportion of fetal blood. However, this concept is no longer tenable because it is now known that there are many maturational

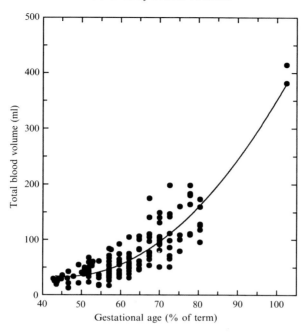

Fig. 3.2. Blood volume of the human fetus as a function of gestational age. (Regression line: $Y = 263.8 - 10.01X + .1088X^2$, $r = .894$, $P < .00001$.)

changes in placental function long after placental weight approaches its maximum near midgestation. Moreover, the early blood volume data are problematic because a plasma label was used for the volume measurements. In addition, younger fetuses have a lower plasma protein concentration and, most likely, a higher capillary permeability to plasma proteins, both of which would promote a greater overestimation of blood volume in the younger fetuses. Data from more recent studies in which a red cell label was used for blood volume measurement in fetal sheep are compared in Fig. 3.3. The blood volumes measured using a red cell label data do not support the concept that weight-normalized blood volume decreases with advancing gestational age in the fetal sheep. Measurements from a number of laboratories in both acutely prepared (Creasy et al., 1970) and chronically catheterized (Morris et al., 1974; Stankewytsch-Janusch et al., 1981; Brace, 1983a) fetal sheep have found blood volume to average 105–115 ml/kg. However, the variability was much greater in the acute than in the chronic preparations (Brace, 1983a).

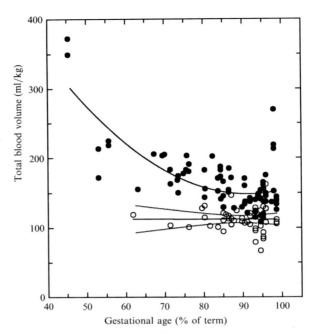

Fig. 3.3. Blood volume normalized for weight as a function of gestational age in the ovine fetus. Filled circles: volumes determined with plasma label or double indicator dilution technique (upper regression line: $Y = 764.7 - 13.49X + .07379X^2$, $r = .741$, $P < .00001$). Open circles: volumes determined with red cell label (lower regression line: $Y = 113.5 - .0155X$, $r = -.0066$, $P = .965$).

Although less data are available for the human, there are suggestions that the weight-normalized fetal blood volume may be higher early in gestation compared to late gestation. Morris et al. (1974) used a plasma label and reported relative volumes averaging 162 ml/kg at 16–22 weeks gestation. Using a red cell label at the time of delivery, Yao et al. (1969) found that the weight normalized fetal blood volume averaged 105 ml/kg whereas Linderkamp (1982) found a volume of 115 ml/kg using similar techniques. Recently Nicolaides et al. (1987) indirectly estimated blood volume in anaemic human fetuses undergoing packed cell transfusion and found an average of 101 ml/kg, with relative volume decreasing from 117 ml/kg at 18 weeks to 93 ml/kg at 31 weeks gestation. Although these data may be interpreted to indicate a decrease in the relative fetal blood volume with advancing gestational age, there are several potential problems. First, the utilization of a plasma label for the volume measurement is problematic for the reasons noted above. Secondly, a systematic bias could have been introduced into the volumes determined at the time of transfusion because of the indirect way in which fetal weight was estimated. In addition, this method for estimating blood volume at transfusion yields an underestimate of the true volume, with an error increasing with time after the start of the transfusion (Brace, 1989*b*). For example, in the older and thus larger fetuses, larger volumes were transfused, thereby requiring more time and thus systematically producing a greater underestimation of the true blood volume in the larger fetuses. Thirdly, the indirect estimate of 93.1 ml/kg at 31 weeks is significantly less than the volume of 105–115 ml/kg at term (Yao et al., 1969; Linderkamp, 1982), again indicating an underestimation of volume during the transfusion studies.

Overall, a comparison of the data from fetal human and sheep suggests that the relative blood volumes may be 105–115 ml/kg in both species. In addition, there presently exist no good data which firmly support the concept that the weight-normalized fetal blood volume decreases with advancing gestational age in either humans or sheep. This is not meant to imply that such a decrease does not occur but rather is meant to emphasize the lack of rigorous data. On the other hand, based on the above discussion, a decrease in the relative fetal blood volume with increasing gestational age seems unlikely.

Physiological variations in fetal blood volume

Even though average weight-normalized fetal blood volume does not appear to vary with fetal weight, there can be large variations in the relative blood volume in individual animals. For example, in chronically catheterized ovine fetuses under resting conditions, blood volume varied from 93 to 129 ml/kg (Brace, 1983*a*). Using multivariate regression analysis, it was found that blood volume in these animals correlated positively with fetal heart rate, arterial pH, and plasma protein concentration, but negatively with fetal venous pressure (Brace, 1984). It may appear logical that a high blood volume would be associated with a high plasma protein concentration due to the effect of the proteins on plasma colloid osmotic pressure. However, there is no obvious direct mechanism whereby fetal blood volume and either pH or heart rate are interdependent. Instead, these observations show that there are secondary mechanisms whereby the stimuli which produce bradycardia and acidosis also constrict the circulation and thereby cause a reduction in fetal blood volume and vice versa. In addition, the observation that a low blood volume is associated with high venous pressure may seem hard to explain. However, one obvious interpretation is that physiological elevation of fetal venous pressure is produced by constriction of the vasculature rather than by 'overfilling' of the circulation. Thus, physiological explanations may account for much of the variation in fetal blood volume among individuals under resting conditions.

The relative blood volume in the fetus also depends on red cell volume, and plasma volume. As seen in Fig. 3.4, high weight-normalized blood volumes are associated with high red cell volumes and high plasma volumes. The reason for these relationships remains to be established. No comparable data presently exist for the human fetus.

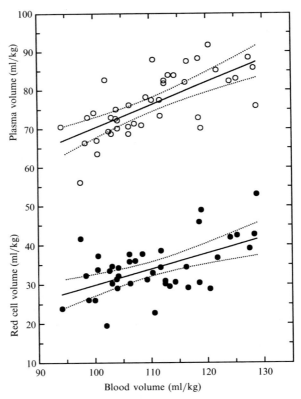

Fig. 3.4. The relationship between the relative blood volume, red cell volume, and plasma volume in the ovine fetus. Filled circles: red cell volume ($Y = -10.46 + .4031X$, $r = .545$, $P = .00023$). Open circles: plasma volume ($Y = 10.46 + .597X$, $P = .693$, $P < .00001$). Dashed lines are 95% confidence intervals.

In pregnant sheep, non-labour uterine contractions, also termed uterine contractures, occur at intervals of approximately 45 min, last 7–8 min, and produce a rise in amniotic fluid pressure of roughly 3 mm Hg. There is accumulating evidence that fetal blood volume decreases transiently during these non-labour uterine contractions. That is, fetal haemoglobin concentration increases significantly (Llanos et al., 1986) as does fetal haematocrit (Brace & Brittingham, 1986). Because there is no releasable pool of non-circulating red blood cells in the ovine fetus (Brace, 1983a), these changes indicate that fetal blood volume decreases by 2–4% during non-labour contractions. The decrease in circulating blood volume is due to a filtration of fluid across the fetal capillaries into the extravascular spaces secondary to the elevation in fetal arterial and venous pressures which occurs during the uterine contractions and are in excess of the rise in amniotic fluid pressure (Brace & Brittingham, 1986). At present, the cause of the rise in fetal vascular pressures is less clear. It had previously been speculated that the elevated vascular pressures may be due to translocation of fetal blood out of the placenta and into the fetal body because a modest expansion of amniotic fluid volume did not eliminate the elevations in fetal vascular pressures during the contractions (Brace & Brittingham, 1986). However, because fetal tracheal (Harding, Hooper & Dickson, 1990) and urinary bladder (unpublished observations) pressures also increase in excess of the rise in amniotic fluid pressure, it is more likely that the rise in fetal vascular pressures and the decrease in blood volume are due to the changes in fetal body position which occur during non-labour uterine contractions (Harding et al., 1990). The time course of the decrease in fetal blood volume during the contractions and of the recovery afterwards has yet to be established.

The neuroendocrine system may also influence fetal blood volume in a number of ways. Autonomic blockade in the ovine fetus causes a small but significant transient rise in fetal blood volume of $3.3 \pm 1.1\%$ (Brace, 1987). Adrenergic receptor blockade also produces a small rise in fetal blood volume (Cheung & Brace, 1988). In addition, the intravascular infusion of arginine vasopressin (AVP) (Tomita et al., 1985), norepinephrine (NE) (Brace & Cheung, 1987), cortisol (Wood, Cheung & Brace, 1987), atrial natriuretic factor (ANF) (Brace, Bayer & Cheung, 1989), and angiotensin II (AII) (Jones, Cheung & Brace, 1991) each reduce fetal blood volume at the high physiological to pharmacological range of plasma concentrations. AVP and NE infusion at low dose both cause a small rise in fetal blood volume (Tomita et al., 1985; Brace & Cheung, 1987), presumably due to a fall in capillary pressure induced by precapillary constriction. For all the above hormones, except ANF, the decrease in blood volume during the physiological to pharmacological infusion rates is associated with elevations in fetal arterial and venous pressures. With ANF infusion, increases in capillary permeability and precapillary dilatation may be involved in mediating the reduction in blood volume (Valentin, Ribstein & Mimran, 1989; Sugimoto et al., 1989). In addition, even small increases in fetal plasma ANF concentration are effective at reducing blood volume and this is independent of renal effects because urine flow was unchanged in several fetuses (Brace et al., 1989). These observations of the effects of vasoactive hormones are important because all of the above hormones are elevated during stress conditions such as acute hypoxia and may play a primary role in mediating any associated changes in vascular volume.

Fetal blood volume responses to hypoxia

A variety of fetal cardiovascular, endocrine, and metabolic responses to acute hypoxia have been studied over many years because hypoxic insult is thought to be a primary cause of fetal and neonatal morbidity and mortality. The fetal blood volume responses to acute hypoxia have been much less studied. In addition, a number of studies have found that the human fetus may undergo a transfusion of blood from the placenta during intrauterine hypoxia (Yao et al., 1969; Linderkamp et al., 1978). Oh et al. (1975) found a similar hypoxia-induced translocation of fetal blood out of the placenta in sheep. However, this translocation does not necessarily indicate that total blood volume was altered. In 1976, Towell suggested that 'protein rich fluid is lost from the fetal vasculature during hypoxia'. Although the evidence supporting this statement is unclear, more recent studies support the concept that fluid is lost from the fetal circulation during acute hypoxia. In 1986, we reported that the total volume of blood circulating in the ovine fetus decreases during acute hypoxia (Brace, 1986). As seen in Fig. 3.5, fetal blood volume decreased rapidly with the onset of hypoxia. The decrease in volume was linearly related to the severity of the acute hypoxia, such that each mm Hg decrease in fetal arterial oxygen tension was associated with a 1% reduction in fetal blood volume. Because the plasma protein concentration increased less than expected ($6.4 \pm 1.7\%$ compared to $10.6 \pm 1.4\%$), it appears that plasma proteins were also lost from the fetal circulation during acute hypoxia. The immature ovine fetus may be even more sensitive to acute hypoxia in that circulating blood volume decreased by an average of 20% (as

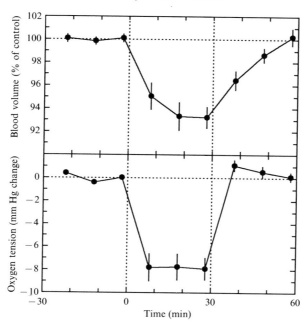

Fig. 3.5. Blood volume response of the ovine fetus to acute hypoxia. Data are
mean ± SE (Brace & Cheung, 1987).

calculated from the rise in fetal haemoglobin concentration) in fetuses
averaging 98 days gestation when oxygen tension was decreased from 23
to 12 mm Hg (Iwamoto et al., 1989). Thus, both fluid and protein are lost
from the circulation of mature and immature fetal sheep during acute
hypoxia. From studies indicating that haemoglobin concentration and/or
haematocrit is elevated in human fetuses subjected to acute hypoxia and/
or asphyxia (Yao et al., 1969; Yao & Lind, 1972; Towell, 1976; Linderkamp, 1982), it is clear that human fetal blood volume also decreases
during hypoxic insults. However, neither the extent nor the time course
can be discerned from available data.

These hypoxia-induced decreases in fetal blood volume are due to a
rise in fetal capillary pressure in conjunction with a high filtration capacity
of the fetal capillaries (Brace & Gold, 1984; Brace, 1986). During mild
hypoxia in the late gestation ovine fetus, the rise in capillary pressure
appears to be due, in part, either to an increased capillary surface area as
fetal vascular pressures are unchanged, or to a vasodilatation in some
organs (Brace, 1986; Cheung & Brace, 1988a). During more severe

hypoxia in late gestation ovine fetuses, arterial and venous pressures are both elevated (Brace, 1986; Cheung & Brace, 1988b) and thus contribute to the reduction in blood volume by further augmenting the rise in capillary pressure. In the immature fetus, large decreases in blood volume occurred even though arterial pressure was unchanged (Iwamoto et al., 1989), again suggesting that either a vasodilatation occurred in some organs or a redistribution of vascular resistances within organs which would then produce the elevation in fetal capillary pressures.

The large increase in fetal plasma catecholamine concentrations during hypoxia has frequently been suggested as a primary mediator of fetal cardiovascular responses to acute hypoxia (Jones, 1980; Cohen, Piasecki & Jackson, 1982; Reuss et al., 1982; Iwamoto, 1983; Brace & Cheung, 1987; Cheung, 1989) and thus may be a mediator of the hypoxia-induced reduction in blood volume. This concept is supported by the observation that intravascular infusions of norepinephrine in ovine fetuses lead to dose-dependent decreases in blood volume (Cheung & Brace, 1988a). In addition, the observation that combined α plus β receptor blockade was effective at preventing the 4–5% fall in ovine fetal blood volume during mild hypoxia (Brace & Cheung, 1987) further suggests the catecholamines may mediate the hypoxia-induced reduction in fetal blood volume. However, the adrenergic receptor blockade unmasked a fall in fetal arterial pressure during the mild hypoxic episodes (Brace & Cheung, 1987). During more severe hypoxia in which fetal arterial oxygen tension was reduced by 10 mm Hg, combined α plus β receptor blockade delayed but did not prevent the increase in fetal vascular pressures, and had no effect on either the time course or the extent of the decrement in fetal blood volume (Brace & Cheung, 1987). Thus, catecholamines do not mediate the large decrease in fetal blood volume which occurs during more severe acute hypoxia. In addition, AVP does not appear to be a primary mediator of the decrease in fetal blood volume because blockade of the vascular receptors for AVP does not alter the blood volume response to acute hypoxia (Piacquadio, Brace & Cheung, 1990). Recent studies also suggest that atrial natriuretic factor (ANF) may be involved in producing the loss of fluid from the fetal circulation during severe acute hypoxia. The evidence for this is twofold: first, severe hypoxia causes a large increase in ovine fetal plasma ANF concentration (Cheung & Brace, 1988b). Secondly, infusion of exogenous ANF to produce plasma concentrations equivalent to those observed during severe fetal hypoxia caused a decrease in fetal blood volume which was of the same magnitude as occurred during hypoxia (Brace et al., 1989). Whether the changes in ANF are causally related or merely occur concomitantly has yet to be determined.

As seen in Fig. 3.5, the decrease in fetal blood volume during acute hypoxia occurs rapidly in that it appears to reach a steady state in roughly 10–15 min. This rapidity has been attributed to the high filtration capacity of the capillaries in the fetal body (Brace, 1986; Cheung & Brace, 1988*b*). Fig. 3.5 also shows that the restoration of blood volume occurs less rapidly but is complete within 30 min after returning to normoxia. This suggests that, once fluid passes acutely into the extravascular space, it can be reabsorbed into the vascular compartment, again suggesting a high filtration capacity of the fetal capillaries.

The effects of long-term hypoxia on fetal blood volume are far less clear. Prystowsky et al. (1960) reported that fetuses of sheep in the high mountains of Peru had a plasma volume the same as animals near sea level but had a greater haematocrit, so total blood volume was elevated. However, the data are difficult to interpret because the plasma label which was used for the volume measurement has methodological errors, as noted above, and the magnitude of the error may change with chronic hypoxia. In 1989, Kitanaka et al., reported that fetal sheep which were exposed to a low oxygen environment for 21 days had an elevated red cell mass and blood volume. These data are also difficult to interpret because the normoxic control fetuses had a weight-normalized blood volume which was 50% greater than found by several others using the same measurement technique (Morris et al., 1974; Stankewytsch-Janusch et al., 1981; Brace, 1983*a*). Thus, although currently available data collectively suggest that chronic hypoxia may lead to an increase in fetal blood volume relative to body weight in sheep, the extent of the increase cannot be determined because of methodological problems with the blood volume measurement.

In humans, the effects of chronic hypoxia on fetal blood volume also are unclear. It has long been believed that fetal polycythaemia may be due to chronic in utero hypoxia (Towell, 1976). Further, Teramo et al., (1987) reported that fetuses of diabetic or hypertensive women have elevated plasma haemoglobin concentrations and/or haematocrits, suggesting an increase in red cell mass and thus fetal blood volume. However, an alternative interpretation is that the polycythaemia and elevated haemoglobin levels are due to a reduction in plasma volume, implying that blood volume may have been reduced.

Effects of anaemia

Even though fetal anaemia develops in humans under a number of different disease states and has been induced in a number of studies in experimental animals, relatively little is known about the acute or chronic effects of anaemia on fetal blood volume. In 1987, Nicolaides et al. estimated blood volume in anaemic fetuses undergoing packed cell transfusions and found that volume was not a function of the severity of the anaemia. This is in agreement with a number of observations in fetal sheep. First, as seen in Fig. 3.6, the weight-normalized blood volume of fetal sheep under basal conditions does not vary significantly with haematocrit over the range of 19 to 43%. Secondly, when ovine fetuses had 20–40% of their initial blood volume removed over 2 h, blood volume returned to normal within 3–4 h of the end of the haemorrhage and remained normal 24 h after the haemorrhage even though haematocrit remained significantly reduced (Brace & Cheung, 1986). In addition, if anaemia in human fetuses was so severe that hydrops fetalis developed, fetal blood volume also appeared to be unaltered (Nicolaides et al., 1987). Thus, available data collectively support the concept that fetal

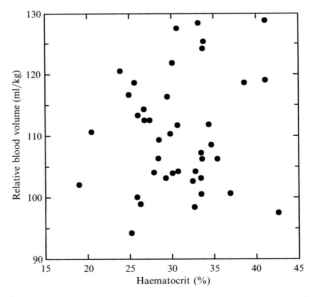

Fig. 3.6. Graph of haematocrit vs weight-normalized blood volume in the fetal sheep ($r = .128$, $P = .425$).

anaemia does not lead to alterations in fetal blood volume, suggesting that blood volume regulatory mechanisms in the fetus must be very powerful.

The effects of haemorrhage on fetal blood volume

There presently exist no data on the effects of haemorrhage on blood volume in the human fetus. In experimental animals, a great number of studies have explored the effects of fetal haemorrhage on a variety of cardiovascular, metabolic and endocrine variables, including fetal blood volume changes.

In 1983, a series of studies were begun to explore the regulation of blood volume in the ovine fetus. It was found that, following rapid haemorrhage of 5 to 25% of the initial blood volume over 5 min, an average of 53% of the lost volume was restored within 30 min (Brace, 1983c). This is remarkable in comparison with the adult which restores only about 20% of the lost volume under comparable conditions. In addition, the protein concentration of the fluid entering the fetal circulation during and after haemorrhage was over 50% of the plasma protein concentration. Because plasma proteins do not cross the placenta, the latter observation suggests that the rapid posthaemorrhagic volume restoration in the fetus was due to a translocation of fluid and protein from the fetal interstitial space (Brace, 1983c). In fetuses subjected to slow haemorrhage of 20–40% of their initial blood volume over 2 h, blood volume returned to normal with 3 h and remained at this level for the subsequent 24 h (Brace & Cheung, 1986). Fetal osmolality was unchanged during slow haemorrhage and blood volume returned to normal only as the plasma protein mass (i.e. concentration × volume) returned to normal (Brace, 1989c). Thus, plasma proteins play an extremely important role in the restoration and maintenance of fetal blood volume and this needs exploration.

The involvement of the neuroendocrine system in the restoration of fetal blood volume after haemorrhage has been explored in a few studies. In fetuses in which the autonomic nervous system was inhibited pharmacologically by a ganglionic blocker, blood volume restoration 30 min after a rapid haemorrhage was only 74% of that in normal fetuses (Brace, 1987). In adrenalectomized ovine fetuses (Ray et al., 1988), haematocrit and blood volume changes during 5 h following rapid haemorrhage were the same as those in non-adrenalectomized fetuses, suggesting fetal blood volume restoration is not dependent upon endocrine support from the fetal adrenal glands. It is clear that a much greater endocrine response occurs following rapid than slow haemorrhage of comparable magnitude.

Vascular volume loading

In the anaemic human fetus, expansion of vascular volume occurs during transfusion of packed red blood cells. Blood volume in these fetuses prior to transfusion has been calculated based on the assumption that the circulating blood volume at the end of the transfusion equals the initial blood volume plus that transfused (Nicolaides et al., 1987). However, in anaemic and non-anaemic fetal sheep, measured blood volume increases by only about half the transfused volume due to a loss of plasma from the circulation during and after transfusion (Brace, 1989*b*). Fluid from the plasma space undoubtedly is lost from the human fetus undergoing transfusion, but the extent and time course of the loss has yet to be determined.

Several studies indicate that the increase in ovine fetal blood volume following intravascular infusion of isotonic fluids is much less than in the adult. One half hour after the infusion of isotonic saline, only 6–7% of the infused volume remained in the fetal circulation (Brace, 1983*b*) compared to an average of 30% in the adult. Fetal blood volume was increased transiently for less than 1 hour after an injection of hypertonic NaCl into the fetal circulation even though 200 ml of water would have had to cross the placenta to restore fetal osmolality (Woods & Brace, 1986). Following infusion of 6% dextran 70 (Brace, 1983*b*), blood volume was expanded by only 50% of the infused volume whereas blood volume in the adult would have increased by 200% of the infused volume because 6% dextran 70 is hyperoncotic in the adult. Three factors contribute to these differences between the fetus and the adult: (1) transcapillary fluid movements in the fetus are much more rapid than in the adult because the capillary filtration coefficient in the fetus is five times that in the adult relative to body weight (Brace & Gold, 1984), (2) the transcapillary fluid movements in the fetus are much more extensive than in the adult because fetal interstitial compliance averages ten times adult values (Brace & Gold, 1984), and (3) the rapid transcapillary protein movements in the fetus noted above and the small volume response to dextran 70 occurs because the fetal capillaries are 15 times more permeable to plasma proteins and have a lower reflection coefficient for the plasma proteins (Gold & Brace, 1988). Thus the observed fetal vascular volume changes during mild to moderate rapid volume expansion are predictable based on a quantitative knowledge of the fluid compartments and capillary membranes.

An understanding of the fetal blood volume responses to vascular volume loading also provides a basis for interpretation of urine flow responses to volume loading. It long has been known that the neonate, and presumably the fetus, is less efficient than the adult at excreting a volume load. This was thought to be due to an immature kidney. However, when fetal and adult sheep were volume loaded with equivalent volumes of saline over 10 min, weight-normalized urine flow increased in the fetus to the same extent as in the adult (Brace et al., 1988). However, urine flow in the fetus returned to normal within 20–30 min whereas urine flow in the adult remained elevated for a prolonged time (Brace et al., 1988). This difference in urine flow response is attributable to differences in blood volume responses, in that the blood volume remained elevated in the adult and thus provided a prolonged elevation of vascular pressures and a prolonged stimulus for AVP and AII to be suppressed and ANF to be elevated (Brace et al., 1988), all of which promote a diuresis. The reduced excretory capacity in the fetus, and presumably the newborn, compared to the adult is attributed to the higher capillary filtration coefficient and permeability in combination with a greater interstitial compliance.

In response to large intravascular infusions (i.e. 1 litre/hour for 4 h), fetal blood volume increased by only 4–5% and 500 ml/h crossed the placental into the maternal circulation (Brace & Moore, 1991). Fetal urine flow also increased to as much as 8 ml/min by the end of the infusion (Brace & Moore, 1991). These observations are important because they demonstrate (i) a great ability of the fetus to maintain its blood volume near normal, (ii) in late gestation the fetal kidney can excrete enormous volumes of fluid with only modest increases in vascular pressures, and (iii) that small increases in fetal vascular pressures can produce almost a 100-fold increase in the filtration capacity of the ovine placenta (Brace & Moore, 1991). Thus, the capillary filtration coefficient in the placenta is a dynamic variable which changes with conditions and these changes may play an important role in regulating fetal blood volume.

There are small, but none the less highly significant increases in ovine fetal blood volume during long-term vascular volume loading. Consecutive intravascular infusions of 1, 2, and 4 litres/day of physiological saline (i.e. 0.7, 1.4, & 2.8 ml/min with increments at 24 hour intervals) increased fetal blood volume by only 5% (roughly 15–20 ml), increased urine flow rate by more than the infusion rate, and resulted in a large majority of infused fluid passing to the maternal compartment (Brace, 1989a). A 3 day infusion of 5 M NaCl at a rate of 10 mM/hour (i.e. 80% of fetal body content of Na^+ & Cl^- per day), caused fetal blood volume to increase by only 3%, urine flow rate to increase by 3.5 litres/day, and amniotic fluid volume to fall in 7 of 8 animals after 24 h (Powell & Brace, 1991). In addition, infusion of physiological saline into the amniotic compartment of fetal sheep over 3 days produced a 3% increase in fetal blood volume while the majority of infused fluid was transferred to the maternal compartment (Gilbert & Brace, 1988). Collectively, these studies show that both excess fluid and excess salt are transferred very efficiently from the fetal/amniotic space to the maternal compartment over a period of days. However, mechanism(s) responsible for this fetal-to-maternal transfer is (are) unclear and the experimental data contradict predictions based on theoretical considerations (Wilbur, Power & Longo, 1978; Faber & Anderson, 1990; Powell & Brace, 1991).

Several recent studies suggest a resolution of these problems may be near. It has been demonstrated that amniotic water is rapidly absorbed into the fetal circulation which perfuses the fetal placenta and perfuses the space between the amnion and chorion in sheep (Gilbert & Brace, 1989). This is illustrated in Fig. 3.7 which shows that an infusion of distilled water into the amniotic cavity induced a rapid absorption of amniotic water into the fetal circulation, and occurs even when the fetal oesophagus was ligated. The pathway for direct exchange of fluid and solutes between the amniotic fluid and fetal blood is referred to as the 'intramembranous pathway' partly to distinguish it from the 'transmembranous pathway' whereby fluid may cross both the amnion and chorion (Gilbert & Brace, 1988). In these studies, the authors have consistently failed to find significant movement of fluid across the transmembranous pathway. However, the filtration coefficient of the intramembranous pathway is sufficiently high and the reflection coefficients sufficiently low for large quantities of fluid and small molecular weight solutes to move from the amniotic space, through the intramembranous pathway, and directly into the fetal circulation each day (Gilbert & Brace, 1990). In addition, ligation of the fetal oesophagus caused the conductance of the intramembranous pathway to double (Gilbert & Brace, 1989) providing an explanation for the observation that polyhydramnios does not develop following oesophageal ligation even though fetal urine flow rate remains normal (Wintour et al., 1978; Lumbers, Smith & Stevens, 1985; Gilbert & Brace, 1989). Thus when fluid is infused into the fetus, urine flow increases; when it is infused into the amniotic space, large volumes are

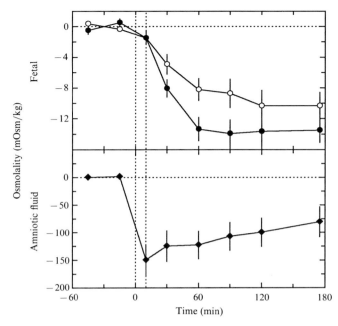

Fig. 3.7. Changes in fetal blood and amniotic fluid osmolality in response to injection of distilled water into amniotic cavity of pregnant sheep at time 0. Open circles, fetuses with oesophagus intact; filled circles, fetuses with oesophagus ligated.

absorbed across the intramembranous pathway. This may be associated with large increases in placental permeabilities and large volumes of fluids and salt are transferred to the maternal circulation (Brace & Moore, 1991). This hypothesis is consistent with our observations that long-term infusions of either isotonic solutions or hypertonic NaCl into either the ovine fetus or amniotic fluid causes neither fetal oedema nor polyhydramnios, even though there may be large increases in fetal urine flow rate (Gilbert & Brace, 1988; Brace, 1989a; Powell & Brace, 1991).

Fetal blood volume responses to changes in maternal osmolality

Physiological changes in maternal osmolality occur with normal eating and drinking, and large increases in maternal osmolality may occur with water deprivation and/or dehydration. Each 1 mOsm/kg change in osmolality in the mother may generate almost 20 mm Hg of osmotic pressure across the placenta. For example, a 1% decrease in osmolality from a normal value of approximately 300 mOsm/kg could potentially generate a transplacental osmotic pressure of 60 mm Hg. Yet, present data from pregnant sheep suggest that changes in maternal osmolality have either no or only transient effects on fetal blood volume. In 1985, Bell and Wintour reported that fetal blood volume in ewes subjected to 4 days of water restriction remained unaffected. In 1986, it was found that fetal blood volume decreased by 11% following a 16% increase in maternal osmolality, produced by a bolus injection of 9% NaCl, but returned to normal within 1 hour and was slightly elevated thereafter (Woods & Brace, 1986). In recent studies, it was found that large decreases in maternal osmolality, produced by intravascular infusion of hypotonic saline, produced no change in fetal blood volume (Powers & Brace, 1991). Collectively, the presently available data suggest that, although increases or decreases in maternal osmolality are accompanied by parallel changes in fetal osmolality, there do not appear to be concomitant changes in fetal blood volume except for short-term transients lasting up to 1 hour.

In humans, changes in maternal osmolality are also accompanied by similar changes in fetal osmolality (Battaglia et al., 1960). However, it is not known whether there are simultaneous changes in fetal blood volume. In addition, although a number of observations suggest that maternal volume restoration or volume expansion may promote an increase in amniotic fluid volume (Goodlin, Anderson & Gallagher, 1983; Sherer et al., 1990), it has not been determined whether there are associated fetal blood volume changes.

Effects of labour and delivery

Several pieces of evidence suggest that the volume of blood circulating in the fetus may decrease during labour, with a further decrease during delivery. In 1972, Comline and Silver reported the haematocrit of the fetal sheep to be increased by 15–20% 15 min before delivery (Comline & Silver, 1972). Because the ovine fetus has a small spleen (Faber, Green & Thornburg, 1974; Towell, 1976; Brace, 1987) and does not have a releasable pool of non-circulating red blood cells (Brace, 1987), the increase in haematocrit reflects a 13–17% decrease in fetal blood volume. Presumably this is due to transcapillary filtration of fluid into the fetal interstitial space secondary to a rise in fetal vascular pressures. In the human fetus, there is a gradual rise in fetal haematocrit during the course of gestation (Soothill, 1989). This reflects haemopoiesis rather than a decrease in circulating blood volume. During delivery by Caesarean section, human fetal haematocrit averages 44% if there has been no labour and 51% if labour was present or with vaginal delivery (Yao et al., 1969; Yao & Lind, 1972; Towell, 1976; Linderkamp, 1982; Teramo et al., 1987), suggesting a 14% decrease in fetal blood volume due to the loss of plasma.

Conclusion

The above analyses suggest: (i) Circulating blood volume in both human and sheep fetuses appears to average 105–115 ml/kg of fetal body weight and does not appear to change over the last 60% of gestation. (ii) Blood volume changes in the fetus can be both rapid and extensive due to the high filtration coefficient of the fetal capillaries and to the high compliance of the fetal interstitial space. (iii) Acute hypoxia is associated with a reduction in fetoplacental blood volume. (iv) The fetus returns its blood volume to normal following haemorrhage in one-tenth of the time required in the adult. (v) Fetal blood volume is within the normal range during mild to severe anaemia. (vi) The fetus is very efficient at maintaining its blood volume near normal during acute and long-term volume loading. (vii) The intramembranous pathway is a very important component of the volume regulatory mechanisms in the fetus. (viii) Placental permeability is a dynamic variable and only small increases in fetal vascular pressures may cause large increases in the permeability characteristics of the placenta. (ix) Changes in maternal osmolality may induce short-term, but do not appear to induce long-term, changes in fetal blood volume. (x) The fetal endocrine system may play a role in regulating fetal blood volume under basal and stress conditions. (xi) Labour and delivery are associated with a reduction in fetal blood volume which is secondary to the transcapillary filtration of fluid into the fetal interstitial space.

References

Barcroft, J., Barron, D. H. & Windle, W. F. (1937). Acquisition of blood by the foetus from the placenta at birth. *Journal of Physiology,* **87**, 73.

Barcroft, J. & Kennedy, J. A. (1939). The distribution of blood between the foetus and the placenta in sheep. *Journal of Physiology,* **95**, 173–86 .

Battaglia, F., Prystowsky, H., Smisson, C., Hellegers, A. & Bruns, P. (1960). Fetal blood studies. XIII. The effect of administration of fluids intravenously to mothers upon the concentrations of water and electrolytes in plasma of human fetuses. *Pediatrics,* **125**, 2–10.

Bell, R. J. & Wintour, E. M. (1985). The effect of maternal water deprivation on ovine fetal blood volume. *Quarterly Journal of Experimental Physiology,* **70**, 95–9.

Brace, R. A. (1983*a*). Blood volume and its measurement in the chronically catheterized sheep fetus. *American Journal of Physiology,* **244**, H487–94.

Brace, R. A. (1983*b*). Fetal blood volume responses to intravenous saline solution and dextran. *American Journal of Obstetrics and Gynecology,* **147**, 777–81.

Brace, R. A. (1983*c*). Fetal blood volume responses to acute fetal hemorrhage. *Circulation Research,* **52**, 730–4.

Brace, R. A. (1984) Blood volume in the fetus and methods for its measurement. In *Animal Models in Fetal Medicine,* ed P. W. Nathanielsz, pp. 19–36, Perinatology Press: New York.

Brace, R. A. (1986). Fetal blood volume responses to acute fetal hypoxia. *American Journal of Obstetrics and Gynecology,* **155**, 889–93.

Brace, R. A. (1987). Fetal blood volume responses to fetal haemorrhage: autonomic nervous contribution. *Journal of Developmental Physiology,* **9**, 97–103.

Brace, R. A. (1989*a*). Fetal blood volume, urine flow, swallowing, and amniotic fluid volume responses to long-term intravascular infusions of saline. *American Journal of Obstetrics and Gynecology,* **161**, 1049–54.

Brace, R. A. (1989*b*). Ovine fetal cardiovascular responses to packed red blood cell transfusions. *American Journal of Obstetrics and Gynecology,* **161**, 1367–74.

Brace, R. A. (1989*c*). Mechanisms of fetal blood volume restoration following slow fetal hemorrhage. *American Journal of Physiology,* **256**, R1040–44.

Brace, R. A., Bayer, L. A. & Cheung, C. Y. (1989). Fetal cardiovascular, endocrine, and fluid responses to atrial natriuretic factor infusion. *American Journal of Physiology,* **257**, R580–7.

Brace, R. A. & Brittingham, D. S. (1986). Fetal vascular pressure and heart rate responses to nonlabor uterine contractions. *American Journal of Physiology,* **251**, R409–16.

Brace, R. A. & Cheung, C. Y. (1986). Fetal cardiovascularand endocrine responses to prolonged fetal hemorrhage. *American Journal of Physiology,* **251**, R417–24.

Brace, R. A. & Cheung, C. Y. (1987). Role of catecholamines in mediating fetal blood volume decrease during acute hypoxia. *American Journal of Physiology,* **253**, H927–32.

Brace, R. A. & Cheung, C. Y. (1990). Fetal blood volume restoration following rapid fetal hemorrhage. *American Journal of Physiology,* **259**, H567–73.

Brace, R. A. & Gold, P. S. (1984). Fetal whole body interstitial compliance, vascular compliance, and capillary filtration coefficient. *American Journal of Physiology,* **247**, R800–5.

Brace, R. A., Miner, L. K., Siderowf, A. D. & Cheung, C. Y. (1988). Fetal and adult urine flow and ANF responses to vascular volume expansion. *American Journal of Physiology,* **255**, R846–50.

Brace, R. A. & Moore, T. R. (1991). Transplacental, amniotic, urinary and fetal fluid dynamics during very large volume fetal intravenous infusions. *American Journal of Obstetrics and Gynecology,* **164**, 907–16.

Caton, D., Wilcox, C. J., Abrams, R. & Barron, D. H. (1975). The circulating plasma volume of the foetal lamb as an index of its weight and rate of weight gain (g/day) in the last third of gestation. *Quarterly Journal of Experimental Physiology,* **60**, 45–54.

Cheung, C. Y. (1989). Direct adrenal medullary catecholamine response to hypoxia in fetal sheep. *Journal of Neurochemistry,* **52**, 148–53.

Cheung, C. Y. & Brace, R. A. (1988). Norepinephrine effects on fetal cardiovascular and endocrine systems. *American Journal of Physiology,* **254**, H734–41.

Cheung, C. Y. & Brace, R. A. (1988). Fetal hypoxia elevates plasma atrial natriuretic factor concentration. *American Journal of Obstetrics and Gynecology,* **159**, 1263–8.

Cohen, W. R., Piasecki, G. J. & Jackson, B. T. (1982). Plasma catecholamines during hypoxemia in fetal lamb. *American Journal of Physiology,* **243**, R520–5.

Comline, R.S. & Silver, M. (1972). The composition of foetal and maternal blood during parturition in the ewe. *Journal of Physiology,* **222**, 233–56.

Creasy, R. K, Drost, M., Green, M. V. & Morris, J. A. (1970). Determination of fetal, placental and neonatal blood volumes in the sheep. *Circulation Research,* **27**, 407–94.

Faber, J. J. & Anderson, D. F. (1990). Model study of placental water transfer and causes of fetal water disease in sheep. *American Journal of Physiology,* **258**, R1257–70.

Faber, J. J., Green, T. J. & Thornburg, K. L. (1974). Arterial blood pressure in the unanaesthetized fetal lamb after changes in fetal blood volume and haematocrit. *Quarterly Journal of Experimental Physiology,* **59**, 241–55.

Gilbert, W. M. & Brace, R. A. (1988). Increase in fetal hydration during long-term intra-amniotic isotonic saline infusion. *American Journal of Obstetrics and Gynecology,* **159**, 1413–17.

Gilbert, W. M. & Brace, R. A. (1989). The missing link in amniotic fluid volume regulation: intramembranous absorption. *Obstetrics and Gynecology,* **74**, 748–54.

Gilbert, W. M. & Brace, R. A. (1990). Novel determination of filtration coefficient of ovine placenta and intramembranous pathway. *American Journal of Physiology,* **259**, R1281–8.

Gold, P. S. & Brace, R. A. (1988). Fetal whole-body permeability-surface area product and reflection coefficient for plasma proteins. *Microvascular Research,* **36**, 262–74.

Goodlin, R. C., Anderson, J. C. & Gallagher, T. F. (1983). Relationship between amniotic fluid volume and maternal plasma volume expansion. *American Journal of Obstetrics and Gynecology,* **146**, 505–11.

Harding, R., Hooper, S. B. & Dickson, K. A. (1990). A mechanism leading to reduced lung expansion and lung hypoplasia in fetal sheep during oligohydramnios. *American Journal of Obstetrics and Gynecology,* **163**, 1904–13.

Iwamoto, H. S., Kaufman, T., Keil, L. C. & Rudolph, A. M. (1989). Responses to acute hypoxemia in fetal sheep at 0.6–0.7 gestation. *American Journal of Physiology,* **256**, H613–20.

Jones, C. T. (1980). Circulating catecholamines in the fetus, their origin, actions and significance. In *Biogenic Amines in Development,* eds H. Parves & S. Parves, pp. 63–86, Elsevier/North Holland Biomedical Press.

Jones, O. W. III, Cheung, C. Y. & Brace, R. A. (1991). Dose-dependent effects of angiotensin II on the ovine fetal cardiovascular system. *American Journal of Obstetrics and Gynecology,* **165**, 1524–33.

Kitanaka, T., Alonso, J. G., Gilbert, R. D., Siu, B. L., Clemons, G. K. & Longo, L. D. (1989). Fetal responses to long-term hypoxemia in sheep. *American Journal of Physiology*, **256**, R1348–54.

Linderkamp, O. (1982). Placental transfusion: determinants and effects. *Clinics in Perinatology*, **9**, 559–92.

Linderkamp, O., Versmold, H. T., Messow-Zahn, K., Muller-Holve, W., Riegel, K. P. & Betke, K. (1978). The effect of intra-partum and intra-uterine asphyxia on placental transfusion in premature and full-term infants. *European Journal of Pediatrics*, **127**, 91–9.

Llanos, A. J., Court, D. J., Block, B. S., Germain, A. M. & Parer, J. T. (1986). Fetal cardiorespiratory changes during spontaneous prelabor uterine contractions in sheep. *American Journal of Obstetrics and Gynecology*, **155**, 893–7.

Lumbers, E. R., Smith, F. G. & Stevens, A. D. (1985). Measurement of net transplacental transfer of fluid to the fetal sheep. *Journal of Physiology*, **364**, 289–99.

Morris, J. A., Morgan, C. A. & Gobuty, A. (1974). Measurement of fetoplacental blood volume in the human previable fetus. *American Journal of Obstetrics and Gynecology*, **118**, 927–31.

Nicolaides, K. H., Clewell, W. H. & Rodeck, C. H. (1987). Measurement of human fetoplacental blood volume in erythroblastosis fetalis. *American Journal of Obstetrics and Gynecology*, **157**, 50–3.

Oh, W., Omori, K., Emmanouilides, G. C. & Phelps, D. L. (1975). Placenta to lamb fetus transfusion in utero during acute hypoxia. *American Journal of Obstetrics and Gynecology*, **122**, 316–22.

Piacquadio, K. M., Brace, R. A. & Cheung, C. Y. (1990). Role of vasopressin in mediating fetal cardiovascular responses to acute hypoxia. *American Journal of Obstetrics and Gynecology*, **163**, 1294–300.

Powell, T. L. & Brace, R. A. (1991). Fetal fluid responses to long-term 5 M NaCl infusion: where does all the salt go? *American Journal of Physiology*, in press.

Powers, D. R. & Brace, R. A. (1991). Fetal cardiovascular and fluid responses to maternal volume loading with lactated Ringer's or hypotonic solution. *American Journal of Obstetrics and Gynecology*, in press.

Prystowsky, H., Hellegers, A., Meschia, G., Metcalfe, J., Huckabee, W. & Barron, D. H. (1960). The blood volume of fetuses carried by ewes at high altitude. *Quarterly Journal of Experimental Physiology*, **45**, 292–7.

Ray, N. D., Turner, C. S., Rawashdeh, N. M. & Rose, J. C. (1988). Ovine fetal adrenal gland and cardiovascular function. *American Journal of Physiology*, **254**, R706–10.

Reuss, M. L., Parer, J. T., Harris, J. L. & Krueger, T. R. (1982). Hemodynamic effects of alpha-adrenergic blockade during hypoxia in fetal sheep. *American Journal of Obstetrics and Gynecology*. **142**, 410–15.

Sherer, D. M., Cullen, J. B. H., Thompson, H. O. & Woods, J. R. Jr. (1990). Transient oligohydramnios in a severely hypovolemic gravid woman at 35 weeks' gestation, with fluid reaccumulating immediately after intravenous maternal hydration. *American Journal of Obstetrics and Gynecology*, **162**, 770–1.

Soothill, P. W. (1989). Cordocentesis: Role of assessment of fetal condition. *Clinics in Perinatology*, **16**, 755–70.

Stankewytsch-Janusch, B., Scroop, G. C., Marker, J. D. & Seamark, R. (1981). Measurement of blood volume in fetal and neonatal sheep using red blood cells labeled with 99m technetium. *Journal of Developmental Physiology*, **3**, 245–54.

Sugimoto, E., Shigemi, K., Okuno, T., Yawata, T. & Morimoto, T. (1989). Effect of ANP on circulating blood volume. *American Journal of Physiology*, **257**, R127–31.

Teramo, K. A., Widness, J. A., Clemons, G. K., Voutilainen, P., Mckinlay, S. & Schwartz, R. (1987). Amniotic fluid erythropoietin correlates with umbilical plasma erythropoietin in normal and abnormal pregnancy. *Obstetrics and Gynecology*, **69**, 710–16.

Tomita, H., Brace, R. A., Cheung, C. Y. & Longo, L. D. (1985). Vasopressin dose-response effects on fetal vascular pressures, heart rate, and blood volume. *American Journal of Physiology*, **249**, H974–80.

Towell, M. E. (1976). Blood volume of the fetus and the newborn infant. In *Perinatal Medicine: The Basic Science Underlying Clinical Practice*, ed. J. W. Goodwin, J. O. Godden & G. W. Chance. pp. 209–222. Williams & Wilkinson, Baltimore.

Valentin, J. P., Ribstein, J. & Mimran, A. (1989). Effect of nicardipine and atriopeptin on transcapillary shift of fluid and proteins. *American Journal of Physiology*, **257**, R174–9.

Wilbur, W. J., Power, G. G. & Longo, L. D. (1978). Water exchange in the placenta a mathematical model. *American Journal of Physiology*, **235**, R181–99.

Wintour, E. M., Barnes, A., Brown, E. H., Hardy, K. J., Horacek, I., Mcdougall, J. G. & Scoggins, B.A. (1978). Regulation of amniotic fluid volume and composition in the ovine fetus. *Obstetrics and Gynecology*, **52**, 689–93.

Wood, C. E., Cheung, C. Y. & Brace, R. A. (1987). Fetal heart rate, arterial pressure, and blood volume responses to cortisol infusion. *American Journal of Physiology*, **253**, R904–9.

Woods, L. L. & Brace, R. A. (1986). Fetal blood volume, vascular pressure, and heart rate responses to fetal and maternal hyperosmolality. *American Journal of Physiology*, **251**, H716–21.

Yao, A. C. & Lind, J. (1972). Blood volume in the asphyxiated term neonate. *Biology of the Neonate*, **21**, 199–209.

Yao, A. C., Moinian, M., & Lind, J. (1969). Distribution of blood between infant and placenta after birth. *Lancet*, **ii**, 871–3.

4

Local and endocrine factors in the control of the circulation

CHARLES E. WOOD

Introduction

Both neural and endocrine systems maintain fetal blood pressure relatively constant and support flow through the umbilical–placental circulation. The autonomic nervous system and the endocrine systems control blood pressure and flow in the late-gestation fetus. For example, fetal sheep respond to injections of α and β adrenergic antagonists with changes in blood pressure and heart rate, respectively, as early as 85 days' gestation (Cassin et al., 1964; Vapaavouri et al., 1973) and late-gestation fetal sheep respond to infusions of arginine vasopressin and angiotensin II with increases in arterial pressure (Ismay, Lumbers & Stevens, 1979; Iwamoto et al., 1979; Yoshimura, Magness & Rosenfeld, 1990a). This chapter will review the mechanisms controlling blood flow through the cerebral, pulmonary, umbilical–placental, adrenal and myocardial circulations in the fetus. After descriptions of local and endocrine controllers of blood flow through these individual circulations, therefore, the coordinated responses of the vascular beds to hypoxia will be discussed.

The cerebral circulation

The ovine fetal cerebral circulation exhibits autoregulation (Fig. 4.1) within the range of arterial pressures of approximately 45–80 mm Hg (Purves & James, 1969; Tweed et al., 1983; Papile, Rudolph & Heymann, 1985). In the newborn dog, cerebral blood flow is maintained constant between approximately 30 and 80 mm Hg (Hernandez, Brennan & Bowman, 1980). Because the late-gestation fetus maintains arterial blood pressure between approximately 40 and 55 mm Hg, a fall in arterial blood pressure below the normally regulated level results in a decrease in cerebral blood flow. Thus, autoregulation of cerebral blood flow in the

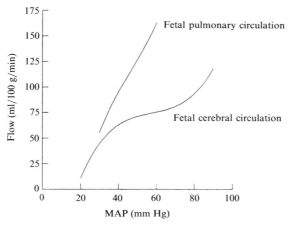

Fig. 4.1. Pressure–flow relationships in the fetal lung and in the fetal brain. (Data are redrawn from Cassin et al., 1964 and from Papile, Rudolph and Heymann, 1985.)

fetus does not maintain flow during episodes of hypotension. Therefore, although 15% haemorrhage (which results in mild hypotension) does not decrease cerebral blood flow (Toubas et al., 1981; Itskovitz, Goetzman & Rudolph, 1982), it is likely that greater degrees of hypotension associated with larger haemorrhage might decrease cerebral blood flow. Autoregulation maintains constant cerebral blood flow during increased arterial blood pressure such as that produced by infusion of arginine vasopressin (Iwamoto et al., 1979).

Prostanoids are important modulators of cerebral blood flow, and may play a central role in the autoregulation of blood flow through the brain. Although there are no published data concerning prostanoid control of autoregulation in the fetus, several studies have been performed in newborn piglets. During hypotensive haemorrhage which lowers arterial blood pressure approximately 35%, cerebral blood flow is maintained constant and net cerebral production of 6-keto-PGF$_{1\alpha}$ is increased (Leffler et al., 1986). Pretreatment of the piglets with indomethacin blocked the increase in 6-keto-PGF$_{1\alpha}$ and allowed cerebral blood flow to decrease approximately 40%. Since 6-keto-PGF$_{1\alpha}$ is a metabolite of PGI$_2$, a potent vasodilator, these data suggest that production of PGI$_2$ maintains cerebral blood flow during periods of hypotension. Adrenergic mechanisms do not by themselves, or in combination with prostanoids, modulate cerebral blood flow during haemorrhage (Armstead et al., 1988).

Cerebral blood flow in the adult animal is influenced by changes in arterial PO_2 and PCO_2. Decreases in P_aO_2 and increases in P_aCO_2 increase cerebral blood flow, although changes in P_aCO_2 are somewhat more potent. In the fetus, the influence of blood gases on cerebral blood flow is similar (Lucas, Kirschbaum & Assali, 1966; Purves & James, 1969; Jones et al., 1978). During maternal ventilatory hypoxia with exposure to various levels of CO_2 in the mother's inspired gas an inverse relationship exists in the fetus between carotid arterial oxygen content (C_aO_2) and cerebral blood flow, and a positive linear relationship exists between carotid arterial P_aCO_2 and cerebral blood flow (Jones et al., 1978). During periods of hypoxia, the cerebral vasculature of the fetus does not autoregulate; that is, during hypoxia there is a linear relationship between arterial pressure and cerebral blood flow in the range of blood pressures in which autoregulation can normally be demonstrated (Tweed et al., 1983).

Fetal cerebral blood flow can best be described as a function of both the arterial pressure and the arterial blood gases. The changes in cerebral blood flow during periods of hypoxia depend in part, therefore, on the systemic reflexes controlling blood pressure. Jansen et al. (1989) found that blood flow to the cerebrum, midbrain, medulla, pons, and cerebellum increased during acute isocapnic hypoxia and that sino-aortic denervation (a surgical procedure which removes afferent fibers from the arterial chemo- & baroreceptors) partially blocked the increase in flow to these areas.

Fetal cerebral blood flow is also a function of the metabolic activity of the fetal brain. High-voltage electrocorticogram (ECoG) activity without eye movements, the equivalent of non-REM (NREM) sleep in the postnatal animal, is associated with a lower rate of cerebral oxidative metabolism and a lower cerebral blood flow than during low-voltage ECoG activity, the equivalent of REM sleep in the postnatal animal (Richardson et al., 1989; Abrams et al., 1990). An increase in cerebral blood flow during REM sleep in the fetus is found during periods of fetal breathing movements (Jansen et al., 1989).

During hypoxia, there is a redistribution of fetal blood flow to defend the delivery of oxygen to the fetal heart and brain. While the blood flow in the cerebral circulation is increased during hypoxia (Jansen et al., 1989), the magnitude of the increase is insufficient to prevent the delivery of oxygen being compromised (Rurak et al., 1990). During sustained hypoxia, the delivery of oxygen is progressively decreased, averaging 78% of prehypoxia levels at 1.6 h and 29% at 7.9 h (Rurak et al., 1990).

Prolonged severe hypoxia (reduction of P_aO_2 from 3.0 to 0.6 mmol/l for 7.2 h) reduces cerebral oxygen consumption, as well (Richardson et al., 1989).

In summary, cerebral blood flow is adjusted physiologically to defend delivery of oxygen to cerebral tissues during periods of increased metabolic demand or periods of reduced substrate supply. This defence is limited, leaving the fetal brain vulnerable to severe or prolonged hypoxia or hypotension.

The pulmonary circulation

The pulmonary circulation maintains a high vascular resistance in fetal life, receiving approximately 8% of the combined ventricular output (for review see Todd & Cassin, 1991). Pulmonary blood flow increases as a function of fetal gestational age, with the flow per unit mass of tissue remaining relatively constant, but the mechanisms maintaining high vascular tone are not completely understood. However, evidence suggests that tone is regulated such that the blood flow is matched to the metabolic demands of the tissue. Occlusion of the pulmonary artery produces dilation of the pulmonary vasculature, suggesting reactive hyperaemia in this vascular bed (Todd & Cassin, 1991). Occlusion of the ductus arteriosus produces an increase in pulmonary arterial pressure and flow; flow then slowly declines, suggesting a time-dependent vasoconstriction (Abman & Accurso, 1989). However, it is clear that fetal pulmonary vasculature does not autoregulate flow as readily as that in the renal or cerebral circulations. The relationship between pulmonary arterial pressure and pulmonary blood flow (Fig. 4.1) is almost linear between 40 and 70 mm Hg (Cassin et al., 1964; Abman & Accurso, 1989).

Pulmonary blood flow is influenced by several local factors, including eicosanoids, endothelium-derived relaxation factor, endothelin, and blood gases. The mechanism responsible for maintaining high pulmonary vascular tone is controversial (Todd & Cassin, 1991); however, the reduction in vascular tone at birth is likely to be mediated by increased production of prostacyclin (Leffler, Hessler & Green, 1984). The effect of other vasoactive substances on tone is dependent upon the initial tone. For example, acetylcholine dilates the fetal pulmonary vasculature but does not alter tone in the adult in which pulmonary vascular tone is already low (Shepard, Blankenship & Stahlman, 1967; Dawes, 1968). Endothelin-1, a powerful vasoconstrictor in systemic vascular tissue in postnatal animals (Tomobe et al., 1988; Uchida et al., 1988; Yanagisawa et al., 1988), dilates the fetal pulmonary circulation (Cassin et al., 1991). However, if the pulmonary vascular bed is dilated initially by ventilation of the lungs, endothelin-1 acts as a constrictor (Cassin et al., 1991). The tone-dependency of pulmonary vascular response to endothelin-1 has prompted Cassin and coinvestigators to suggest an interaction between endothelin-1 and endothelium-derived relaxation factor (Furchgott & Zawadski, 1980; Leffler et al., 1984).

Increases in pulmonary arterial PO_2 dilate and decreases in PO_2 constrict the pulmonary circulation (Morin et al., 1988). Inflation of the lungs also dilates the vasculature (Iwamoto, Teitel & Rudolph, 1987). Therefore, the reduction in pulmonary vascular resistance at the time of birth is a function of an interaction between blood gases, prostacyclin and mechanical factors.

The control of blood flow through the fetal lung is therefore appropriate for the function of the organ in utero. Since the fetal lung is not an organ of gas exchange, it is advantageous to maintain a high vascular resistance, so that most of the blood ejected from the right ventricle is diverted through the ductus arteriosus into the systemic circulation. The metabolic needs of the pulmonary tissue are met by mechanisms matching the blood flow to the metabolic demands.

The umbilical–placental circulation

The umbilical–placental circulation is a low resistance circuit through which nearly 50% of the fetal combined ventricular output flows. Changes in arterial pressure play an important role in the determination of umbilical–placental blood flow. While this vascular circuit is not innervated, several hormonal and locally produced constrictor and dilator agents can alter resistance in this system. Umbilical–placental vascular bed resistance increases in response to various vasoconstrictors, such as angiotensin II, norepinephrine, phenylephrine, and vasopressin (AVP). Prostaglandin $F_{2\alpha}$ and thromboxane A_2 constrict, and prostacyclin I_2 dilates, the umbilical–placental vasculature. Interestingly, prostaglandin E_2 (PGE$_2$) (which is known to be a dilator in most vascular beds) constricts the umbilical–placental bed (Parisi & Walsh, 1986). The response of the umbilical–placental circulation to various vasoconstrictors is weak relative to the action of these vasoconstrictors in other vascular beds. Therefore, constrictors (such as AVP and phenylephrine) tend to redistribute blood flow into the umbilical–placental circulation from the systemic circulation.

Vasoconstrictors act at various sites within the umbilical–placental circulation to modulate flow. In a recent report, Adamson and coworkers (1989) found that both angiotensin II and norepinephrine constrict this vascular bed; angiotensin II constricts mainly the umbilical artery and norepinephrine constricts mainly the vessels downstream from the cotyledonary vascular segments. Recent evidence suggests that angiotensin II stimulates PGE_2 and prostacyclin production, while phenylephrine does not (Yoshimura et al., 1990a). The mechanism by which angiotensin-stimulated production of prostaglandins, which are known to be both constrictors and dilators, produces a net vasoconstriction is not presently understood.

The oxygen tension of umbilical arterial blood also influences blood flow through the umbilical–placental circulation. Increases (Nyberg & Westin, 1957; Assali, Kirschbaum & Dilts, 1968; Lewis, 1968) and decreases (Nyberg & Westin, 1957) in oxygen tension increase and decrease, respectively, the vascular tone in the umbilical vessels. The importance of changes in oxygen tension in the control of umbilical flow in the fetus in utero is not known; however, constriction of the umbilical artery at birth must be, in part, caused by exposure to the increased oxygen content.

Blood flow through the umbilical–placental circulation is greatly affected by changes in the fetal arterial blood pressure. Vasoconstrictors infused into the fetal circulation often increase umbilical–placental blood flow because the constrictor actions are weak in the umbilical vessels relative to the constrictor actions elsewhere. For example, intravenous infusion of AVP into the fetus (Fig. 4.2) constricts the vasculature in the fetal peripheral circulation and redistributes fetal combined ventricular output towards the placenta (Iwamoto et al., 1987). Intravenous injection of sar[1],ala[8]-angiotensin II into the fetus (Fig. 4.3) lowers arterial blood pressure and reduces umbilical-placental blood flow, shunting flow from the placenta towards the fetal peripheral circulation (Iwamoto & Rudolph, 1979). Infusion of phenylephrine intravenously into baroreceptor-denervated fetuses subjected to slow haemorrhage increases arterial blood pressure, decreases arterial PCO_2 and increases arterial PO_2, suggesting that blood flow is shunted towards the umbilical–placental circulation (Chen & Wood, 1992).

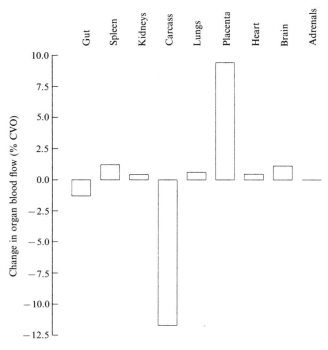

Fig. 4.2. Mean changes in the percentage distribution of fetal combined ventricular output during intravenous infusion of arginine vasopressin. (Data are redrawn from Iwamoto et al., 1979.)

The adrenal gland

Blood flow through the adrenal gland is often increased during periods of 'stress': that is, times during which adrenal secretion of cortisol is increased above the levels expected in unstimulated fetuses of the same gestational age. For example, both haemorrhage (Toubas et al., 1981) and hypoxia (Cohn et al., 1974) increase adrenal blood flow. The variables controlling blood flow through this organ are not known, although it is clear that there is active control of vascular tone. In the adult animal, the rate of secretion of cortisol by the adrenal gland is a function of the plasma ACTH concentration and the rate of adrenal blood flow (Nelson & Hume, 1955). It seems likely that the increase in adrenal blood

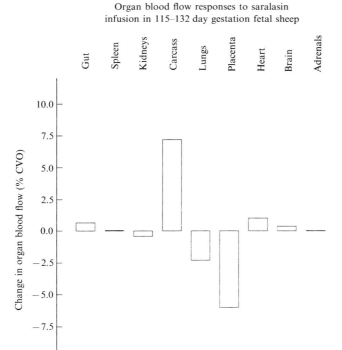

Fig. 4.3. Mean changes in the percentage distribution of fetal combined ventricular output during intravenous infusion of sar^1–ala^8 angiotensin II. (Data are redrawn from Iwamoto & Rudolph, 1979.)

flow during hypoxia or other stimuli to cortisol secretion is one factor important in the control of cortisol secretion.

Myocardial circulation

Little is known about the mechanisms controlling the myocardial circulation in the fetal animal. Myocardial oxygen consumption in fetal sheep (115–121 days' gestation) is similar to that in adult, but is significantly higher in newborn (4–25 days) sheep (Fisher, Heymann & Rudolph, 1980). The oxygen content of coronary sinus blood is equal at all three ages. However, the higher oxygen content of arterial blood in the adult is reflected in a larger arteriovenous difference in oxygen content when compared to the fetus or newborn. Myocardial blood flow, expressed as a flow per unit mass per minute (Fisher, Heymann & Rudolph, 1981), is greatest in the myocardium of the newborn sheep, slightly less in the fetal sheep, and lowest in the adult sheep (201 ± 21, 156 ± 11, and 82 ± 8 ml/min per 100 g left ventricle, respectively). Myocardial blood flow is likely to be closely related to the metabolic demands of the myocardium. During hypoxia, or after exchange transfusion with maternal blood to reduce fetal arterial blood oxygen content, myocardial blood flow is increased to maintain delivery of oxygen to the myocardium (Peeters et al., 1979; Itskovitz et al., 1984). Fisher, Heymann, and Rudolph (1981) speculated that increased oxygen consumption in the newborn reflected a greater work rate of the myocardium at that age. They suggested that the product of the heart rate and the blood pressure, which is higher in newborn sheep, is a useful correlate of the myocardial oxygen consumption because it reflects myocardial work (Fisher et al., 1981).

The coordinated cardiovascular response to hypoxia

Many physiological experiments designed to investigate the fetal response have involved compression of the umbilical cord, reduction of blood flow to the uterus or, more commonly, production of ventilatory hypoxia by reduction of the content of oxygen in the mother's inspired gases. These experiments performed in the chronically catheterized, unanesthetized fetal sheep provide an illustration of the coordinated response to a stimulus which alters cardiovascular function both directly and reflexly. Furthermore, since asphyxia is the most common form of fetal stress, the cardiovascular responses to hypoxia and/or hypercapnia are perhaps the most important adaptive responses responsible for maintaining fetal homeostasis.

Hypoxia stimulates homeostatic cardiovascular responses which are coordinated to maintain blood flow to organs important for maintenance of life, such as the fetal heart and brain. During hypoxia, therefore, blood flow is shunted away from the fetal carcass or peripheral circulation and redirected towards the fetal heart, brain, and placenta (Fig. 4.4; see Cohn et al., 1974). This response is homeostatic in that the tissues which can withstand a short-term reduction in oxygen delivery, including the gastrointestinal tract, lungs, and peripheral circulation, suffer reduced flow to allow greater flow to the placenta (to maximize the uptake of oxygen from the maternal circulation) and to allow greater flow to the heart and brain.

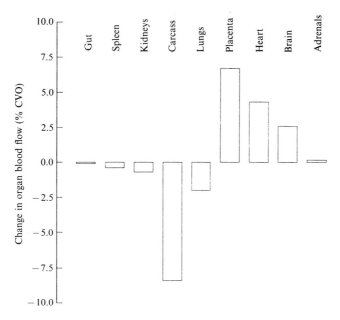

Fig. 4.4. Mean changes in the percentage distribution of fetal combined ventricular output during ventilatory hypoxia. (Data are redrawn from Cohn et al., 1974.)

Decreased P_aO_2 directly constricts the vasculature of the lung (Todd & Cassin, 1991). In other vascular beds, such as the cerebral and myocardial circulation, decreased P_aO_2 dilates the vasculature (Reuss et al., 1982; Gilbert et al., 1990) to maintain constant delivery of oxygen and other required metabolic substrates. Without neural and endocrine reflex adjustments during hypoxia, therefore, peripheral vasodilatation would tend to reduce blood pressure with consequent fall in placental perfusion. Hypoxia results in reflex increases in vasomotor tone and increases in the rate of secretion of vasoconstrictor hormones which constrict the peripheral vasculature and increase arterial blood pressure above that observed during normoxia (Cohen et al., 1982). Severe hypoxia directly stimulates the fetal adrenal medulla to secrete epinephrine (Comline & Silver, 1961). Catecholamines, vasopressin, and angiotensin generally increase vascular tone in the peripheral circulation of the fetus but do not constrict the myocardium or brain vascalature (Iwamoto & Rudolph, 1979; Iwamoto et al., 1979; Reuss et al., 1982), where blood flow is matched to the metabolic demand. The increase in total peripheral resistance increases arterial blood pressure and secondarily increases umbilical–placental flow. The net result of this process is a redistribution of fetal combined ventricular output towards the placenta. Gas exchange at the placenta depends on the flow of blood through it; therefore, shunting of the fetal combined ventricular output towards the placenta improves the uptake of oxygen from the maternal circulation and improves the excretion of carbon dioxide into the maternal circulation.

Not all of these responses are equally sensitive to hypoxia, and not all of the endocrine or neural responses play equivalent roles in the redistribution of combined ventricular output to the placenta. For example, plasma renin activity and plasma angiotensin II concentration are high in the fetus compared to the nonpregnant adult sheep (Broughton-Pipkin et al., 1974). The high circulating concentrations of angiotensin II tonically constrict the fetal systemic vasculature and therefore are partially responsible for maintaining umbilical-placental flow and maintaining exchange of blood gases between the fetal and maternal circulations (Iwamoto & Rudolph, 1979). Renin secretion is increased during periods of hypoxia and asphyxia; however, the magnitude of the response of the renin–angiotensin system is small compared to other constrictor systems. When the effects of hypoxia and hypercapnia are considered separately, hypercapnia is a more potent stimulus to renin secretion than is hypoxia (Wood, Kane & Raff, 1990). The responses to hypercapnia are blocked by sinoaortic denervation, which interrupts afferent fibers from the peripheral chemoreceptors (Wood, Kane & Raff, 1990).

Vasopressin circulates in low plasma concentrations in the fetus. Plasma vasopressin concentrations increase greatly during periods of hypoxia (Alexander et al., 1973; Rurak, 1978). Increases in fetal plasma vasopressin concentrations, equal to those produced by hypoxia, have been shown to increase fetal blood pressure and redistribute fetal combined ventricular output towards the placenta (Iwamoto et al., 1979). For this reason, some investigators have speculated that these vasopressin responses are of primary importance in the cardiovascular adaptations to hypoxia (Iwamoto et al., 1979; Perez et al., 1989). However, there is some disagreement on this point, in that some investigators found (Perez et al., 1989), whilst others did not find (Piacquado, Brace & Cheung, 1990), a significant effect of blockade of vasopressin receptors on the increase in blood pressure and maintenance of fetal blood gases during hypoxia.

Hypoxia is a more potent stimulus to vasopressin secretion than is hypercapnia, and there is a large synergism between hypoxia and hypercapnia in the stimulation of vasopressin secretion (Raff, Kane & Wood, 1991). Denervation of the peripheral chemoreceptors does not affect the fetal vasopressin response to either hypoxia or hypercapnia (Raff, Kane & Wood, 1991). Therefore, it is likely that vasopressin is controlled by a 'chemoreceptor' located elsewhere, probably within the central nervous system itself.

It is interesting that peripheral chemodenervation blocks the increase in mean arterial blood pressure and decrease in heart rate observed during hypoxia, but does not alter the magnitude of the vasopressin response. This is inconsistent with the notion that vasopressin is primarily responsible for the cardiovascular responses to hypoxia. The increase in blood pressure during hypoxia is clearly, therefore, mediated by factors (such as vasomotor tone) other than the increased vasopressin concentration. While it is clear that vasopressin alone can increase fetal blood pressure and redistribute flow towards the placenta, it is possible that during hypoxia other influences (perhaps tissue hypoxia & hyperaemia) modulate the vasoconstrictor actions of vasopressin.

The decrease in heart rate observed during hypoxia is also a response to peripheral chemoreceptor stimulation and not a direct effect of vasopressin on the heart. Several investigators have suggested that vasopressin has a direct effect on the myocardial circulation to decrease heart rate. This suggestion is based on the observation that during vasopressin infusions heart rate decreases before there is a quantifiable increase in arterial blood pressure (Iwamoto et al., 1979). Also, attempts to servocontrol blood pressure during vasopressin infusions have not been successful in blocking the decrease in fetal heart rate (Harper & Rose, 1988). However, the observation that peripheral chemodenervation abolishes the bradycardia, but not the vasopressin response to hypoxia, suggests that the stimulus to bradycardia in previous experiments was not adequately quantified (Iwamoto et al., 1979) or controlled (Harper & Rose, 1988). The redistribution of blood flow during hypoxia is therefore most likely dependent upon increased vasomotor tone. Dawes and coworkers (1968) demonstrated a neural mechanism that contributed to the increase in vascular tone during hypoxia.

Overview and conclusions

A complete understanding of the mechanisms controlling changes in resistance and flow through the circulatory system of the fetus requires detailed information concerning the local effectors of changes in tone within specific vascular beds, and the coordination of these local systems by neural and endocrine systems. The redistribution of fetal combined ventricular output during disturbances of the system such as hypoxia, therefore, is a function of changes in tone in all vascular beds, changes in fetal combined ventricular output, and changes in arterial blood pressure.

There is a long way to go before the local and endocrine factors controlling the circulation in the fetus are fully understood. A better understanding of local control will lead to a better understanding of coordinated homeostatic adjustments to hypoxia and haemorrhage. More importantly, a better understanding of this problem will improve our understanding of the pathophysiology of conditions which are fatal or debilitating in the newborn. While significant advances in this area have been made, more information is required before we understand fully the mechanisms and causes of conditions such as persistent pulmonary hypertension of the newborn, or patent ductus arteriosus.

References

Abman, S. H. & Accurso, F. J. (1989). Acute effects of partial compression of ductus arteriosus on fetal pulmonary circulation. *American Journal of Physiology,* **257**, H626–34.

Abrams, R. M., Post, J. C., Burchfield, D. J., Gomez, K. J., Hutchison, A. A. & Conlon, M. (1990). Local cerebral blood flow is increased in rapid-eye-movement sleep in fetal sheep. *American Journal of Obstetrics and Gynecology,* **162**, 278–81.

Adamson, S. L., Morrow, R. J., Bull, S. B. & Langille, B. L. (1989). Vasomotor responses of the umbilical circulation in fetal sheep. *American Journal of Physiology,* **256**, R1056–62.

Alexander, D. P., Britton, H. G., Nixon, D. A., Ratcliffe, J. G. & Redstone, D. (1973). Corticotrophin and cortisol concentrations in the plasma of the chronically catheterised sheep fetus. *Biology of the Neonate,* **23**, 184–92.

Armstead, W. M., Leffler, C. W., Busija, D. W., Beasley, D. G. & Mirro, R. (1988). Adrenergic and prostanoid mechanisms in control of cerebral blood flow in hypotensive newborn pigs. *American Journal of Physiology,* **254**, H671–7.

Assali, N. S., Kirschbaum, T. H. & Dilts, P. V. (1968). Effects of hyperbaric oxygen on uteroplacental and fetal circulation. *Circulation Research,* **22**, 573–88.

Broughton-Pipkin, F., Kirkpatrick, S. M. L., Lumbers, E. R. & Mott, J. C. (1974). Renin and angiotensin-like levels in foetal, new-born, and adult sheep. *Journal of Physiology,* **241**, 575–88.

Cassin, S., Dawes, G. S., Mott, J. C., Ross, B. B. & Strang, L. B. (1964). The vascular resistance of the foetal and newly ventilated lung of the lamb. *Journal of Physiology,* **171**, 61–79.

Cassin, S., Dawes, G. S. & Ross, B. B. (1964). Pulmonary blood flow and vascular resistance in immature foetal lambs. *Journal of Physiology*, **171**, 80–9.

Cassin, S., Kristova, V., Davis, T., Kadowitz, P. & Gause, G. (1991). Tone-dependent responses to endothelin in the isolated perfused fetal sheep pulmonary circulation in situ. *Journal of Applied Physiology*, **70**, 1228–34.

Chen, H.-G. & Wood, C. E. (1992). Reflex control of fetal arterial pressure and hormonal responses to slow hemorrhage. *American Journal of Physiology*, **262**, H225–33.

Cohen, W. R., Piasecki, G. F. & Jackson, B. T. (1982). Plasma catecholamines during hypoxemia in fetal lamb. *American Journal of Physiology*, **243**, R520–5.

Cohn, H. E., Sacks, E. J., Heymann, M. A. & Rudolph, A. M. (1974). Cardiovascular responses to hypoxemia and acidemia in fetal lambs. *American Journal of Obstetrics and Gynecology*, **120**, 817–24.

Comline, R. S. & Silver, M. (1961). The release of adrenaline and noradrenaline from the adrenal glands of the foetal sheep. *Journal of Physiology*, **156**, 424–44.

Dawes, G. S. (1968). *Foetal and Neonatal Physiology*. Year Book Medical Publishers, Chicago.

Dawes, G. S., Lewis, B. V., Milligan, J. E., Roach, M. R. & Talner, N. S. (1968). Vasomotor responses in the hind limbs of foetal and new-born lambs to asphyxia and aortic chemoreceptor stimulation. *Journal of Physiology*, **195**, 55–81.

Fisher, D. J., Heymann, M. A. & Rudolph, A. M. (1980). Myocardial oxygen and carbohydrate consumption in fetal lambs in utero and in adult sheep. *American Journal of Physiology*, **238**, H399–405.

Fisher, D. J., Heymann, M. A. & Rudolph, A. M. (1981). Myocardial consumption of oxygen and carbohydrates in newborn sheep. *Pediatric Research*, **15**, 843–6.

Furchgott, R. F. & Zawadski, J. V. (1980). The obligatory role of endothelial cells in the relaxation of arterial smooth muscle by acetylcholine. *Nature*, **288**, 373–6.

Gilbert, R. D., Pearce, W. J., Ashwal, S. & Longo, L. D. (1990). Effects of hypoxia on contractility of isolated fetal lamb cerebral arteries. *Journal of Developmental Physiology*, **13**, 199–203.

Harper, M. A. & Rose J. C. (1988). Arginine vasopressin infusion stimulates adrenocorticotropic hormone and cortisol release in the ovine fetus. *American Journal of Obstetrics and Gynecology*, **159**, 983–8.

Hernandez, M. J., Brennan, R. W. & Bowman, G. S. (1980). Autoregulation of cerebral blood flow in the newborn dog. *Brain Research*, **184**, 199–202.

Ismay, M. J. A., Lumbers, E. R. & Stevens, A. D. (1979). The action of angiotensin II on the baroreflex response of the conscious ewe and the conscious fetus. *Journal of Physiology*, **288**, 467–79.

Itskovitz, J., Goetzman, B. W., Roman, C. & Rudolph, A. M. (1984). Effects of fetal-maternal exchange transfusion on fetal oxygenation and blood flow distribution. *American Journal of Physiology*, **247**, H655–60.

Itskovitz, J., Goetzman, B. W. & Rudolph, A. M. (1982). Effects of hemorrhage on umbilical venous return and oxygen delivery in fetal lambs. *American Journal of Physiology*, **242**, H543–8.

Iwamoto, H. S. & Rudolph, A. M. (1979). Effects of endogenous angiotensin II on the fetal circulation. *Journal of Developmental Physiology*, **1**, 283–93.

Iwamoto, H. S., Rudolph, A. M., Keil, L.C. & Heymann, M. A. (1979). Hemodynamic responses of the sheep fetus to vasopressin infusion. *Circulation Research*, **44**, 430–6.

Iwamoto, H. S., Teitel, D. & Rudolph, A. M. (1987). Effects of birth-related events on blood flow distribution. *Pediatric Research*, **22**, 634–40.

Jansen, A. H., Belik, J., Ioffe, S. & Chernick, V. (1989). Control of organ blood flow in fetal sheep during normoxia and hypoxia. *American Journal of Physiology*, **257**, H1132–9.

Jones, M. D., Sheldon, R. E., Peeters, L. L., Makowski, E. L. & Meschia, G. (1978). Regulation of cerebral blood flow in the ovine fetus. *American Journal of Physiology*, **235**, H162–6.

Leffler, C. W., Busija, D. W., Beasley, D. G. & Fletcher, A. M. (1986). Maintenance of cerebral circulation during hemorrhagic hypotension in newborn pigs: role of prostanoids. *Circulation Research*, **59**, 562–7.

Leffler, C. W., Hessler, J. R. & Green, R. S. (1984). The onset of breathing at birth stimulates pulmonary vascular prostacyclin synthesis. *Pediatric Research*, **18**, 938–42.

Lewis, B. V. (1968). The response of isolated sheep & human umbilical arteries to oxygen and drugs. *British Journal of Obstetrics and Gynaecology*, **75**, 87–91.

Lucas, W., Kirschbaum, T. & Assali, N. S. (1966). Cephalic circulation and oxygen consumption before and after birth. *American Journal of Physiology*, **210**, 287–92.

Morin, F. C., III, Egan, E. A., Ferguson, W. & Lundgren, C. E. G. (1988). Development of pulmonary vascular response to oxygen. *American Journal of Physiology*, **254**, H542–6.

Nelson, D. H. & Hume, D. M. (1955). Corticosteroid secretion in the adrenal venous blood of the hypophysectomized dog as an assay for ACTH. *Endocrinology*, **57**, 184–92.

Nyberg, R. & Westin, B. (1957). The influence of oxygen tension and some drugs on human placental vessels. *Acta Physiologica Scandinavica*, **39**, 216–27.

Papile, L. A., Rudolph, A. M. & Heymann, M. A. (1985). Autoregulation of cerebral blood flow in the preterm fetal lamb. *Pediatric Research*, **19**, 159–61.

Parisi, V. M. & Walsh, S. W. (1986). Arachidonic acid metabolites and the regulation of placental and other vascular tone during pregnancy. *Seminars in Perinatology*, **10**, 288–98.

Peeters, L. L., Sheldon, R. E., Jones, M. D., Makowski, E. L. & Meschia, G. (1979). Blood flow to fetal organs as a function of arterial oxygen content. *American Journal of Obstetrics and Gynecology*, **135**, 637–46.

Perez, R., Espinoza, M., Riquelme, R., Parer, J. T. & Llanos, A. J. (1989). Arginine vasopressin mediates cardiovascular responses to hypoxemia in fetal sheep. *American Journal of Physiology*, **256**, R1011–18.

Piacquado, K. M., Brace, R. A. & Cheung, C. Y. (1990). Role of vasopressin in mediation of fetal cardiovascular responses to hypoxia. *American Journal of Obstetrics and Gynecology*, **163**, 1294–1300.

Purves, M. J. & James, I. M. (1969). Observations on the control of cerebral blood flow in the sheep fetus and newborn lamb. *Circulation Research*, **25**, 651–67.

Raff, H., Kane, C. & Wood, C. E. (1991). Vasopressin responses to hypoxia and hypercapnia in late-gestation fetal sheep. *American Journal of Physiology*, **260**, R1077–81.

Reuss, M. L., Parer, J. T., Harris, J. L. & Krueger, T. R. (1982).
Hemodynamic effects of alpha-adrenergic blockade during hypoxia in fetal
sheep. *American Journal of Obstetrics and Gynecology*, **142**, 410–15.

Richardson, B. S., Carmichael, L., Homan, J. & Gagnon, R. (1989). Cerebral
oxidative metabolism in lambs during perinatal period: relationship to
electrocortical state. *American Journal of Physiology*, **257**, R1251–7.

Rurak, D. W. (1978). Plasma vasopressin levels during hypoxaemia and the
cardiovascular effects of exogenous vasopressin in foetal and adult sheep.
Journal of Physiology, **277**, 341–57.

Rurak, D. W., Richardson, B. S., Patrick, J. E., Carmichael L. & Homan, J.
(1990). Blood flow and oxygen delivery to fetal organs and tissues during
sustained hypoxemia. *American Journal of Physiology*, **258**, R1116–22.

Shepard, F. M., Blankenship, W. & Stahlman, M. (1967). Cardiovascular
response of the neonatal lamb to acetylcholine. *American Journal of
Physiology*, **213**, 895–8.

Todd, M. L. & Cassin, S. (1991). Fetal and neonatal pulmonary circulation. In
The Lung: Scientific Foundations, ed. R. G. Crystal & J. B. West. pp.
1687–98, Raven Press, New York.

Tomobe, Y., Miyauchi, T., Saito, A., Yanagisawa, M., Kimura, S. Goto, K. &
Masaki, T. (1988). Effects of endothelin on the renal artery from
spontaneously hypertensive and Wistar Kyoto rats. *European Journal of
Pharmacology*, **152**, 373–4.

Toubas, P. L., Silverman, N. H., Heymann, M. A. & Rudolph, A. M. (1981).
Cardiovascular effects of acute hemorrhage in fetal lambs. *American
Journal of Physiology*, **240**, H45–8.

Tweed, W. A., Cote, J., Pash, M. & Lou, H. (1983). Arterial oxygenation
determines autoregulation of cerebral blood flow in the fetal lamb.
Pediatric Research, **17**, 246–9.

Uchida, Y., Ninomiya, H., Saotome, M., Nomura, A., Ohtsuka, M.,
Yanagisawa, M., Goto, K. & Masaki, T. (1988). Endothelin, a novel
vasoconstrictor peptide, a potent broncho-constrictor. *European Journal
of Pharmacology*, **154**, 227–8.

Vapaavouri, E. K., Shinebourne, E. A., Williams, R. L., Heymann, M. A. &
Rudolph, A. M. (1973). Development of cardiovascular responses to
autonomic blockade in intact fetal and neonatal lambs. *Biology of the
Neonate*, **22**, 177–88.

Wiriyathian, S., Porter, J. C., Naden, R. P. & Rosenfeld, C. R. (1983).
Cardiovascular effects and clearance of arginine vasopressin in the fetal
lamb. *American Journal of Physiology*, **245**, E24–31.

Wood, C. E., Kane, C. & Raff, H. (1990). Peripheral chemoreceptor control
of fetal renin responses to hypoxia and hypercapnia. *Circulation Research*,
67, 722–32.

Yanagisawa, M., Kurihawa, H., Kimura, S., Tomobe, Y., Kobayashi, M.,
Mitsui, Y., Yazaki, Y., Goto, K. & Masaki, T. (1988). A novel potent
vasoconstrictor peptide produced by vascular endothelial cells. *Nature*,
332, 411–15.

Yoshimura, T., Magness, R. R. & Rosenfeld, C. R. (1990*a*). Angiotensin II
and alpha-agonist II. Effects on ovine fetoplacental prostaglandins.
American Journal of Physiology, **251**, H473–9.

Yoshimura, T., Magness, R. R. & Rosenfeld, C. R. (1990*b*). Angiotensin II
and alpha-agonist I. Responses of ovine fetoplacental vasculature.
American Journal of Physiology, **259**, H464–72.

5

Fetal placental circulation

ANTHONY M. CARTER

Introduction

The fetal placental circulation is characterized by its low vascular resistance and correspondingly high rate of blood flow. The human placenta receives about 20% of the biventricular cardiac output at term (Eik-Nes, Brubakk & Ulstein, 1980; De Smedt, Visser & Meijboom, 1987). In sheep, placental blood flow before the third trimester accounts for approximately half of the biventricular output, with a gradual decrease throughout the third trimester to about 40% at term (Iwamoto et al., 1989). At this time the placenta contains approximately 20% of fetal blood volume (Creasy et al., 1970). These high rates of blood flow reflect the essential role of the placental circulation in fetal respiration, substrate transfer and the mediation of fetal–maternal signals.

The development and structural organization of the placental vasculature in man is quite well known. Until recently, however, access to the human fetus was limited, and physiological information was restricted to studies of the previable conceptus (Rudolph et al., 1971) and measurements of blood flow in the umbilical cord made after delivery of the infant (Štembera et al., 1965). Combination of real-time ultrasonography with the pulsed Doppler ultrasound technique now enables the estimation of volume flow in the umbilical vein in utero (Gill & Kossoff, 1981; Eik-Nes et al., 1980). Nevertheless, most current knowledge about the physiology of the fetal placental circulation is derived from studies of fetal sheep. Many recent studies employ the microsphere technique introduced by Rudolph & Heymann (1967). Other methods used to measure placental blood flow in sheep have been reviewed elsewhere (Carter, 1975). There has been an evolution towards the study of chronically instrumented sheep preparations, with increasing attention being paid to behavioural

116

state. Studies have usually been performed at >120 days' gestation (term is about 147 days), but important information is beginning to emerge on placental blood flow in mid-pregnancy (Bell et al., 1986; Iwamoto et al., 1989, see Chapter 2).

The existence of a body of experimental data for the sheep fetus has enabled the construction of mathematical models that have furthered our understanding of the placental circulation and its interplay with the rest of the fetal cardiovascular system (Huikeshoven et al., 1985; Longo, 1987). However, extrapolation from the sheep to man is subject to many limitations, including those imposed by differences in the structural organization of the placenta.

Structural organization of the fetal placental vasculature

The human placenta is haemochorial: maternal blood enters the intervillous space from spiral arteries in the basal plate, flows around the fetal villi, and drains through venous openings in the basal plate (Fig. 5.1). The basic structural unit of the fetal placenta, the cotyledon, arises from the

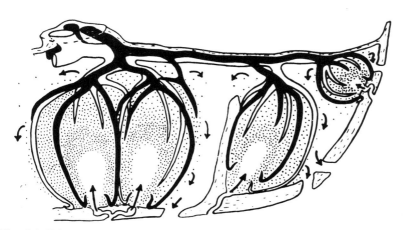

Fig. 5.1. Diagram of the circulation of maternal blood through the intervillous space of the human placenta. The basic structural unit of the fetal placenta, the cotyledon, is formed by repetitive branching of a stem villus to form a villous tree. The relative density of the terminal villi is indicated by stippling and arrows show the direction of flow of the maternal blood. The spiral arteries empty at the centres of the cotyledons, the intralobular spaces, which are relatively free of villi. The blood must then perfuse a densely packed mass of villi to reach the extralobular spaces between the cotyledons and in the subchorial lake. Drainage occurs through venous opening in the basal plate. (From Wigglesworth, 1969.)

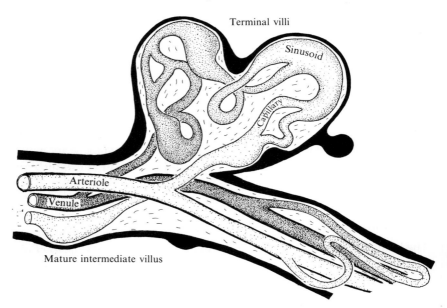

Fig. 5.2. The capillary arrangement in a terminal villus (above) and an intermediate villus of the human placenta. The terminal villi are the final branches of the villous tree and are considered important for maternofetal exchange. The fetal capillaries within the terminal villi form hairpin loops, both limbs of which are thought to participate in placental exchange. (From Kaufmann & Scheffen, 1991.)

chorionic plate and branches to form a villous tree. The bulk of the placenta is made up of about 60 cotyledons of large to medium size, although there are about 200 cotyledons in all (Crawford, 1962). The primary trunk of each cotyledon contains an artery and a vein derived, respectively, from one of the paired umbilical arteries and the umbilical vein. A detailed description of vessel arrangement at various levels of the villous tree can be found in a recent review by Kaufmann, Luckhardt & Leiser (1988). The final branches of the villous trees are the terminal villi (Fig. 5.2), which account for approximately 50% of the surface area in contact with maternal blood, and are considered important for materno-fetal exchange. The terminal villi are connected to more proximal villi by a narrow neck region containing two to four narrow capillaries, but in the bulbous peripheral parts the capillaries are more or less dilated with diameters >10 μm and up to 40 μm. The maternofetal diffusion distance at this point is as little as 4 μm (Kaufmann, 1985; Kaufmann et al., 1988).

In the sheep, tufts of villi develop in apposition to endometrial caruncles that are present in the uterus of the non-pregnant ewe. Thus, instead of a single, discoid placenta, like the human placenta, the maternal and fetal tissues form 40–100 discrete cotyledons. Within these, the integrity of the maternal capillaries is maintained, and the ovine placenta is classified as syndesmochorial (Steven, 1968).

Although the placentas of different species vary greatly in gross form and fine structure (Amoroso, 1952; Steven, 1975; Faber & Thornburg, 1983), the aspect of greatest importance for placental gas exchange is the spatial arrangement of the blood vessels and the relative directions of fetal and maternal placental blood flows (Carter, 1989). In the ovine placenta, exchange occurs between fetal and maternal capillaries with concurrent or crosscurrent flows (Silver, Steven & Comline, 1973). A countercurrent arrangement provides a better basis for exchange, as evidenced by the smaller difference in umbilical and uterine venous PO_2 in the mare compared to that in the sheep (Silver et al., 1973). Counter-current flow was first described for the rabbit placenta (Mossman, 1926) and is also seen in the placenta of the guinea-pig (Kaufmann & Davidoff, 1977). In the human placenta, the terminal villi are arranged at varying angles to the direction of the maternal blood stream. Moreover, the fetal capillaries form hairpin-like loops (Fig. 5.2), both limbs of which are presumed to participate in placental exchange (Kaufmann, 1985).

Fetal placental blood flow

There is a steady increase in fetal placental blood flow in the course of ovine pregnancy (Makowski et al., 1968), although the proportion of fetal cardiac output distributed to the placenta decreases with advancing fetal age (Rudolph & Heymann, 1970). In relation to fetal weight, placental blood flow is much greater at mid-gestation than at term (Bell et al., 1986). The increase in umbilical blood flow between 90 and 115 days is due mainly to a fall in vascular resistance, and between 115 and 140 days to a rise in fetal arterial blood pressure (Dawes, 1962).

An increase in umbilical blood flow with increasing gestation has also been demonstrated for the human fetus (Erskine & Ritchie, 1985; Lingman & Maršál, 1986; Gerson et al., 1987; Fig. 5.3). However, the mean velocity of blood flow in the umbilical vein is constant between 28 weeks and term, leaving only a steady increase in vessel diameter to account for the rise in total blood flow (Erskine & Ritchie, 1985; Lingman & Maršál, 1986). This is not without clinical significance, as blood flow

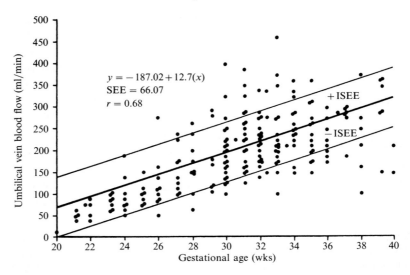

Fig. 5.3. Umbilical blood flow meaurements in the second and third trimesters of human pregnancy plotted against gestational age. Placental blood flow increases as the fetus grows. SEE = standard error of the estimate. (From Gerson et al., 1987.)

velocity can be determined with greater precision than the cross sectional area of the umbilical vein. In relation to fetal weight, umbilical venous blood flow has been reported to fall from 153 ml/min per kg at 20 weeks to 108 ml/min per kg at 40 weeks (Gerson et al., 1987). Lingman & Maršál (1986) also found a decrease in weight-related umbilical blood flow with gestational age.

In sheep there is a wide variation in the rate of fetal placental blood flow at term, from 154 to 444 ml/min per kg body weight in the ovine fetus, without any significant variation in fetal oxygen consumption (VO_2) at these extremes of flow (Clapp, 1978). At low rates of blood flow, the fetus compensates for the reduced oxygen delivery (DO_2) by increasing the fractional extraction of oxygen. This results in a lowering of the O_2 content of the umbilical arterial blood. Most authors are agreed that there is a lower limit for DO_2 of about 0.6 mmol/min per kg fetal weight. If DO_2 falls below this level, VO_2 will fall, as the fetus can no longer maintain oxidative metabolism, and metabolic acidosis will develop (Wilkening & Meschia, 1983; Edelstone, Caine & Fumia, 1985a; Edelstone et al., 1989; Gu, Jones & Parer, 1985; Paulone, Edelstone & Shedd, 1987).

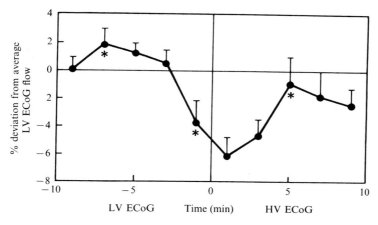

Fig. 5.4. Two min means of umbilical blood flow plotted against time, from 10 min prior to 10 min after the transition from low to high voltage electrocortical activity in the fetal sheep. Flow values are expressed as percentage deviations from the average flow during low voltage electrocortical activity (LV ECoG). An asterisk indicates a significant difference in umbilical blood flow from the previous 2 min period. (From Slotten et al., 1989.)

Some of the observed variation in placental blood flow may reflect diurnal rhythms (Walker et al., 1977), or the alterations in fetal behavioural state that are reflected in the electrocorticogram (ECoG). A low voltage ECoG is associated predominantly with rapid eye movement (REM) sleep, interspersed with periods of active wakefulness, whereas a high voltage ECoG is recognized as non-REM sleep. A decrease in umbilical blood flow precedes the change from low to high voltage electrocortical activity states (Fig. 5.4), but 5 min into the high voltage state blood flow rises again (Slotten, Phernetton & Rankin, 1989). On average, placental blood flow is 12% higher during the low voltage than during the high voltage ECoG state (Slotten et al., 1989), although this difference can be difficult to detect (Jensen et al., 1986). The placenta must suffer a significant vasoconstriction during high voltage ECoG, since arterial blood pressure is higher at this time, with a subsequent vasodilatation during the ensuing low voltage state (Slotten et al., 1989).

Behavioural states in the human fetus have been defined on the basis of fetal body movements, eye movements, and heart rate patterns (Nijhuis et al., 1982). Flow velocity waveforms in the umbilical artery during quiet sleep (state 1F) and active sleep (state 2F) have been analyzed under standardized fetal heart rate conditions (van Eyck et al., 1987) and the results indicate that placental vascular resistance does not change with behavioural state in the human fetus. This observation is of practical importance, since umbilical artery flow velocity waveforms can be studied in late pregnancy without taking fetal behavioural state into account (van Eyck et al., 1987). Interestingly, total resistance to blood flow in the descending aorta does seem to be greater during active sleep, presumably due to increased perfusion of the fetal skeletal muscle, reflecting the higher incidence of body movements associated with this state (van Eyck et al., 1985).

Episodes of rapid, irregular fetal breathing are a normal occurrence in the low voltage ECoG state of the fetal sheep. They result in an increase in fetal oxygen consumption ($\dot{V}O_2$) with a concomitant rise in fetal heart rate, arterial blood pressure, and placental blood flow (Rurak & Gruber, 1983). In the human fetus, too, the velocity of blood flow in the umbilical vein is seen to increase during fetal breathing (Maršál et al., 1984). During large amplitude breathing activity in the ovine fetus, stimulated by hypercapnia, the normal pattern of pulsatile blood flow in the umbilical artery is severely disrupted, and there is a resultant fall in the mean rate of blood flow (Rurak, Cooper & Taylor, 1986). Momentary interruption of flow has also been reported to occur during high amplitude breathing in the human fetus, and it has been recommended that only periods without fetal breathing should be considered when quantifying fetal blood flow (Maršál et al., 1984).

Umbilical blood flow is unaffected by the uterine contractures that occur throughout pregnancy in the ewe, although these are associated with an increase in fetal O_2 uptake due to an increase in fetal muscular activity or tone during the contractures (Llanos et al., 1988). Similarly, human studies have failed to reveal any effect of labour on the rates of blood flow in the fetal descending aorta (Maršál et al., 1984) or umbilical vein (Stuart et al., 1978).

Maternal exercise does not represent a major stressful or hypoxic event to the fetus, although there is a sudden decrease in uterine blood flow at the onset of exercise, and a further decrease with time that results from exercise-induced hyperthermia and respiratory alkalosis (Lotgering, Gilbert & Longo, 1983a). Umbilical blood flow has been reported to fall during exercise of the ewe to exhaustion (Clapp, 1980), but fetal blood gases were unaffected by mild exercise (Chandler & Bell, 1981), and even prolonged exercise at 70% of maximal maternal O_2 consumption did not result in major fetal cardiovascular changes (Lotgering, Gilbert & Longo, 1983b). A fuller account of maternal and fetal responses to exercise during pregnancy is given by Lotgering, Gilbert & Longo (1985).

Fetal placental blood flow may decrease during maternal hyper-thermia, but only if the resultant hyperventilation and respiratory alkalosis goes untreated; if normocapnia is maintained, fetal placental blood flow remains constant (Oakes et al., 1976). It has been known for some time that umbilical blood flow may fall during maternal hypocapnia (Motoyama et al., 1967), although this is but one component of the fetal response to acute respiratory alkalosis (Carter & Grønlund, 1985). Daily exposure of the ewe to high ambient temperatures throughout mid and into late pregnancy, which results in a decrease in placental weight, is associated with a reduction in maternal and fetal placental blood flow and retardation of fetal growth (Bell, Wilkening & Meschia, 1987).

Umbilical blood flow is maintained during acute maternal hypoxia in the near-term fetal sheep (Parer, 1980; Block et al., 1989). In fetuses at 0.6–0.7 gestation, however, umbilical vascular resistance increased during acute hypoxia and fetal placental blood flow decreased, both absolutely and as a percentage of cardiac output (Iwamoto et al., 1989). During prolonged fetal hypoxaemia, secondary to the restriction of uterine blood flow, fetal placental blood flow increased transiently at 1 h, but it did not differ from the control level after 24 h or 48 h of hypoxaemia without acidaemia (Bocking et al., 1988). In contrast, when sustained hypoxaemia, caused by lowering the maternal inspired O_2 concentration, lead to progressive acidaemia, the initial rise in placental blood flow was followed by a decline (Rurak et al., 1990; Fig. 5.5). Fetal responses to hypoxaemia are discussed more fully elsewhere (Chapters 8 and 9).

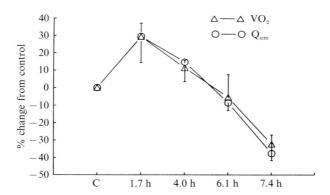

Fig. 5.5. Percentage changes in umbilical blood flow (Q_{um}) and fetal oxygen consumption (VO_2) with time in sheep made hypoxaemic by lowering the O_2 fraction of maternal inspired air to 9–10%. An initial rise in placental blood flow is followed by a fall as the fetus becomes progressively acidaemic. (From Rurak et al., 1990.)

Placental blood flow and fetal oxygen consumption

It has been thought that fetal VO_2 is relatively insensitive to acute changes in fetal placental blood flow and O_2 delivery (DO_2). Thus when placental blood flow is reduced by compression of the umbilical cord (Künzel et al., 1977; Itskovitz, LaGamma & Rudolph, 1983, 1987), by inflating a cuff around the fetal descending aorta (Wilkening & Meschia, 1989), or by inflation of an intravascular catheter (Edelstone, Peticca & Goldblum, 1985b), DO_2 can be reduced to almost half the control value without influencing VO_2 (Fig. 5.6). Likewise, mathematical modelling of partial cord occlusion predicts that fetal VO_2 can be maintained until umbilical blood flow has been reduced by about 50% (Huikeshoven et al., 1985).

In another study it was shown that VO_2 decreased when fetal placental blood flow fell below 150 ml/min per kg with the ewe breathing room air, but that this limit could be extended to 75 ml/min per kg by giving supplemental O_2 to the ewe (Edelstone et al., 1985b).

The dependence of VO_2 on DO_2 becomes relevant as soon as the latter is reduced to an extent that can not be compensated for by increased O_2 extraction. Thus fetal VO_2 falls rapidly following the arrest of uterine blood flow, and both VO_2 and peripheral blood flow is linearly related to arterial oxygen content ($[O_2]a$) during the first minute of asphyxia (Jensen, Hohmann & Künzel, 1987). Fetal skeletal muscle cells in monolayer culture also exhibit a linear relation between VO_2 and PO_2 (Braems & Jensen, 1991). Moreover, when the relation between VO_2 and PO_2 of the intact fetus is studied over a wide range of PO_2 values, achieved by ventilation of the lungs, the data suggest that there is no margin of safety in O_2 supply for a significant fraction of fetal tissues (Asakura, Ball & Power, 1990). Therefore it is important to distinguish between acute moderate hypoxia, in which the whole fetus can sustain oxidative metabolism, and a state of acute severe hypoxia ($[O_2]a$ of 1.0–1.5 mM), in which the VO_2 of some fetal organs is selectively and markedly decreased (Boyle et al., 1990).

Intrauterine growth retardation (IUGR) of the human fetus is associated with a low umbilical venous blood flow (Gill et al., 1984). In sheep, fetal growth can be reduced from 4% per day to 2% per day by computer-controlled restriction of umbilical blood flow for c. 10 days (Anderson & Faber, 1984). In this model of IUGR, a 43% reduction in placental perfusion was accompanied by a 17% fall in VO_2 (Anderson, Parks & Faber, 1986). A reduction in fetal placental blood flow, and thus in DO_2,

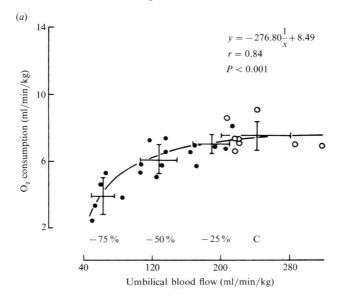

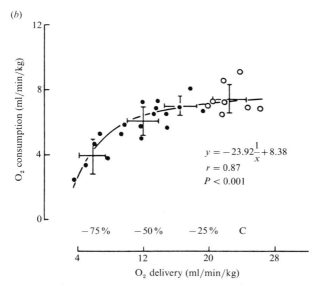

Fig. 5.6. Oxygen consumption (VO_2) by the fetal sheep as a function of umbilical blood flow and O_2 delivery. Fetal placental blood flow was reduced by inflating a balloon occluder around the umbilical cord. Fetal VO_2 was maintained with reduction of blood flow to about 50% of control values. Further reductions were associated with a progressive fall in fetal VO_2. (From Itskovitz et al., 1983.)

is also seen in models of IUGR that rely upon perturbation of the maternal placental circulation by uterine embolization (Clapp et al., 1980) or uterine artery ligation (Carter & Detmer, 1990). When the size of the placenta is limited by the removal of endometrial caruncles prior to conception (Robinson, Falconer & Owens, 1985; Owens, Falconer & Robinson, 1986, 1987*a*) fetal VO_2 is reduced to the same extent as fetal weight. However, there is a smaller margin of safety between supply of and demand for oxygen (Owens et al., 1987*a*), glucose (Owens et al., 1987*b*), and other substrates in the IUGR fetus.

Umbilical venous return

A sizeable fraction of the umbilical venous return passes through the ductus venosus, about 45% in the ovine fetus (Edelstone, Rudolph & Heymann, 1980). Due to streaming of ductus venosus blood flow within the thoracic inferior vena cava, and through the foramen ovale, this highly oxygenated blood is distributed preferentially to the heart and brain (Edelstone & Rudolph, 1979; Reuss, Rudolph & Heymann, 1981). The left hepatic venous blood, which has an O_2 saturation 10–15% higher than blood from the contralateral vein, tends to follow the same pattern of distribution (Rudolph, 1983; Fig. 5.7). This may be important in species such as the guinea pig, that lack a ductus venosus (Carter & Detmer, 1990), but where most umbilical venous blood nevertheless passes through the foramen ovale (Everett & Johnson, 1950).

There has been much discussion about the role of the ductus venosus and the intrahepatic termination of the umbilical vein, the umbilical-portal sinus, in the regulation of placental vascular resistance. Mathematical modelling of the fetal circulation does suggest that a change in resistance of the ductus venosus can have a substantial effect on umbilical blood flow (Huikeshoven et al., 1985). In one study it was found that the vascular resistance of the umbilical sinus was greatly increased during severe hypoxia (Brinkman, Kirschbaum & Assali, 1970), but this observation could not be confirmed when umbilical venous and ductus venosus flows were measured during fetal hypoxaemia in a chronic sheep preparation (Edelstone et al., 1980). A greater fraction of umbilical venous return passed through the ductus following partial cord occlusion, but this seemed to depend upon the relatively greater resistance to blood flow through the liver than in the ductus venosus, as the estimated resistance in the ductus did not change (Edelstone et al., 1980).

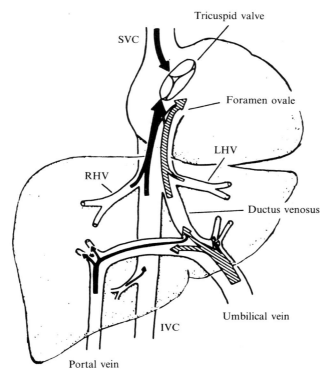

Fig. 5.7. Venous flow patterns in the fetal sheep. The umbilical venous return is distributed to the left lobe of the liver, through the ductus venosus, and to the right lobe of the liver. Portal venous blood passes almost exclusively to the right lobe. Ductus venosus and left hepatic venous blood preferentially pass through the foramen ovale, whereas right hepatic venous and distal inferior vena caval blood are preferentially directed through the tricuspid valve. SVC, superior vena cava; IVC, inferior vena cava; LHV, left hepatic vein; RHV, right hepatic vein. (From Rudolph, 1983.)

Recently, Paulick et al. (1990) re-examined the distribution of vascular resistances between the descending aorta and the inferior vena cava. In normoxaemic fetuses, the umbilical arteries and placental vasculature accounted for 82% of total resistance to fetal placental blood flow, the umbilical veins for 11%, and the ductus venosus and liver for only 7%. During fetal hypoxaemia there was a rise in arterial blood pressure and in the pressure gradient across the umbilical circulation, but no alteration in placental blood flow, indicating an increase in total vascular resistance.

There was no change in resistance across the umbilical arteries and placenta or in the combined resistance of the liver and ductus venosus, but the resistance of the umbilical vein (measured between a peripheral umbilical venous branch & the portal sinus) increased more than twofold.

Control of fetal placental circulation

The umbilical vasculature is not innervated (Reilly & Russell, 1977), so that control of placental vascular resistance must be of an endocrine or paracrine nature. The vascular resistance of the ductus venosus could be subject to neural control, but whether the ductus participates in the regulation of placental blood flow has yet to be resolved. Oscillations in autonomic tone, synchronized with the switch between high and low voltage ECoG states, are apparently responsible for changes in regional blood flow elsewhere in the fetus (Jensen et al., 1986; Slotten et al., 1989).

Local (paracrine) control

In the lung, ventilation–perfusion ratios are subject to local regulation, and it has been suggested that similar mechanisms operate to ensure matching of fetal and maternal blood flows in the placenta (Rankin, 1976). Specifically, it has been proposed that perfusion–perfusion ratios are maintained by local synthesis of a substance, such as prostaglandin E_2, which is vasodilator in the uterine circulation and vasoconstrictor in the umbilical circulation (Rankin, 1976; Rankin & Phernetton, 1976). Mismatching of fetal and maternal blood flows is a significant factor in placental gas exchange, accounting for about 50% of the vein-to-vein PO_2 gradient, which is 17 mm Hg in the sheep (Comline & Silver, 1970). Power, Dale & Nelson (1981) examined the ratio between maternal and fetal blood flows in small pieces of placental cotyledons (cubes about 2–3 mm on edge) after injecting large numbers of microspheres, labelled with different radionuclides, into the fetal and maternal circulations. The maternal-fetal blood flow ratio was <0.5 in 9% of the cotyledon, 0.5–1.5 in 70% and >1.5 in the remaining 21% (Fig. 5.8). A significant correlation was found between maternal and fetal placental blood flows. Using a similar approach, it has been shown that changes in perfusion consequent upon air embolism or noradrenaline infusion are qualitatively matched in the adjacent maternal and fetal circulations (Stock et al., 1989). These results were taken to indicate the presence of a control

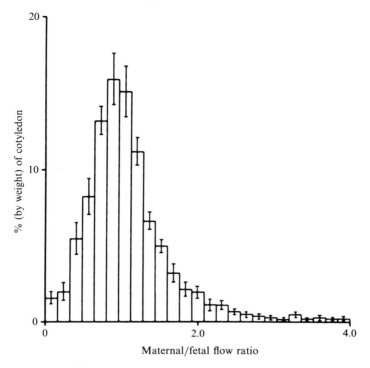

Fig. 5.8. Frequency distribution of the ratio of maternal to fetal blood flow within an average cotyledon of the sheep placenta. The ratio is between 0.5 and 1.5 in 70% of the cotyledon. Matching of maternal and fetal flows is thought to be under paracrine control. (From Power et al., 1981.)

mechanism that acts at the local level to stabilize the distribution of maternal and fetal placental blood flows.

Hormonal effects

The lack of innervation of umbilical blood vessels has prompted speculation that fetal placental blood flow may be subject to endocrine regulation. Thus umbilical vascular resistance was said to increase during hypoxaemia in young fetuses as if the influence of a vasoconstrictor substance had increased or that of a vasodilator substance decreased (Iwamoto et al., 1989). Hypoxaemia increases the plasma concentrations of vasoconstrictive hormones such as catecholamines, vasopressin and angiotensin II, and hormone-mediated constriction is a conceivable mechanism for the increase in resistance of the umbilical veins during hypoxaemia (Paulick et al., 1990). Umbilical vascular resistance fell following administration of triiodothyronine to the fetus, allowing for an increase in fetal placental blood flow coincident with an increase in fetal VO_2 (Lorijn, Nelson & Longo, 1980). However, there is no clear-cut evidence that this or any other hormone participates in the regulation of placental vascular resistance.

Systemic effects

The baro- and chemoreflexes of the fetus are difficult to assess, especially in relation to the complex pattern of changes that occurs in hypoxia or asphyxia (Hanson, 1988; Chapter 1). Recently, Jansen et al. (1989) measured regional blood flows during isocapnic hypoxia in intact, vago-tomized, and sino-aortic denervated fetuses. It was concluded that the aortic and carotid chemoreceptors are involved in the redistribution of blood flow that occurs during hypoxaemia, although there was a residual effect after denervation that could be attributed to catecholamine release or direct vasodilatation of the blood vessels by hypoxia. Fetal placental blood flow was not affected by denervation in normoxaemic fetuses. However, whereas placental perfusion was maintained during hypoxae-mia in fetuses with intact innervation, there were significant decreases in placental blood flow and in the placental fraction of cardiac output during hypoxaemia after denervation.

The observation that placental blood flow falls during hypoxaemia in the chemoreceptor-denervated fetus raises the crucial question of whether or not fetal placental blood flow is under feedback control. Anderson & Faber (1984) concluded that it was not, since neither driving pressure nor resistance responded to chronic reduction of placental blood flow by occlusion of the distal aorta. However, Huikeshoven et al. (1985) have pointed to an interesting discrepancy between experimental findings and model predictions of the response to increased umbilical vascular resistance: mean arterial blood pressure was unaltered when vascular resistance was raised by compression of the umbilical cord (Itskovitz, LaGamma & Rudolph, 1983), whereas mathematical model-ling of the fetal circulation predicts that this manoeuvre should cause a fall in blood pressure. It was therefore suggested that reflex mechanisms may be activated in the intact fetus (Huikeshoven et al., 1985), a hypothesis that deserves further attention.

References

Amoroso, E. C. (1952). Placentation. In *Marshall's Physiology of Reproduction*, vol 2. ed. A.S. Parkes. pp. 127–311. Longmans, London.

Anderson, D. F. & Faber, J. J. (1984). Regulation of fetal placental blood flow in the lamb. *American Journal of Physiology*, **247**, R567–74.

Anderson, D. F., Parks, C. M. & Faber, J. J. (1986). Fetal O_2 consumption in sheep during controlled long-term reductions in umbilical blood flow. *American Journal of Physiology*, **250**, H1037–42.

Asakura, H., Ball, K. T. & Power, G. G. (1990). Interdependence of arterial PO_2 and O_2 consumption in the fetal sheep. *Journal of Developmental Physiology*, **13**, 205–13.

Bell, A. W., Kennaugh, J. M., Battaglia, F. C., Makowski, E. L. & Meschia, G. (1986). Metabolic and circulatory studies of fetal lamb at midgestation. *American Journal of Physiology*, **250**, E538–44.

Bell, A. W., Wilkening, R. B. & Meschia, G. (1987). Some aspects of placental function in chronically heat-stressed ewes. *Journal of Developmental Physiology*, **9**, 17–29.

Block, B. S., Schlafer, D. H., Wentworth, R. A., Kreitzer, L. A. & Nathanielsz, P. W. (1989). Intrauterine growth retardation and the circulatory responses to acute hypoxemia in fetal sheep. *American Journal of Obstetrics and Gynecology*, **161**, 1576–9.

Bocking, A. D., Gagnon, R., White, S. E., Homan, J., Milne, K. & Richardson, B. S. (1988). Circulatory responses to prolonged hypoxemia in fetal sheep. *American Journal of Obstetrics and Gynecology*, **159**, 1418–24.

Boyle, D. W., Hirst, K., Zerbe, G. O., Meschia, G. & Wilkening, R. B. (1990). Fetal hind limb oxygen consumption and blood flow during acute graded hypoxia. *Pediatric Research*, **28**, 94–100.

Braems, G. & Jensen, A. (1991). Hypoxia reduces oxygen consumption of fetal skeletal muscle cells in monolayer culture. *Journal of Developmental Physiology*, **16**, 209–15.

Brinkman, C. R., Kirschbaum, T. H. & Assali, N. S. (1970). The role of the umbilical sinus in the regulation of placental vascular resistance. *Gynecological Investigation*, **1**, 115–27.

Carter, A. M. (1975). Placental circulation. In *Comparative Placentation*, ed. D.H. Steven. pp. 108–160. Academic Press, London.

Carter, A. M. (1989). Factors affecting gas transfer across the placenta and the oxygen supply to the fetus. *Journal of Developmental Physiology*, **12**, 305–22.

Carter, A. M. & Detmer, A. (1990). Blood flow to the placenta and lower body in the growth-retarded guinea pig fetus. *Journal of Developmental Physiology*, **13**, 261–9.

Carter, A. M. & Grønlund, J. (1985). Contribution of the Bohr effect to the fall in fetal PO_2 caused by maternal alkalosis. *Journal of Perinatal Medicine*, **13**, 185–93.

Chandler, K. D. & Bell, A. W. (1981). Effects of maternal exercise on fetal and maternal respiration and nutrient metabolism in the pregnant ewe. *Journal of Developmental Physiology*, **3**, 161–76.

Clapp, J. F. (1978). The relationship between blood flow and oxygen uptake in the uterine and umbilical circulations. *American Journal of Obstetrics and Gynecology*, **132**, 410–13.

Clapp, J. F. (1980). Acute exercise stress in the pregnant ewe. *American Journal of Obstetrics and Gynecology*, **136**, 489–94.

Clapp, J. F., Szeto, H. H., Larrow, R., Hewitt, J. & Mann, L. I. (1980). Umbilical blood flow response to embolization of the uterine circulation. *American Journal of Obstetrics and Gynecology*, **138**, 60–7.

Comline, R. S. & Silver, M. (1970). PO_2, PCO_2 and pH levels in the umbilical and uterine blood of the mare and ewe. *Journal of Physiology*, **209**, 587–608.

Crawford, J. M. (1962). Vascular anatomy of the human placenta. *American Journal of Obstetrics and Gynecology*, **84**, 1543–67.

Creasy, R. K., Drost, M., Green, M. V. & Morris, J. A. (1970). Determination of fetal, placental and neonatal blood volumes in the sheep. *Circulation Research*, **27**, 487–94.

Dawes, G. S. (1962). The foetus, the placenta and umbilical blood flow. *Journal of Physiology*, **163**, 43P.

Dawes, G. S., Mott, J. C. & Widdicombe, J. G. (1954). The foetal circulation in the lamb. *Journal of Physiology*, **126**, 563–87.

De Smedt, M. C. H., Visser, G. H. A. & Meijboom, E. J. (1987). Fetal cardiac output estimated by Doppler echocardiography during mid- and late gestation. *American Journal of Cardiology*, **60**, 338–42.

Edelstone, D. I., Caine, M. E. & Fumia, F. D. (1985*a*). Relationship of fetal oxygen consumption and acid-base balance to fetal hematocrit. *American Journal of Obstetrics and Gynecology*, **151**, 844–51.

Edelstone, D. I., Darby, M. J., Bass, K. & Miller, K. (1989). Effects of reductions in hemoglobin-oxygen affinity and hematocrit level on oxygen consumption and acid-base state in fetal lambs. *American Journal of Obstetrics and Gynecology*, **160**, 820–8.

Edelstone, D. I., Peticca, B. B. & Goldblum, L. J. (1985*b*). Effects of maternal oxygen administration on fetal oxygenation during reductions in umbilical blood flow in fetal lambs. *American Journal of Obstetrics and Gynecology*, **152**, 351–8.

Edelstone, D. I. & Rudolph, A. M. (1979). Preferential streaming of ductus venosus blood to the brain and heart in fetal lambs. *American Journal of Physiology*, **237**, H724–9.

Edelstone, D. I., Rudolph, A. M. & Heymann, M. A. (1980). Effects of hypoxemia and decreasing umbilical flow on liver and ductus venosus blood flows in fetal lambs. *American Journal of Physiology*, **238**, H656–63.

Eik-Nes, S. H., Brubakk, A. O. & Ulstein, M. K. (1980). Measurement of human fetal blood flow. *British Medical Journal*, **ii**, 283–4.

Erskine, R. L. A. & Ritchie, J. W. K. (1985). Quantitative measurements of fetal blood flow using Doppler ultrasound. *British Journal of Obstetrics and Gynaecology*, **92**, 600–4.

Everett, N. B. & Johnson, R. J. (1950). Use of radioactive phosphorus in studies of fetal circulation. *American Journal of Physiology*, **162**, 147–52.

Eyck, J. van, Wladimiroff, J. W., Noordam, M. J., Tonge, H. M. & Prechtl, H. F. R. (1985). The blood flow velocity waveform in the fetal descending aorta: its relationship to fetal behavioural states in normal pregnancy at 37–38 weeks. *Early Human Development*, **12**, 137–43.

Eyck, J. van, Wladimiroff, J. W., Wijngaard, J. A. G. W. van den, Noordam, M. J. & Prechtl, H. F. R. (1987). The blood flow velocity waveform in the fetal internal carotid and umbilical artery; its relation to fetal behavioural states in normal pregnancy at 37–38 weeks. *British Journal of Obstetrics and Gynaecology*, **94**, 736–41.

Faber, J. J. & Thornburg, K. L. (1983). *Placental Physiology,* Raven Press, New York.

Gerson, A. G., Wallace, D. M., Stiller, R. J., Paul, D., Weiner, S. & Bolognese, R. J. (1987). Doppler evaluation of umbilical venous and arterial blood flow in the second and third trimesters of normal pregnancy. *Obstetrics and Gynecology*, **70**, 622–6.

Gill, R. W. & Kossoff, G. (1981). Pulsed Doppler combined with B-mode imaging for blood flow measurement. *Contributions to Gynecology and Obstetrics*, **6**, 139–41.

Gill, R. W., Kossoff, G., Warren, P. S. & Garrett, W. J. (1984). Umbilical venous flow in normal and complicated pregnancy. *Ultrasound in Medicine and Biology*, **10**, 349–63.

Gu, W., Jones, C. T. & Parer, J. T. (1985). Metabolic and cardiovascular effects on fetal sheep of sustained reduction of uterine blood flow. *Journal of Physiology*, **368**, 109–29.

Hanson, M. A. (1988). The importance of baro- and chemoreflexes in the control of the fetal cardiovascular system. *Journal of Developmental Physiology*, **10**, 491–511.

Huikeshoven, F. J., Hope, I. D., Power, G. G., Gilbert, R. D. & Longo, L. D. (1985). Mathematical model of fetal circulation and oxygen delivery. *American Journal of Physiology*, **249**, R192–202.

Itskovitz, J., LaGamma, E. F. & Rudolph, A. M. (1983) The effect of reducing umbilical blood flow on fetal oxygenation. *American Journal of Obstetrics and Gynecology*, **145**, 813–18.

Itskovitz, J., LaGamma, E. F. & Rudolph, A. M. (1987) Effects of cord compression on fetal blood flow distribution and O_2 delivery. *American Journal of Physiology*, **252**, H100–9.

Iwamoto, H. S., Kaufman, T., Keil, L. C. & Rudolph, A. M. (1989). Responses to acute hypoxemia in fetal sheep at 0.6–0.7 gestation. *American Journal of Physiology*, **256**, H613–20.

Jansen, A. H., Belik, J., Ioffe, S. & Chernick, V. (1989). Control of organ blood flow in fetal sheep during normoxia and hypoxia. *American Journal of Physiology*, **257**, H1132–9.

Jensen, A., Bamford, O. S., Dawes, G. S., Hofmeyr, G. & Parkes, M. J. (1986). Changes in organ blood flow between high and low voltage electrocortical activity in fetal sheep. *Journal of Developmental Physiology*, **8**, 187–94.

Jensen, A., Hohmann, M. & Künzel, W. (1987). Dynamic changes in organ blood flow and oxygen consumption during acute asphyxia in fetal sheep. *Journal of Developmental Physiology*, **9**, 543–59.

Kaufmann, P. (1985). Basic morphology of the fetal and maternal circuits in the human placenta. *Contributions to Gynecology and Obstetrics*, **13**, 5–17.

Kaufmann, P. & Davidoff, M. (1977). The guinea-pig placenta. *Advances in Anatomy, Embryology, and Cell Biology*, **53**, (2), 1–91.

Kaufmann, P., Luckhardt, M. & Leiser, R. (1988). Three-dimensional representation of the fetal vessel system in the human placenta. *Trophoblast Research*, **3**, 113–37.

Kaufmann, P. & Scheffen, I. (1991). Placental development. In *Neonatal and Fetal Medicine*, ed. Polin & Fox. Saunders, Orlando.

Künzel, W., Mann, L. I., Bhakthavathsalan, A., Airomlooi, J. & Liu, M. (1977). The effect of umbilical vein occlusion on fetal oxygenation, cardiovascular parameters, and fetal electroencephalogram. *American Journal of Obstetrics and Gynecology*, **128**, 201–8.

Lingman, G. & Maršál, K. (1986). Fetal central blood circulation in the third trimester of normal pregnancy – a longitudinal study. I. Aortic and umbilical blood flow. *Early Human Development*, **13**, 137–50.

Llanos, A. J., Block, B. S. B., Court, D. J., Germain, A. M. & Parer, J. T. (1988). Fetal oxygen uptake during uterine contractures. *Journal of Developmental Physiology*, **10**, 525–9.

Longo, L. D. (1987). Respiratory gas exchange in the placenta. In *Handbook of Physiology. Section 3. The Respiratory System. Volume IV. Gas Exchange*, pp. 351–401. American Physiological Society, Bethesda.

Lorijn, R. H. W., Nelson, J. C. & Longo, L. D. (1980). Induced fetal hyperthyroidism: cardiac output and oxygen consumption. *American Journal of Physiology*, **239**, H302–7.

Lotgering, F. K., Gilbert, R. D. & Longo, L. D. (1983a). Exercise responses in pregnant sheep: oxygen consumption, uterine blood flow, and blood volume. *Journal of Applied Physiology*, **55**, 834–41.

Lotgering, F. K., Gilbert, R. D. & Longo, L. D. (1983b). Exercise responses in pregnant sheep: blood gases, temperatures, and fetal cardiovascular system. *Journal of Applied Physiology*, **55**, 842–50.

Lotgering, F. K., Gilbert, R. D. & Longo, L. D. (1985). Maternal and fetal responses to exercise during pregnancy. *Physiological Reviews*, **65**, 1–36.

Makowski, E. L., Meschia, G., Droegemueller, W. & Battaglia, F. C. (1968). Measurement of umbilical arterial blood flow to the sheep placenta and fetus in utero. *Circulation Research*, **23**, 623–31.

Maršál, K., Lindblad, A., Lingman, G. & Eik-Nes, S. H. (1984). Blood flow in the fetal descending aorta; intrinsic factors affecting fetal blood flow, i.e., fetal breathing movements and cardiac arrhythmia. *Ultrasound in Medicine and Biology*, **10**, 339–48.

Mossman, H. W. (1926). The rabbit placenta and the problem of placental transmission. *American Journal of Anatomy*, **37**, 433–97.

Motoyama, E. K., Rivard, G., Acheson, F. & Cook, C. D. (1967). The effect of changes in maternal pH and PCO_2 on the PO_2 of fetal lambs. *Anesthesiology*, **28**, 891–903.

Nijhuis, J. G., Prechtl, H. F. R., Martin, C. B. & Bots, R. S. G. M. (1982). Are there behavioural states in the human fetus? *Early Human Development*, **6**, 177–95.

Oakes, G. K., Walker, A. M., Ehrenkranz, R. A., Cefalo, R. C. & Chez, R. A. (1976). Uteroplacental blood flow during hyperthermia with or without alkalosis. *Journal of Applied Physiology*, **41**, 197–201.

Owens, J. A., Falconer, J. & Robinson, J. S. (1986). Effect of restriction of placental growth on umbilical and uterine blood flows. *American Journal of Physiology*, **250**, R427–34.

Owens, J. A., Falconer, J. & Robinson, J. S. (1987a). Effect of restriction of placental growth on oxygen delivery to and consumption by the pregnant uterus and fetus. *Journal of Developmental Physiology*, **9**, 137–50.

Owens, J. A., Falconer, J. & Robinson, J. S. (1987b). Effect of restriction of placental growth on fetal and utero-placental metabolism. *Journal of Developmental Physiology*, **9**, 225–38.

Parer, J. T. (1980). The effect of acute maternal hypoxia on fetal oxygenation and the umbilical circulation in the sheep. *European Journal of Obstetrics, Gynecology and Reproductive Biology,* **10**, 125–36.

Paulick, R. P., Meyers, R. L., Rudolph, C. D. & Rudolph, A. M. (1990). Venous responses to hypoxemia in the fetal lamb. *Journal of Developmental Physiology,* **14**, 81–8.

Paulone, M. E., Edelstone, D. I. & Shedd, A. (1987). Effects of maternal anemia on uteroplacental and fetal oxidative metabolism in sheep. *American Journal of Obstetrics and Gynecology,* **156**, 230–6.

Peeters, L. L. H., Sheldon, R. E., Jones, M. D., Makowski, E. L. & Meschia, G. (1979). Blood flow to fetal organs as a function of arterial oxygen content. *American Journal of Obstetrics and Gynecology,* **135**, 637–46.

Power, G. G., Dale, P. S. & Nelson. P. S. (1981). Distribution of maternal and fetal blood flow within cotyledons of the sheep placenta. *American Journal of Physiology,* **241**, H486–96.

Rankin, J. H. G. (1976). A role for prostaglandins in the regulation of the placental blood flows. *Prostaglandins,* **11**, 343–53.

Rankin, J. H. G. & Phernetton, T. M. (1976). Effect of prostaglandin E_2 on ovine maternal placental blood flow. *American Journal of Physiology,* **231**, 754–9.

Reilly, F. D. & Russell, P. T. (1977). Neurohistochemical evidence supporting an absence of adrenergic and cholinergic innervation in the human placenta and umbilical cord. *Anatomical Record,* **188**, 277–86.

Reuss, M. L., Rudolph, A. M. & Heymann, M. A. (1981). Selective distribution of microspheres injected into the umbilical veins and inferior venae cavae of fetal sheep. *American Journal of Obstetrics and Gynecology,* **141**, 427–32.

Robinson, J. S., Falconer, J. & Owens, J. A. (1985). Intrauterine growth retardation: Clinical and experimental. *Acta Paediatrica Scandinavica Supplementum,* **319**, 135–42.

Rudolph, A. M. (1983). Hepatic and ductus venosus bloodflows during fetal life. *Hepatology,* **3**, 254–8.

Rudolph, A. M. & Heymann, M. A. (1967). The circulation of the fetus in utero. Methods for studying distribution of blood flow, cardiac output and organ blood flow. *Circulation Research,* **21**, 163–84.

Rudolph, A. M. & Heymann, M. A. (1970). Circulatory changes during growth in the fetal lamb. *Circulation Research,* **26**, 289–99.

Rudolph, A. M., Heymann, M. A., Teramo, K. A. W., Barrett, C. T. & Räihä, N. C. R. (1971). Studies on the circulation of the previable human fetus. *Pediatric Research,* **5**, 452–65.

Rurak, D. W., Cooper, C. C. & Taylor, S. M. (1986). Fetal oxygen consumption and PO_2 during hypercapnia in pregnant sheep. *Journal of Developmental Physiology,* **8**, 447–59.

Rurak, D. W. & Gruber, N. C. (1983). Increased oxygen consumption associated with breathing activity in fetal lambs. *Journal of Applied Physiology,* **54**, 701–7.

Rurak, D. W., Richardson, B. S., Patrick, J. E., Carmichael, L. & Homan, J. (1990). Oxygen consumption in the fetal lamb during sustained hypoxemia with progressive acidemia. *American Journal of Physiology,* **258**, R1108–15.

Silver, M., Steven, D. H. & Comline, R. S. (1973). Placental exchange and morphology in ruminants and the mare. In *Foetal and Neonatal Physiology,* ed. K. W. Cross. pp. 245–271. Cambridge University Press, Cambridge.

Slotten, P., Phernetton, T. M. & Rankin, J. H. G. (1989). Relationship between fetal electrocorticographic changes and umbilical blood flow in the near-term sheep fetus. *Journal of Developmental Physiology,* **11**, 19–23.

Štembera, Z. K., Hodr. J. & Janda, J. (1965). Umbilical blood flow in healthy newborn infants during the first minutes after birth. *American Journal of Obstetrics and Gynecology,* **91**, 568–74.

Steven, D. H. (1968). Placental vessels of the foetal lamb. *Journal of Anatomy,* **103**, 539–52.

Steven, D. H. (1975). Anatomy of the placental barrier. In *Comparative Placentation,* ed. D. H. Steven. pp. 25–57. Academic Press, London.

Stock, M. K., Reid, D. L., Phernetton, T. M. & Rankin, J. H. G. (1989). Matching of maternal and fetal flow ratios in the sheep placenta. *Journal of Developmental Physiology,* **11**, 29–35.

Stuart, B., Drumm, J., Fitzgerald, D. E. & Duignon, N. M. (1978). Fetal blood velocity waveforms in uncomplicated labour. *British Journal of Obstetrics and Gynaecology,* **88**, 865–9.

Walker, A. M., Oakes, G. K., McLaughlin, M. K., Ehrenkranz, R. A., Alling, D. W. & Chez, R. A. (1977). 24-hour rhythms in uterine and umbilical blood flows of conscious pregnant sheep. *Gynecological Investigation,* **8**, 288–98.

Wigglesworth, J. S. (1969). *Journal of Obstetrics and Gynaecology of the British Commonwealth,* **76**, 979–89.

Wilkening, R. B. & Meschia, G. (1983). Fetal oxygen uptake, oxygenation, and acid-base balance as a function of uterine blood flow. *American Journal of Physiology,* **244**, H749–55.

Wilkening, R. B. & Meschia, G. (1989). Effect of umbilical blood flow on transplacental diffusion of ethanol and oxygen. *American Journal of Physiology,* **256**, H813–20.

6

Growth and development of the heart

KENT L. THORNBURG AND MARK J. MORTON

Introduction

Until just a few years ago, studies of cardiac development were based primarily on anatomical insight. But with the advent of new molecular and cellular techniques, the study of cardiac development now strives to determine the chemical basis of morphological transformations and physiological function of primitive organs. Through the fusion of new techniques with knowledge of structure, there will be major leaps in understanding of normal and aberrant cardiac development, leaps which will undoubtedly lead to innovative modes of treatment and prevention of congenital heart disease.

The formation of the heart requires a number of complex processes which include cell division, cell enlargement, cell death and massive cell migration. By these processes, the heart goes through a number of stages, developing from an amorphous mass of undifferentiated cells in the early embryo to a fully formed miniature heart in the late embryo. Developmental progress can be monitored morphologically for the purpose of understanding normal ontogenetic patterns and in pin-pointing pathological change. A number of staging schemes have been devised to aid in this process but few are useful for interspecies comparisons. However, there are several general periods that describe development of the heart in most vertebrates (van Mierop, 1979; Hirakow & Gotoh, 1980; Icardo, 1984; Reller, Gerlis & Thornburg, 1991).

Early development of the heart

The first developmental period is *precardiogenesis*, before the heart proper is actually formed. At the cephalic end of the early embryo before gastrulation, there are two lateral areas of mesoderm which contain cells

137

that will become the heart (Fig. 6.1(*a*)). These fold underneath the embryo along with tissue that is forming the primitive gut. The *fusion* stage is characterized by the formation of a single tubular heart by the fusion of the aforementioned lateral mesodermal cells which meet in the midline beneath the embryo (Fig. 6.1(*b*)(*c*)). This primitive heart becomes functional soon after its formation and is composed of three concentric layers – two cellular layers and a middle layer of amorphous

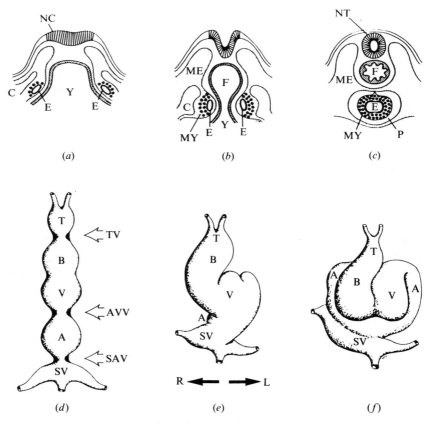

(*a*)   (*b*)   (*c*)

(*d*)   (*e*)   (*f*)

Fig. 6.1. Diagrammatic representation of the developing embryo heart. (*a*), (*b*) and (*c*) are transverse sections of the early embryo. (*d*), (*e*) and (*f*) show the looping process and the arrangement of the chambers just prior to separation. C: celomic cavity, E: endocardial tubes, F: forgut, ME: mesoderm, MY: myocardium, P: pericardial cavity, NC: neural crest, NT: neural tube, Y: yolksac, A: atrium, B: bulbus cordis, SV: sinus venosus, T: truncus arteriosus, AVV: atrioventricular valve, SAV: sinoatrial valve, TV: truncal valve. (From Reller, Gerlis and Thornburg, 1991, with permission.)

cardiac jelly (Icardo, 1984). The heart tube then undergoes a change in shape so that it bulges rightward and continues to bend until a C-shaped loop is formed. This is the *looping* stage (Fig. 6.1(*d*)(*e*)(*f*)). The mechanical processes that underlie the movement of the heart during looping are not understood but the process is complete when the primitive atria are adjacent to the primitive ventricular outlet region (bulbus cordis). The visceral pericardium is formed at this stage as mesenchymal cells, of sinus venosus origin, migrate over the surface of the heart (Icardo, 1984).

The ventricular myocardium, the outer layer of the tube, undergoes several transitional changes during the looping period and takes on a characteristic appearance with an inner loosely organized spongy zone and an outer denser compact zone. The endocardium invaginates into the cardiac jelly and the spongy zone of myocardium forming a labyrinthine network of trabeculae. The coalescence of these trabeculae is involved in the formation of papillary muscle and a portion of the interventricular septum during later stages.

Following the looping manoeuvre, the heart is in position to form its chambers and outflow vessels. This is accomplished by *septation* of the heart which is very complex and involves the formation of the atrial septum, the interventricular septum, the atrioventricular canal and the conotruncal septum which divides the primitive outflow tract into the aorta and pulmonary artery. In the region separating the primitive atria from ventricular chambers, cardiac jelly-derived thickenings in the wall protrude into the atrioventricular canal. These specialized tissues are called the dorsal and ventral endocardial cushions and are crucial structures in the formation of separate atrioventricular valves. After septation the general structural features of the fetal heart are present.

Development of the myocyte

The myocyte does not differentiate immediately into a miniature version of the adult working heart cell (Challice & Viragh, 1973). In fact, when first capable of contraction, the immature myocyte has few features that resemble its adult counterpart. The adult cell is characterized by its high level of organization and efficiency. Most of its volume comprises the contractile machinery in the form of myofibrils (Simpson, Rayns & Ledingham, 1973). Each myofibril is composed of alternating light and dark bands which lend a striated appearance under the microscope. Each light zone is bisected by a very dense 'Z' line to which the contractile protein, actin, is attached. The darker bands are composed of myosin and

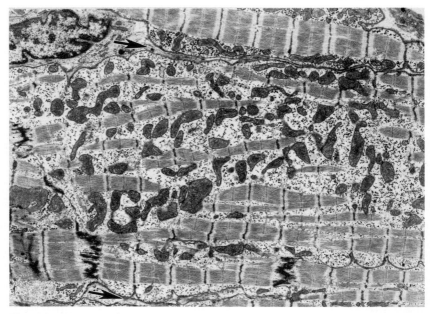

Fig. 6.2. Electron micrograph from 135 day fetal sheep heart. Myocyte boundaries are shown by large arrows. Note myofibrils along cell periphery. Mytochondria are scattered among myofibrils and cytoplasm. Pepper-like background in cytoplasm shows presence of glycogen particles. Magnification 6500×.

overlapping actin along with the other contractile proteins that are invisible, even by electron microscopy. Each contractile unit between Z lines is known as a sarcomere. Juxtaposed to myofibrils are rows of mitochondria that provide the metabolic fuel for the contractile machinery (Fig. 6.2 shows a near term fetal heart with features intermediate between embryonic and adult).

The central portion of the adult cell is occupied by two or more nuclei and other organelles including the Golgi apparatus and ribosome-studded endoplasmic reticulum. These structures are involved in the manufacture of cell proteins. The adult cell contains two other organelles that are prerequisite to an understanding of developing heart function – the transverse tubular system (T-tubules) and the sarcoplasmic reticulum (SR). The T-tubules are extensions of the outer plasma membrane (sarcolemma) that invaginate into the inner regions of the cell. With every beat, the T-tubules carry the action potential deep into the cell interior to the level of the Z line of each sarcomere. The SR is a vast intracellular membranous network found throughout the cell but with regional variations in composition and function. The SR releases calcium into the cytoplasm when stimulated by the action potential thereby causing contraction. The SR then re-acquires intracellular calcium to bring about relaxation. Its subsarcolemmal cisternae, which form in intimate proximity to the sarcolemma, are thought to participate in the transduction of the action potential signal and the stimulated release of calcium.

The embryonic myocyte is characterized by its roundish shape, prominent single nucleus and sparse organellar structure. As one would expect, contractile material is present when the heart first beats. However, the myofibrils are few in number at this stage and are scattered along the cell periphery. Most curiously, they are often placed at odd angles with one another in the same cell. From appearances, one would not predict that contraction is possible. Conspicuous by its absence is the SR at this early developmental stage. Because the sarcoplasmic reticulum is involved in the uptake and release of calcium during the adult cardiac cycle, one must assume that these functions are performed by the sarcolemma.

T-tubules appear as the myocytes become mature, another process related to maturation of the fetus in general (Smolich, 1987). T-tubules are found before birth in some species, such as guinea pigs, monkeys, sheep, and humans but develop after birth in small rodents, rabbits, cats and dogs. The SR is detectable within the sheep cardiomyocyte by 51 days of gestation (Brook et al., 1983) and gradually increases in volume fraction until reaching adult levels after birth.

The regulation of myocyte growth is interesting. It appears that the heart grows primarily by hyperplasia (cell division) until after birth in most species (Oparil, 1985). During this period, heart cells maintain a relatively constant size. But after a critical period of postnatal time (which depends on species), the cells stop dividing and grow only by hypertrophy. This means that all adult working myocardial cells are the same cells that were present during the postnatal period; the heart has continued to 'grow' only through the enlargement of individual myocytes (hypertrophy). Other non-myocyte cell types in the heart continue to grow by hyperplasia. How this transition in the role of growth occurs is not known.

Development of the autonomic control

The autonomic nervous system innervates the adult heart and plays an important role in adjusting cardiac output in response to moment-by-moment changes in activity. Precocious animals (e.g. guinea pig) tend to have greater autonomic maturity at birth than altricial animals such as the rat (Anderson, 1990). Because each species has a different level of maturity when offspring are born, birth itself is not a good indicator of cardiac or nervous system maturity. The staging scheme proposed by Witschi is particularly useful for the comparison of species differences because it uses developmental landmarks for determining maturity levels rather than gestational age or time related to postnatal life (Witschi, 1956; Hirakow & Gotoh, 1980).

In the rat, five postnatal weeks are required for the myocardium to reach adult levels of norepinephrine concentration, whereas the guinea pig myocardium shows near adult levels at birth (DeChamplain et al., 1970; Lipp & Rudolph, 1972). Norepinephrine concentrations are believed to reflect the presence of mature adrenergic nerves since cardiac norepinephrine is avidly taken up and stored by adrenergic nerve endings. Myocardial nerves are found by mid-gestation in sheep (Lebowitz et al., 1972) and norepinephrine concentrations increase with gestational age and are at adult levels by three postnatal days of age (Friedman, 1972a). In the rabbit, both adrenergic and cholinergic terminals are found by the 24th day of gestation (Papka, 1981).

In spite of the fact that β-adrenergic and cholinergic blockade do not significantly affect heart rate or blood pressure in near term fetal sheep (Thornburg & Morton, 1983), the response to administration of exogenous catecholamines is enhanced in late fetal life. In fact, the myocardium of the sheep appears to be more sensitive during the perinatal period than in the adult (Friedman, 1972b). The dog myocardium appears, however, to be less sensitive (Rockson et al., 1981). β-adrenergic receptor density becomes greater with increasing gestational age in most mammals studied whereas α-adrenergic receptor density is highest during the perinatal period. The role of the α-receptor has great significance during the developmental period because of its putative role in regulation of cell growth by hypertrophy during this period (Simpson, 1985). α-receptor density increases during development until birth and declines thereafter. The adult heart has very few α-adrenergic receptors.

Function of the embryonic heart

The function of the embryonic heart has been studied most thoroughly in chick and rat. The chick embryo heart contracts sporadically after as little as 36 h incubation time. The rate increases with development until the looping stage at which time the rate may exceed 200/min. As nervous system control is established it slows again before hatching. Nakazawa et al. (1988) found that the embryonic heart rate of rats also increased with age, being about 100, 125, 175 and 200 beats/min at 11, 12, 13, and 15 days of postcoital age. Heart weights increased from 0.16 to 1.4 mg during that period.

The heart makes beating motions before the circulation is fully formed. Once the vasculature is complete, the heart is able to generate pressure and move blood properly through the circulation in spite of the absence of true valves. This is evidently possible because interchamber wall thickenings function as valves in the early heart. Nakazawa et al. (1988) were able to demonstrate (with great skill) that the embryonic rat heart is able to generate mean arterial pressures in the umbilical artery ranging from about 0.2 mm Hg at day 11 to about 2.5 mm Hg by day 15. Chick embryos of the same weight showed similar pressures (Clark & Hu, 1982).

Determinants of fetal cardiac output

The fetus has different needs from the adult. It must devote its energies to the process of growth much more than to activities that require exercise or even cognition. Therefore, it is not surprising that the fetus may have different regulatory priorities from the adult. The fetus consumes oxygen at twice the rate of the adult per unit weight. Therefore, fetal cardiac output is likely to be very high. In fact, cardiac output per kg body wt is some three to four times higher in sheep fetuses than in their adult counterparts (Walker, 1987).

The fetal circulation is characterized by four shunts which are not present in the adult (Dawes, 1968). The *placental circulation* is a relatively low resistance circulatory bed which lies between the descending aorta and the inferior vena cava. In most mammalian species (but not all), oxygenated blood returning from the placenta through the umbilical vein joins the inferior vena cava via the *ductus venosus* at the level of the liver. The *foramen ovale* allows blood to flow between the atria according to the kinetic energies of the caval blood flows and their respective pressures in the right and left atria (Faber et al., 1985). The *ductus arteriosus* connects the pulmonary artery and the aortic arch so that the outputs of both ventricles contribute to the lower fetal body blood flow. Two haemodynamic features that result from the presence of these shunts should be kept in mind. 1) The right and left ventricles have common atrial filling pressures and common arterial outflow pressures. 2) The ventricles pump in parallel which means that the sum of the outputs of the two ventricles becomes the fetal cardiac output.

The determinants of ventricular stroke volume in the adult are known to be *preload, afterload, contractility,* and *chamber size.* The product of stroke volume and heart rate determines ventricular output. In the adult with its separate pulmonary and systemic circulations in series, the stroke volumes are equal. But, because the fetal ventricles pump in parallel, the stroke volumes are not necessarily equal. However, the above mentioned factors that determine the output of the adult ventricles also determine the output of fetal ventricles. Before these regulatory features are discussed for the immature heart, two basic concepts must be reviewed, ventricular wall stress and the pressure–volume relation.

Wall stress

Stress in the wall of the ventricle is defined as the force per unit cross sectional area. This is the force that must be overcome during diastole to distend the heart and fill it. During systole, this is the force that the myofibrils must produce to generate pressure and shorten. Thus, wall stress at end diastole is preload and wall stress during systole is afterload. Transmural pressure and geometry dominate but are not the only determinants of wall stress. A thin walled spherical model consisting of incompressible material which distributes force equally in all directions is a gross over simplification of a ventricle but provides information regarding the most important determinants of wall stress. According to the law of Laplace:

$$S_w = \tfrac{1}{2}(Pr/h) \tag{1}$$

where S_w = wall stress in the circumferential direction (pascals); P = transmural pressure (pascals); r is the radius of curvature (mm); and h is the wall thickness (mm). This equation shows that the anatomical features of the heart chambers as well as the transmural pressures determine the wall stress of the ventricular chamber.

The fetal ventricles are anatomically different in that the right ventricle has a larger equatorial radius of curvature but thinner wall thickness and therefore a larger radius to wall thickness ratio than does the left. The above equation predicts that the fetal right ventricle will therefore have the higher wall stress when transmural pressures are equal.

Pressure–volume relations

The relationship between pressure across the ventricular wall and volume in the ventricular chamber is usually described by generating a pressure–volume curve in a freshly excised but relaxed heart. This method can be criticized because the in vitro heart does not mimic precisely the behaviour of the beating heart in vivo. However, the technique offers great insight into passive heart function. Fig. 6.3 shows pressure–volume curves from a near-term sheep fetus (Pinson, Morton & Thornburg, 1987). Romero, Covell & Friedman (1972) showed that the pressure–volume curves for both ventricles shift progressively to the right with development, but that the right ventricular pressure–volume curve is always positioned to the right of the left ventricular curve. This indicates that the fetal right ventricle is normally larger than the left at the same transmural pressure. The curves in Fig. 6.3 also show that the volume of the ventricle is dependent on both the presence of the pericardium (3(a)) and on the pressure in the contralateral ventricle (3(b)). The volume in both ventricles is increased if pericardial restraint is lost and such hearts have larger stroke volumes (Riemenschneider, 1990). When the pericardium is present, the volume of either ventricle is larger if the pressure in the opposite ventricle is low. This indicates that the two ventricles compete for space in the pericardium and that ventricular interaction is an important mechanical feature of heart function in the fetus (Versprille et al., 1978).

Ventricular chamber transmural pressure is difficult to measure. Most investigators do not measure pericardial pressure for technical reasons. Instead, they refer intracardiac pressures referenced to amniotic fluid pressure. Pericardial pressures, when measured with a soft catheter with side holes, gave values similar to those obtained using a flat balloon if there was adequate fluid in the pericardium (>1 ml) (Morton & Thornburg, 1987). In the absence of adequate fluid, the pericardium provides localized restraint which is underestimated by fluid–filled catheters.

Preload

Preload is the stress in the ventricular chamber wall just before contraction begins. Isolated myocardial muscle strips display a relationship between muscle length (beyond its resting length) and active generation of tension by the muscle. In other words, heart muscle is able to generate

Kent L. Thornburg and Mark J. Morton

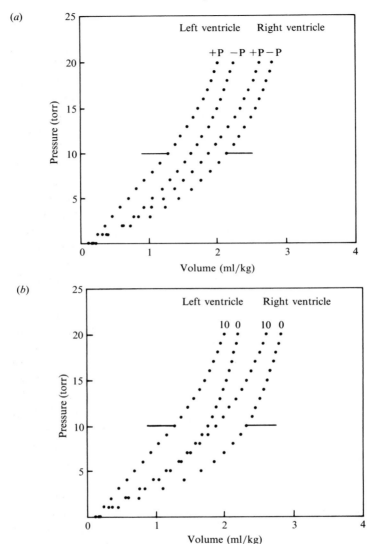

Fig. 6.3. Pressure–volume curves from eight K^+–arrested fetal ventricles are shown with and without the pericardium in place (upper panel) and during changes in contralateral ventricular pressure (lower panel). (Upper panel) The pressure–volume curve of each ventricle was determined with the opposite ventricle at 10 mm Hg and the pericardium in place (+P) or removed (−P). The horizontal lines at 10 mm Hg are standard error bars. (Lower panel) The pressure–volume curve of each ventricle was determined with the pericardium in place and the opposite ventricle at either 0 or 10 mm Hg. (From Pinson, Morton and Thornburg, 1987, with permission.)

increasing amounts of tension as it is stretched within the physiological range. This translates to the whole ventricle as a larger stroke volume when end-diastolic chamber volume is increased. This is the so-called Frank–Starling relationship or Starling's Law of the Heart. The traditional view that Starling's Law is due solely to the advantageous alignment of overlapping actin and myosin filaments is currently debated. Recent evidence indicates that muscle fibre length somehow alters the sensitivity of the contractile units to Ca^{2+} and that such a biochemical alteration underlies the Law (Opie, 1991).

Preload has been studied in fetal sheep but it is difficult to quantify. End-diastolic wall tension is especially difficult to estimate in the right ventricle where the chamber shape defies mathematical description. Instead, preload is usually estimated using 'mean filling pressure' (mean ventricular end-diastolic pressure or mean atrial pressure) as an index of wall tension and therefore preload. End-diastolic volume is a better index of preload than filling pressure but is less often used for technical reasons.

The rationale for using mean atrial pressure for preload is as follows. If the ventricular pressure–volume relationship is unique and the relationship between mean atrial pressure and ventricular end-diastolic pressure constant, then each mean atrial pressure will define a unique ventricular transmural end diastolic pressure and volume. If the relationship between volume and geometry is also constant, then the determinants of wall stress, transmural pressure and geometry can be expressed by mean atrial pressure. To study the role of preload as a determinant of stroke volume, the ventricular function curve has been used to good effect (Bishop, Stone & Guyton, 1964). The function curve is a representation of the relationship between the stroke volume of a ventricle and an index of preload (mean transmural filling pressure). But one must understand the assumptions that underlie the use of the function curve before interpreting it. For example, the position of the curve is influenced directly by changes in afterload and contractility and by factors which effect the relationship between mean atrial pressure and end-diastolic wall stress such as the pericardium, heart rate and rhythm and filling of the contralateral ventricle. However, if these factors are constant or accounted for, function curves yield useful information regarding the role of preload in affecting stroke volume.

Fig. 6.4 shows right and left ventricular function curves from eight fetuses where filling pressures were altered by rapidly withdrawing and reinfusing blood (pericardium intact & sealed). First, notice the shape of the curves with their ascending and plateau limbs. The fetal heart

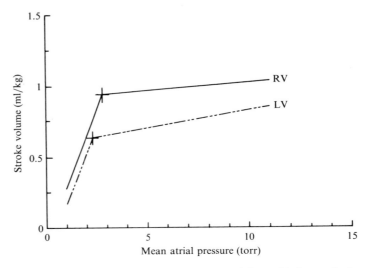

Fig. 6.4. Simultaneous function curves showing right and left ventricular stroke volume of near term fetuses during alterations of mean right atrial pressure produced by rapid hemorrhage and rapid re-infusion. The function curve consists of a steep ascending limb and a plateau limb at elevated atrial pressures. The star on each curve represents the standard deviation of stroke volume and mean atrial pressure at the computer derived breakpoint of the curve ($n = 12$). (From Reller, Morton, Reid and Thornburg, 1987, with permission.)

normally operates at the break in the curves at a mean transmural pressure of about 3 mm Hg. From this position, the fetus will rapidly lose stroke volume if the filling pressure is reduced, but will gain only little in the way of stroke volume if filling is increased. Thus it is very difficult for the fetus to increase its stroke volume by increasing intravascular volume yet the output of the ventricles is quite vulnerable to a fall in filling pressure.

One explanation is that afterload increases during blood volume expansion, offsetting any gain in stroke volume due to increased preload. This might occur either because of ventricular distention with increased r/h ratio (Equation 1) or because of increased arterial pressure, or both (Ross, 1976; Hawkins et al., 1989). Another explanation is pericardial restraint with inadequate estimation of the transmural pressure with a fluid-filled catheter (Grant et al., 1989). Clearly, from Fig. 6.3 the volume of the ventricle can be increased at a constant filling pressure by removing the pericardium or reducing the volume of the contralateral ventricle. The extent to which either of these manipulations might affect stroke

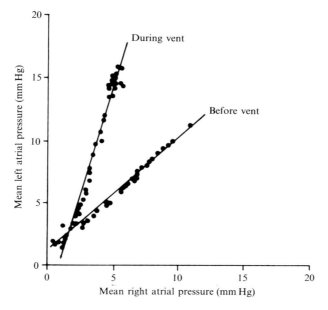

Fig. 6.5. Mean left atrial pressure of a single near-term sheep fetus plotted as a function of mean right atrial pressure before (control) and during ventilation in utero with oxygen. Pressures were varied by rapidly withdrawing and reinfusing fetal blood. Note that while the lungs are being ventilated with oxygen, left atrial pressure is always greater than right atrial pressure. (From Morton, Pinson and Thornburg, 1987, with permission.)

volume in a healthy fetus is uncertain. The mechanism for the plateau of the function curve remains controversial and requires further investigation.

A second feature of the function curves is also important. The stroke volume of the right ventricle is larger than the stroke volume of the left ventricle at all physiological filling pressures. This can be explained by the fact that the volume of the right ventricle at equal filling pressure is significantly larger than the volume of the left ventricle (Fig. 6.3). It is known that the fetal right and left ventricles ordinarily have equal filling pressures over a wide range of pressures (Fig. 6.5). As far as is known, only atrial ventricular valve stenosis, premature closure of the foramen ovale and ventilation in utero (Fig. 6.5) can disrupt this relationship.

The foregoing uncertainty notwithstanding, simply increasing filling pressures in the fetus will not raise fetal stroke volume to neonatal levels. It has been shown that ventilation in utero will increase left ventricular stroke volume dramatically (Morton, Pinson & Thornburg, 1987). Since this procedure is accompanied by a left to right interatrial pressure gradient it is possible that fetal left ventricular stroke volume is increased at birth by increased preload made available, for the first time, by decompression of the right ventricle (Fig. 6.5). The mechanism for right ventricular stroke volume increase at birth is unlikely to involve preload for the same reasons.

Afterload

Afterload is the stress in the ventricular wall during the contraction phase of the cardiac cycle. The wall stress during contraction is a determinant of how much blood will be ejected during a beat based on the finding in isolated muscle that the extent and velocity of contraction are inversely related to muscle tension. Intuitively wall stress during the ejection phase would be a function of the 'difficulty' of ejecting the blood into the arterial tree. This 'difficulty factor' is determined by the impedance of the vascular tree and is mostly a function of the arterial vascular resistance and arterial compliance. Since mean arterial pressure is the product of vascular resistance and cardiac output, and pulse pressure is largely determined by the quotient of stroke volume and arterial compliance, we see how impedance in the vascular tree is coupled to the ventricle through systolic pressure to become a major determinant of afterload. Equation 1 shows that systolic pressure is proportional to wall stress and therefore afterload. Accordingly, as vascular resistance is increased by a vascular occlusion or by vasoconstrictor drugs, arterial pressure is increased and stroke volume is reduced, proportional to the increase in wall stress.

As mentioned above, geometry is also an important determinant of wall stress and therefore afterload. The fetal right ventricle has a larger circumferential radius of curvature and thinner wall than does the left and because of this anatomical disadvantage, the right ventricle is less able to eject a 'full' stroke volume with increasing arterial pressure. This is shown in Fig. 6.6. Notice that, while both the right and left ventricular stroke volumes decrease as the ventricles beat against increasing resistances (generated by gradually occluding the descending aorta with an inflatable cuff), right ventricular stroke volume is reduced by nearly 40% with a mere 20 mm Hg increase in mean arterial pressure. Left ventricular stroke volume is decreased by less than 10% by the same change in arterial pressure.

Because the right ventricle is more sensitive to increases in arterial pressure, even small increases in pressure will adversely affect right

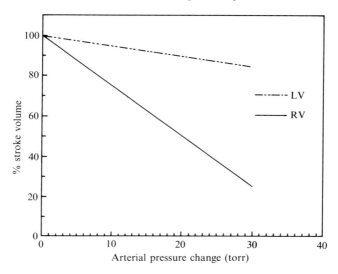

Fig. 6.6. Simultaneous right ventricular and left ventricular stroke volumes from nine fetuses are shown during stepwise increase in arterial pressure produced by inflation of an occluder on the descending aorta. Stroke volume is expressed as a percentage of control value and arterial pressure as the increase above control. The linear regression coefficient for each ventricle was calculated and the average slope forced through 100% on the *Y* axis and the lines extended through the pressure range studied. (From Reller, Morton, Reid and Thornburg, 1987, with permission.)

ventricular output. Examples are: 1) In sheep fetuses that were subjected to hypoxaemia by having the ewe breathe reduced oxygen mixtures, reductions in cardiac output were found only in fetuses that demonstrated a hypertensive response to the hypoxaemia. Furthermore, in fetuses that became hypertensive, reductions in right ventricular output accounted for most of the decrease in cardiac output (Reller et al., 1989). 2) Fetal cardiac output was lower in sheep fetuses reared at altitude. These fetuses had near normal oxygen tensions but were hypertensive and showed reductions in right ventricular stroke volume which accounted for most of the decrease in fetal output. From these studies it is concluded that the immature right ventricle is particularly vulnerable to a rise in arterial pressure. Conversely, when arterial pressure or vascular resistance drop such as at birth or during profound anaemia, right ventricular function might be augmented as a result of its sensitivity to changes in afterload.

It appears, however, that the right ventricle can be 'conditioned' to become better able to eject against increased arterial pressure. A mean pressure load of 10 mm Hg was imposed on the right ventricle of sheep fetuses near term by inflating an occluder around the main pulmonary artery for about 10 days (Pinson, Morton & Thornburg, 1991). After the loading period, the free wall of the right ventricle was thickened and the radius to wall thickness ratio was smaller and closer to the left ventricular value. Correspondingly, the effect of increased arterial pressure on right ventricular function was reduced making it similar to the normal left ventricle (Fig. 6.7). In the laboratory of Gilbert et al., where fetuses were exposed to chronic maternal hypoxaemia, both ventricles became conditioned and were less sensitive to increased arterial pressure than were their control counterparts (Kitanaka et al., 1984; Alonso et al., 1989; Kamitomo et al., 1991). These data indicate that pressure loading (or even hypoxaemia itself) may condition the ventricle so that it is less likely to fail under conditions of increased pressure load.

Nevertheless, there may be limits to the adaptability of the right ventricle to chronic pressure load. Ventricular dysfunction and failure is

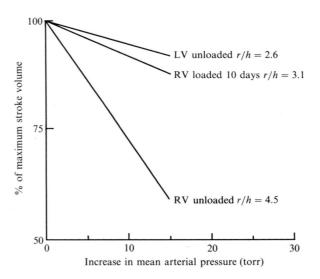

Fig. 6.7. Percentage change in right ventricular stroke volume of fetuses plotted as a function of increase in pulmonary artery pressure. The normal relationships between stroke volume and mean arterial pressure for the unloaded right ventricle (RV unloaded) and the unloaded left ventricle (LV unloaded) are taken from Fig. 6.6. The relationship between stroke volume and pulmonary arterial pressure after 10 days of mild pressure loading is shown as 'RV loaded 10 days'. Each curve is shown with its respective radius to wall thickness ratios which affect wall tension as shown in Equation 1.

common in adults with congenitally 'corrected' transposition of the great vessels in whom the ventricle supplying the systemic circulation is morphologically a right ventricle. This contrasts with the right ventricle of severe congenital pulmonary stenosis which usually retains its function at normal levels despite being exposed to systemic or greater pressures. Perhaps the time of loading, in utero for congenital pulmonary stenosis vs after birth for corrected transposition, is important for sufficient adaptation to occur. Such factors as myocyte number, size and coronary vascularity may play important roles in this distinction.

Contractility

Contractility (or inotropic state) is a description of the relative contractile strength of the myocardium in the absence of changes in preload or afterload. This has been well reviewed by Anderson (1990) for the fetal heart. Factors known to affect contractility are cytosolic calcium ion concentration, sensitivity of the contractile elements to calcium ion, the inherent ability of myosin to act as an ATPase, and other vaguely defined biochemical alterations of the proteins associated with the contractile machinery. Drugs which augment contractility are known as inotropic agents. Generally, any agent which increases cyclic AMP production (e.g. adrenergic agonists) or decreases its breakdown (e.g. phosphodiesterase inhibitors) will increase contractility. Digitalis is an inotropic agent which probably acts by increasing sodium–calcium exchange through an increase in intracellular sodium caused by the blockade of the sodium-potassium ATPase pump. Heart rate is also related to increased intracellular calcium.

Friedman found in 1972 that developed tension, as well as velocity of shortening at constant tension, were less in fetal lambs than adult sheep. While these findings support the idea of decreased contractility in the fetus, the velocity of shortening at very low levels of afterload was similar in fetal and adult sheep. Because the fetal heart was composed of only 30% myofibrils as opposed to the adult heart with 60%, Friedman suggested that the contractility of individual sarcomeres was similar in fetal and adult hearts, but there was simply more contractile material in adult hearts. Subsequent years have brought a wealth of understanding regarding contractile protein chemistry, sarcoplasmic reticulum development and adrenergic receptor development but have not greatly altered Friedman's prescient conclusions.

Anderson et al. (1984) using both in vivo and in vitro techniques, studied post extrasystolic potentiation as an index of contractility. They argued that the ratio of potentiated dF/dt or dP/dt to baseline values in isolated muscle and in vivo respectively are independent of the amount of contractile protein. In these studies, there is a clear increase in contractility from 93 days gestation to 62 days of postnatal life. However, the increase in contractility does not translate into increased cardiac performance; the fractional shortening is constant from approximately 120 days gestation to 122 days of age except for a transient increase at birth. Anderson speculated that the increase in contractility represented the development of a reserve that the fetus could utilize for the stresses of birth and neonatal life.

One might argue that the near-term fetal lamb is relatively mature and that maturational changes in contractility might be more apparent in a species less developed at birth. Nakanishi & Jarmakani (1984) studied rabbits from 0.58 gestation (18 days) through late gestation neonatal and adult periods. Between 18 days gestation and 5 days of age, heart weight increased 69 fold. Maximal developed tension of isolated heart muscle increased 3.8 fold when normalized per g of myocardium but only 1.2 fold when developed tension was also normalized for myofibril content. Thus, there are subtle increases in contractility with the development of the myocyte. However, the progressive, orderly compaction of myofibrils within the myocyte, with their associated connections to the sarcolemma and the ready availability of calcium from the SR, appears to be the dominant factor increasing the strength of myocyte contraction during development.

Despite the overwhelming importance of the amount of contractile protein for cardiac function, the mechanism of cardiac contraction and relaxation changes dramatically during development. Perhaps the most fundamental change is in excitation–contraction coupling. Ryanodine, which selectively inhibits sarcoplasmic uptake and release of calcium has little effect on 18 and 21 day fetal rabbit hearts but reduces adult and newborn contraction almost 50%. Conversely, lanthanum, which inhibits sarcolemmal calcium transport, almost completely eliminates contraction in 18 day fetuses, having a progressively lesser effect with increasing development. These pharmacological changes parallel the morphological development of the sarcoplasmic reticulum in the rabbit. Thus, Nakanishi proposed the schema of excitation–contraction coupling where, early in development, all of the calcium necessary to initiate contraction enters through the sarcolemma (Nakanishi & Jarmakani, 1984). This is in stark contrast to the adult where calcium crosses the sarcolemma in relatively small quantities but triggers release of larger amounts of calcium from the sarcoplasmic reticulum. Again the degree of maturity of the SR at birth is species-dependent. In the cat, the anatomical maturity of T-tubules and the SR correlates with functional maturity between the newborn and adult stages (Maylie, Thornburg & Faber, 1978). In species that mature after birth, there is a transition period where both the sarcolemma and the SR apparently contribute to the intracellular activator calcium, the former becoming increasingly less important with maturity.

Heart rate

The role of heart rate vs preload in regulating stroke volume has been controversial though it now appears that opinions about the role of heart rate are sufficiently unified to allow general conclusions to be drawn (Rudolph, 1987; Anderson, 1990). Under experimental conditions where heart rate is increased in fetal sheep by pacing, output is not generally increased because of a concomitant decrease in preload. Furthermore, the decrement in output depends upon which atrium is being paced (Rudolph & Heymann, 1973; Anderson et al., 1987). This means that stroke volume falls as heart rate increases in spite of increases in contractile strength that accompany the tachycardia. However, it is likely that compensatory increases in heart rate that occur spontaneously will also be accompanied by inotropic support so that under such circumstances stroke volume may increase along with rate (Anderson, 1990).

Battaglia and Meschia (1986) noted that heart rate is relatively constant among very young fetuses of different species over a considerable range of body size unlike the heart rate of adult animals which tends to be inversely related to body size. They speculated that this relates to the fact that embryonic and early fetal tissues have about the same metabolic rate across species and that heart size to body size ratio is constant across species. Since metabolic rate is nearly constant across species (per unit mass), cardiac output which supplies the oxygen necessary for metabolism is by necessity linked to body mass. Thus, heart size (and therefore stroke volume) increases proportionately with body mass and so heart rate need not vary across species despite even large differences in mass. Rather, for the fetus, differences in heart output are met by regulation of heart size both within the growing fetus and across species lines. Battaglia and Meschia speculated further that the decrease in heart rate of large mammals near term (in contrast to the increase in small mammals) may be related to a reduction in weight-specific metabolic rate. Decreases in heart rate are due to the increasing 'tone' from the maturing parasympathetic nervous system.

Conclusion

For short-term circulatory regulation, the fetus appears to have two major mechanisms to increase cardiac output: increased rate and contractility. However, for either to be effective, preload must be maintained. To increase output from day to day, the fetus relies on cardiac growth. The mystery of birth-related increases in cardiac output remains incompletely understood, but probably includes hormonal changes. Differential changes in right and left ventricular preload and afterload accompany the abolition of fetal shunts and the progressive reduction in pulmonary vascular resistance.

Reference

Alonso, J. G., Okai, T., Longo, L. D. & Gilbert, R. D (1989). Cardiac function during long term hypoxemia in fetal sheep. *American Journal of Physiology,* **257**, H581–9.

Anderson, P. A. W., Killam, A. P., Mainwaring, R. D. & Oakeley, A. E. (1987). *In utero* right ventricular output in the fetal lamb: the effect of heart rate. *Journal of Physiology,* **387**, 297–316.

Anderson, P. A. W. (1990). Myocardial development. In *Fetal and Neonatal Cardiology,* ed. W. A. Long. pp. 17–38. W. A. Saunders, London.

Anderson, P. A. W., Glick, K. I., Manring, A. & Crenshaw, Jr C. (1984). Developmental changes in cardiac contractility in fetal and postnatal sheep: in vitro and in vivo. *American Journal of Physiology,* **247**, H371–9.

Battaglia, F. C. & Meschia, G. (1986). *An Introduction to Fetal Physiology.* Academic Press. New York, pp. 197–8.

Bishop, V. S., Stone, H. L. & Guyton, A. C. (1964). Cardiac function curves in conscious dogs. *American Journal of Physiology,* **207**, 677–82.

Brook, W. H., Connell, S., Cannata, J., Maloney, J. E. & Walker, A. M. (1983). Ultrastructure of the myocardium during development from early fetal life to adult life in sheep. *Journal of Anatomy,* **137**, 729–41.

Challice, C. E. & Viragh, S. (1973). The embryologic development of the mammalian heart. In *Ultrastructure in Biological Systems,* Academic Press, **6**, 91–126.

Clark, E. B. & Hu, N. (1982). Developmental hemodynamic changes in the chick embryo from stage 18 to 27. *Circulation Research,* **51**, 810–15.

Dawes, G. S. (1968). *Foetal and Neonatal Physiology: A comparative study of the changes at birth.* Chicago, Year Book Medical Publishers.

DeChamplain, J., Malmfors, T., Olson L. & Sachs, C. H. (1970). Ontogenesis of peripheral adrenergic neurons in the rat: pre- and postnatal observations. *Acta Physiologica Scandinavica,* **80**, 276–88.

Faber, J. J., Anderson, D. F., Morton, M. J., Parks, C. M., Pinson, C. W. & Thornburg, K. L. (1985). Hemodynamics of shunts in the fetal lamb. In *Cardiovascular Shunts, Alfred Benzon Symposium 21*, ed. K. Johanson & W. W. Burggren. Munksgaard, Copenhagen.

Friedman, W. F. (1972*a*). The intrinsic physiologic properties of the developing heart. *Progress in Cardiovascular Diseases*, **15**, 87–111.

Friedman, W. F. (1972*b*). Neuropharmacologic studies of perinatal myocardium. *Cardiovascular Clinics*, **4**, 43–57.

Grant, D. A., Maloney, J. E., Tyberg, J. V. & Walker, A. M. (1989). Modulation of the fetal left ventricular function curve by the thoracic tissues. *Society for the Study of Fetal Physiology*, 16th Meeting, July 2–4, p. F12.

Hawkins, J., Van Hare, G. F., Schmidt, K. G. & Rudolph, A. M. (1989). Effects of increasing afterload on left ventricular output in fetal lambs. *Circulation Research*, **65**, 127–34.

Hirakow, R. & Gotoh, T. (1980). Ontogenetic implication of the myocardial ultrastructure in the development of mammalian heart. In *Etiology and Morphogenesis of Congenital Heart Disease*, ed. R. Van Praagh & A. Takao, pp. 99–108, Futura Publishing Co.

Icardo, J. M. (1984). The growing heart: an anatomical perspective. In *Growth of the Heart in Health and Disease*, ed. R. Zak. pp. 41–79. Raven Press, New York.

Kamitomo, M., Browne, V. A., Longo, L. D. & Gilbert, R. D. (1991). Right and left ventricular function in fetal sheep exposed to long-term hypoxia. *Society for Gynecologic Investigation*, 38th Annual Meeting, San Antonio, Texas, March 20–23, p. 116.

Kitanaka, T., Alonso, J. G., Gilbert, R. D., Siu, B. L., Clemons, G. K. & Longo, L. D. (1984). Fetal responses to long-term hypoxemia in sheep. *American Journal of Physiology*, **256**, R1348–54.

Lebowitz, E. A., Novick, J. S. & Rudolph, A. M. (1972). Development of myocardial sympathetic innervation in the fetal lamb. *Pediatric Research*, **6**, 887–93.

Lipp, J. A. & Rudolph, A. M. (1972). Sympathetic nerve development in the rat and guinea-pig heart. *Biology of the Neonate*, **21**, 76–82.

Maylie, J. G., Thornburg, K. L. & Faber, J. J. (1978). Force-frequency relations of the neonatal cat heart. In *Fetal and Newborn Cardiovascular Physiology*, vol. 1, ed. L. D. Longo & D. D. Reneau. pp. 391–398. Garland STPM Press, New York & London.

Morton, M. J. & Thornburg, K. L. (1987). The pericardium and cardiac transmural filling pressure in the fetal sheep. *Journal of Developmental Physiology*, **9**, 159–68.

Morton, M. J., Pinson, C. W. & Thornburg, K. L. (1987) In utero ventilation with oxygen augments left ventricular stroke volume in lambs. *Journal of Physiology*, **383**, 413–24.

Nakanishi, T. & Jarmakani, J. M. (1984). Developmental changes in myocardial mechanical function and subcellular organelles. *American Journal of Physiology*, **246**, H615–25.

Nakazawa, M., Miyagawa, S., Ohno, T., Miura, S. & Takao, A. (1988). Developmental hemodynamic changes in rat embryos at 11 to 15 days of gestation: normal data of blood pressure and the effect of caffeine compared to data from chick embryo. *Pediatric Research*, **23**, 200–5.

Oparil, S. (1985). Pathogenesis of ventricular hypertrophy. *Journal of the American College of Cardiology,* **5**, 57–65.

Opie, L. H. (1991). *The Heart: Physiology and Metabolism.* Raven Press, New York.

Papka, R. E. (1981). Development of innervation to the ventricular myocardium of the rabbit. *Journal of Molecular and Cellular Cardiology,* **13**, 217–28.

Pinson, C. W, Morton, M. J. & Thornburg, K. L. (1991). Mild pressure loading alters right ventricular function in fetal sheep. *Circulation Research,* No. 4, **68**, 947–57.

Pinson, C. W., Morton, M. J. & Thornburg, K. L. (1987). An anatomic basis for fetal right ventricular dominance and arterial pressure sensitivity. *Journal of Developmental Physiology,* **9**, 253–69.

Reller, M. D., Gerlis, L. M. & Thornburg, K. L. (1991). Cardiac embryology: basic review and clinical correlations. *Journal of the Society of Echocardiology.* (In Press).

Reller, M. D., Morton, M. J., Giraud, G. D., Reid, D. L. & Thornburg, K. L. (1989). The effect of acute hypoxemia on ventricular function during beta-adrenergic and cholinergic blockade in the fetal lamb. *Journal of Developmental Physiology,* **11**, 263–9.

Reller, M. D., Morton, M. J., Reid, D. L. & Thornburg, K. L. (1987). Fetal lamb ventricles respond differently to filling and arterial pressures and to in utero ventilation. *Pediatric Research,* **22**, 621–6.

Riemenschneider, T. A. (1990). Pericardial development. In *Fetal and Neonatal Cardiology,* ed. W. A. Long. pp. 39–42. Saunders, London.

Rockson, S. G., Homcy, C. J., Quinn, P., Manders, T., Haber, E. & Vatner, S. (1981). Cellular mechanisms of impaired adrenergic responsiveness in neonatal dogs. *Journal of Clinical Investigation,* **67**, 319–27.

Romero, T., Covell, J. & Friedman, W. F. (1972). A comparison of pressure–volume relations of the fetal, newborn, and adult heart. *American Journal of Physiology,* **222**, 1285–90.

Ross, J. Jr. (1976). Afterload mismatch and preload reserve: a conceptual framework for the analysis of ventricular function. *Progress in Cardiovascular Disease,* **18**, 255.

Rudolph, A. M. (1987). Regulation of Fetal Cardiac Output. In *Perinatal Development of the Heart and Lung,* ed. J. Lipshitz, J. Maloney, C. Nimrod & G. Carson. pp. 73–82. Perinatology Press, New York.

Rudolph, A. M. & Heymann, M. A. (1973). Control of the foetal circulation. In *Foetal and Neonatal Physiology.* University Press, Cambridge.

Simpson, F. O., Rayns, D. G. & Ledingham, J. M. (1973). The ultrastructure of ventricular and atrial myocardium. In *Ultrastructure in Biological Systems.* Academic Press, **6**, 1–41.

Simpson, P. (1985). Stimulation of hypertrophy of cultured neonatal rat heart cells through an α_1-adrenergic receptor and induction of beating through an α and β_1 receptor interaction: evidence for independent regulation of growth and beating. *Circulation Research,* **56**, 884–94.

Smolich, J. J. (1987). The morphology of the developing myocardium. In *Research in Perinatal Medicine (V). Perinatal Development of the Heart and Lung,* ed. J. Lipshitz, J. Maloney, C. Nimrod & G. Carson. pp. 1–22. Perinatology Press, New York.

Thornburg, K. L. & Morton, M. J. (1983). Filling and arterial pressures as determinants of RV stroke volume in the sheep fetus. *American Journal of Physiology,* **244**, H656–63.

Thornburg, K. L. & Morton, M. J. (1986). Filling and arterial pressures as determinants of left ventricular stroke volume in unanesthetized fetal lambs. *American Journal of Physiology,* **251**, H961–8.

Van Mierop, L. H. S. (1979). Morphological development of the heart. In *Handbook of Physiology, Section 2 The Cardiovascular System, vol I The Heart,* ed. R. M. Berne, N. Sperelakis & S. R. Geiger. pp. 1–28. American Physiology Society.

Versprille, A., Jansen, J. R. C., Harinck, C. J. van Nie & de Neef, K. J. (1978). Functional interaction of both ventricles at birth and the changes during the neonatal period in relation to the changes of geometry. In *Fetal and Newborn Cardiovascular Physiology Vol 1,* ed. L. D. Longo & D. D. Reneau. pp. 391–398. Garland STPM Press, New York & London.

Walker, A. M. (1987). Developmental aspects of cardiac physiology and morphology. In *Perinatal Development of the Heart & Lung,* ed. J. Lipshitz, J. Maloney, C. Nimrod & G. Carson. pp. 73–82. Perinatology Press, New York.

Witschi, E. (1956). *Development of Vertebrates.* Philadelphia, WB Saunders.

7

Circulatory transitions at birth and the control of the neonatal circulation

ADRIAN M. WALKER

Introduction

'in the foetus . . . whilst the blood is not passing through the lungs, . . . but flowing by the foramen ovale and ductus arteriosus, directly from the vena cava into the aorta, whence it is distributed to the whole body, both ventricles have the same office to perform . . . It is only when the lungs come to be used and it is requisite that the passages indicated should be blocked up . . . (that) the right has only to throw the blood through the lungs, whilst the left has to impel it through the whole body.'

William Harvey (1578–1657)

William Harvey's observations on the perinatal circulation emphasize the central role that changes in the lung play in the cascade of events which begins with the first air breath and ends with the transformation of the circulation from the fetal to the neonatal form. Beginning with the fetal circulation, this chapter describes the important circulatory changes which follow the onset of air breathing at birth and the mechanisms by which they are accomplished, giving emphasis to the pulmonary circulation. As significant maturation of the cardiovascular system occurs in late gestation, in preparation for birth, there is substantial potential for the normal transitional process to be disrupted by preterm delivery. Therefore this chapter also examines the perinatal and postnatal changes in the circulation which follow preterm birth.

Fetal circulation

Ventricular outputs

In the adult circulation, the right heart, the lungs, the left heart and the systemic circulation are arranged in series. Blood flow through each of these elements is identical, and equals the cardiac output. In the fetal circulation, the left and right ventricle each pump blood into the arterial circulation in parallel (Fig. 7.1). Thus it has become customary to consider cardiac output in the fetus as the sum of the right and left ventricular outputs, the combined ventricular output. In the fetal lamb near term, combined ventricular output is about 450 ml/min per kg of body weight (Table 7.1). Working in parallel, the right ventricle ejects two-thirds of this (300 ml/min per kg) and the left ventricle one-third (150 ml/min per kg). In the preterm fetal lamb, combined ventricular output is greater (approximately 550 ml/min per kg; Iwamoto et al., 1989). These outputs significantly exceed the resting cardiac output of about 100 ml/ min per kg of body weight in the adult. Calculation of ventricular stroke volumes using a representative fetal heart rate of 150 beats/min at term yields values of 2 ml/kg for the right ventricle and 1 ml/kg for the left ventricle. These may be compared to values of 1 ml/kg for each of the adult ventricles working in series (Table 7.1). Thus an elevated heart rate together with an elevated stroke volume (of the right ventricle) explains the impressive pumping performance of the fetal heart in comparison with the adult heart. Associated with this high basal performance, the fetal heart has no apparent capacity to increase its output in response to factors such as hypoxia or volume infusions which increase cardiac output in adults (Rudolph, 1985). Remarkably, however, ventricular outputs do increase dramatically at birth. The stroke volume of the newborn is twice the adult stroke volume, and because the newborn heart rate is twice the adult rate, cardiac output in the newborn immediately after birth is four times greater (Table 7.1).

Venous return

The outstanding anatomical feature of the fetal circulation is the presence of vascular shunts, the foramen ovale on the venous side and the ductus arteriosus on the arterial side (Fig. 7.1), which ensure that most blood flow bypasses the lung. Instead, blood flow is directed to the organ of gas exchange, the placenta. In late gestation, 40% of fetal combined ven-

Table 7.1. *Haemodynamics during development in sheep*

Developmental stage	Cardiac output (ml/min per kg)	Heart rate (beats/min)	Ventricular output (ml/min per kg)		Stroke volume (ml/kg)	
			Left	Right	Left	Right
Fetus (at term)	450	150	150	300	1	2
Newborn (at birth)	400	200	400	400	2	2
Adult	100	100	100	100	1	1

Source: Data from Heymann et al., 1981; Klopfenstein & Rudolph, 1978; Peeters et al., 1979; Berman & Musselman, 1979; Sidi et al., 1983; Smolich, 1986.

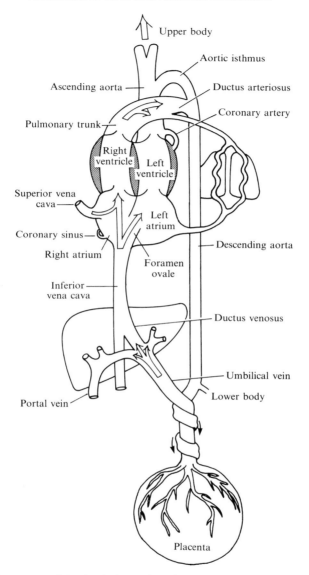

Fig. 7.1. The course of the fetal circulation. (Based on Rudolph, 1974; Teitel et al., 1987; Teitel, 1988.)

164   *Adrian M. Walker*

tricular output is directed to the placenta (Fig. 7.2). Earlier in gestation
the ratio of placental to fetal weight is greater and proportionally more of
the combined ventricular output goes to the placenta. Oxygenated blood
returns from the placenta to the fetus via the umbilical veins to the fetal
liver, where it joins blood flowing in the portal venous system. Umbilical

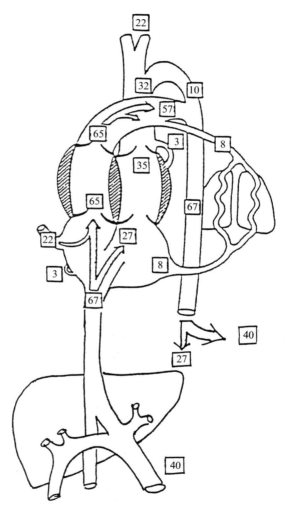

Fig. 7.2. The distribution of combined ventricular output (the sum of left and right
ventricular outputs) in the fetal lamb. The numbers represent the percentage of
combined ventricular output ejected by each ventricle and flowing through the
major arterial and venous pathways identified in Fig. 7.1. (Modified from
Rudolph, 1974; Teitel et al., 1987; Teitel, 1988.)

venous blood can then pass directly to the inferior vena cava via the ductus venosus or enter the hepatic microcirculation and flow to the inferior vena cava via the hepatic veins. The ductus venosus, which is part of the liver vasculature, is one of the vascular shunts unique to the fetal circulation, and to the transitional newborn circulation. In some species (the pig and the horse) the ductus venosus is absent in the mature fetus (Edelstone, 1980). In the fetal lamb, about 50% of umbilical venous flow passes through the ductus venosus, and the balance is distributed to the left and right lobes of the liver through the portal venous system (Edelstone, Rudolph & Heymann, 1978). The ductus venosus also acts as a bypass for a small portion (10%) of portal venous flow from the gastrointestinal tract; the remainder passes to the right lobe of the liver.

The pattern of blood flow in the great thoracic veins and heart has been quantified in the fetal lamb (Fig. 7.2). Inferior vena caval return represents 67% of the combined ventricular output and the superior vena caval return 22%; the flow from the lungs (8%) and heart (3%) together make up the remainder. Superior vena caval flow is returned to the right ventricle; only minimal amounts normally cross the foramen ovale to the left ventricle, although this may increase in fetal asphyxia (Dawes, 1968). Inferior vena caval flow is divided between the right and left ventricles. 40% of inferior vena caval flow passes through the foramen ovale into the left atrium; the balance combines with superior vena caval blood in the right atrium. Blood flow shunted through the foramen ovale is influenced by changes in pulmonary vascular resistance; as pulmonary blood flow increases, the proportion of inferior vena caval return entering the left atrium falls (Rudolph, 1977). Superior vena caval return represents a greater proportion of venous return in the monkey and baboon fetus (and this is probably also true in the human fetus) than in the lamb fetus in which the brain is smaller (Paton et al., 1973).

Blood in the thoracic inferior vena cava is not homogeneous in its composition and ultimate arterial distribution (Edelstone & Rudolph, 1979). One-third of the thoracic vena caval flow is derived from umbilical venous flow crossing the ductus venosus, and two-thirds from abdominal inferior vena caval flow. Umbilical venous blood is relatively well oxygenated with a saturation of about 85%, while abdominal venous blood is poorly oxygenated. These blood streams remain unmixed in the thoracic inferior vena cava, and in the fetal lamb obvious streams of well-oxygenated and poorly oxygenated blood are visible through the thin-walled vena cava. Streaming of umbilical venous blood in the thoracic inferior vena cava and through the foramen ovale results in preferential distribution of oxygenated blood to the heart and brain (Reuss & Rudolph, 1980). Oxygen saturation in the left ventricle and ascending aorta averages about 60%, exceeding the levels in the right ventricle and pulmonary trunk (53%) and descending aorta (55%).

Regional circulations

In the fetal circulation both the left ventricle and the right ventricle eject blood into the arterial circuit, but distribution of the two ventricular outputs in the fetal body differs. Most blood ejected by the left ventricle perfuses the upper body; less than one-third (10% of combined ventricular output) flows through the aortic isthmus to the descending aorta, and then to the lower body and placenta (Fig. 7.2). 90% of blood ejected by the right ventricle bypasses the lungs and flows via the ductus arteriosus to the lower body and placenta. Thus the upper body is perfused exclusively by the left ventricle, whereas the lower body and placenta are largely perfused by the right ventricle, with just a small contribution from the left ventricle.

Average percentages of combined ventricular output distributed to various organs in the fetal lamb are the following: placenta, 40; lungs, 8; gastrointestinal tract, 5; brain, 4; myocardium, 3; kidneys, 3; spleen, 1; liver, 0.3; and adrenal glands, 0.1 (Cohn et al., 1974; Longo et al., 1978; Peeters et al., 1979). The balance of the flow (35%) is distributed principally to the bones, skin and skeletal muscle.

In primates (Behrman et al., 1970; Paton et al., 1973) and previable man (Rudolph et al., 1971), the proportional distribution of cardiac output to fetal organs is similar to that seen in the lamb, with the exception of brain flow which is 15% of the cardiac output in the primate and human fetus.

Changes in the circulation at birth

Closure of the ductus venosus

In the fetus, umbilical venous blood flow provides greater than 95% of the total ductus venosus flow, with portal flow constituting the remainder (Edelstone, Rudolph & Heymann, 1978). After birth, when umbilical flow ceases, there is a very large fall in blood flow through the ductus venosus. However a portion of portal venous flow may continue to pass through the ductus venosus for several days after birth in newborn lambs, decreasing gradually until functional closure occurs (Zink & Van Petten,

1980). In the human newborn, the ductus venosus is functionally closed within hours of birth, although it remains potentially patent for many days (Walsh, Myer & Lind, 1974). Functional closure appears to occur passively as a result of the decrease of blood flow and blood pressure in the portal sinus, leading to retraction and narrowing of the inlet of the ductus venosus (Meyer & Lind, 1966). Neural or chemical mechanisms are not likely to participate in ductal closure. A muscular sphincter with autonomic innervation has been described at the junction of the umbilical vein with the ductus venosus, but the structural evidence is controversial (Walsh et al., 1974) and blood flow studies indicate that the nervous system exerts little effect upon the ductus venosus in the fetus or newborn (Edelstone, 1980). The ductus venosus is relaxed by PGE_2 and PGI_2, and it contracts in response to compounds such as indomethacin which inhibit prostaglandin synthesis (Adeagbo, Coceani & Olley, 1982). However, as these responses are weak (much less than those of the ductus arteriosus) it is unlikely that prostaglandins play a role in fetal patency or newborn closure of the ductus venosus. Permanent obliteration of the ductus venosus occurs by proliferation of connective tissue which fills the lumen. This process begins a few days after birth and is completed by 20 days of age in human infants (Meyer & Lind, 1966).

Closure of the foramen ovale

In the fetal circulation, the foramen ovale is a pathway for venous blood to flow directly into the left side of the heart, effectively bypassing the pulmonary circulation. Anatomically and functionally the foramen ovale is a channel between the inferior vena cava and left atrium, not an opening between the two atria. The inferior vena cava bifurcates at the heart, forming two channels: the foramen ovale on the left side and the inferior vena cava inlet to the right atrium on the right side. Blood flowing into the heart in the inferior vena cava is divided into left and right streams by the crista dividens, an extension of the upper part of the interatrial septum which protrudes into the inferior vena cava.

On the left atrial end, the foramen ovale terminates in a one-way valve, only permitting flow from right to left. The valve is usually depicted as a 'flap' but in the lamb takes the form of a 'wind-sock' (Anderson et al., 1985) bulging toward the inferior vena cava when closed. A large positive hydrostatic pressure difference does not keep the foramen ovale open in the fetus, as mean pressures in the inferior vena cava, right atrium and left atrium are very similar, approximately 3 mm Hg (Anderson et al., 1985;

Teitel, Iwamoto & Rudolph, 1987). Although blood pressure in the inferior vena cava is low, the flow is high, more than two-thirds of the total venous return. Of the two forces which determine blood flow through the foramen ovale, the hydrostatic pressure difference between inferior vena cava and left atrium and the kinetic energy of the blood stream, it is the kinetic energy which is far larger and which maintains the foramen ovale in the open position (Anderson et al., 1985).

At birth the foramen ovale closes in two stages. The first, which can occur extremely rapidly in association with the first breaths (Walsh et al., 1974), is a functional closure as haemodynamic changes hold the valve closed. The second is anatomical when the valve becomes fixed to the interatrial septum. The two important haemodynamic changes that result in closure are the increase in pulmonary blood flow and the cessation of the placental circulation. Increasing blood flow through the lung increases pulmonary venous return and elevates left atrial pressure to approximately 7 mm Hg, closing the valve of the foramen ovale. As more than half of the inferior vena cava flow is derived from umbilical venous return, removal of the placental circulation results in a marked fall in blood returning to the heart, also favouring closure.

Although functional closure of the foramen ovale occurs immediately after the onset of air breathing, or shortly thereafter, right-to-left shunting may persist for several days. It can be induced by pathophysiological conditions, which increase pulmonary vascular resistance and reduce pulmonary blood flow, and normal behaviours such as crying and straining. A small left-to-right shunt due to an incompetent valve is often present for several months after birth (Rudolph, 1974). Anatomical closure of the foramen ovale is a slow process which normally does not occur before the end of the first year of life. A small opening persists into adult life in about 25% of adults (Walsh et al., 1974) without shunting and with no functional handicap.

Closure of the ductus arteriosus

The ductus arteriosus is a muscular artery connecting the main pulmonary artery and the descending aorta which is widely patent in fetal life. Structurally, the ductus arteriosus differs from the two vessels it joins in that its wall is largely smooth muscle, while that of the pulmonary artery and aorta consists predominantly of elastic tissue (Walsh et al., 1974).

Patency of the ductus arteriosus in the human fetus and many animals is an active process effected by a prostaglandin. In lamb fetuses PGE_2 is believed to be the primary prostaglandin maintaining ductal patency, because it is the most potent ductus arteriosus-relaxing agent known; its action may be complemented by PGI_2, which is the major prostaglandin released by the ductus arteriosus (Coceani & Olley, 1980). Because local production of prostaglandins may not be adequate at fetal oxygen levels, circulating PGE_2 controls the ductus arteriosus (Clyman, 1987). PGE_2 concentrations are high in the fetal circulation, three to five times adult levels, due to low pulmonary blood flow and therefore low clearance, as well as to placental production (Challis et al., 1976). Pharmacological inhibition of prostaglandin synthesis constricts the fetal ductus in vitro and in vivo. This effect is more marked in immature lambs and, even in mature lambs, pharmacological constriction of the ductus arteriosus is almost equal to the powerful oxygen-induced constriction (Coceani & Olley, 1980).

At birth, increasing blood oxygen tension is the stimulus for closure of the ductus arteriosus. Postnatally, its calibre appears to be determined by a balance between oxygen-induced vasoconstriction on the one hand and the vasodilator effects of prostaglandins on the other (Heymann, 1985). Sensitivity to constriction by oxygen develops over the last third of gestation (Clyman, 1987). At the same time, the sensitivity to dilatation by PGE_2 and PGI_2 decreases with gestational age. At normal birth, the clearance of circulating PGE_2 is enhanced as pulmonary blood flow increases, favouring closure. Catabolism of PGE_2 by the fetal lung increases with gestational age (Clyman et al., 1981), so that pulmonary clearance is less and circulatory PGE_2 levels greater in the immature infant. Failure of the ductus arteriosus to close after birth in preterm infants may therefore reflect immaturity of pulmonary clearance and a greater sensitivity to dilatation by prostaglandins.

The fall in pulmonary artery pressure that normally occurs at birth may also facilitate closure, as the ductal constriction is more prominent at the pulmonary (low pressure) end than the aortic end of the vessel (Clyman et al., 1989). If pulmonary vascular resistance does not fall normally at birth, persistently elevated pulmonary artery pressure may oppose ductus constriction and preserve responsiveness to PGE_2.

In full-term infants and animals the ductus arteriosus begins to constrict soon after the onset of air breathing. The rate of this functional closure varies among species, from a few minutes in guinea pigs and rabbits to 15 h in humans (Clyman, 1987). In lambs, the functional closure is complete at 1 hour although a narrow anatomical patency may persist at 4 h (Smolich et al., 1991). In preterm infants, ductal patency frequently persists for several days.

Continuing patency of the ductus arteriosus has important consequences for the distribution of cardiac output and pulmonary blood flow. When pulmonary vascular resistance falls and while the ductus remains patent after normal birth, left ventricular output passes to the lung via a left-to-right ductal shunt, as well as to the systemic circulation. In these circumstances right ventricular output equals the effective blood flow through the systemic circulation, and is substantially less than left ventricular output (Emmanouilides et al., 1970; Gessner et al., 1965). In the preterm infant the 'steal' of a substantial portion of left ventricular output from the systemic to the pulmonary circulation may compromise blood flow to tissues such as the myocardium, diaphragm, and abdominal organs (Clyman, 1990).

Changes in the pulmonary circulation

The pulmonary circulation develops uniquely in utero, having on the one hand to develop a vascular bed large enough to accommodate the increase in blood flow at birth, while on the other to maintain a level of vascular resistance high enough to limit pulmonary blood flow and fetal cardiac output before birth. In the fetus, pulmonary blood flow under normal conditions of oxygenation averages about 150 ml/minute per 100g of lung tissue (Cohn et al., 1974; Iwamoto, Teitel & Rudolph, 1987), a level which is 'low' by comparison with postnatal flow but comparable to flow to other fetal organs such as the brain, an organ which is considered to be highly perfused in fetal life (Jones & Traystman, 1984; Szymonowicz et al., 1988).

'Low' pulmonary blood flow in the fetus is the result of high pulmonary vascular resistance, sustained by constriction of highly muscular, small pulmonary arteries. Fetal pulmonary vessels are highly reactive to a range of physiological stimuli from as early as 0.5 gestation. Constriction is stimulated by hypoxaemia, acidaemia, α-adrenergic catecholamines and sympathetic nerve stimulation, whereas dilatation is produced by oxygen, acetylcholine, β-adrenergic catecholamines, histamine, prostacyclin (PGI_2), and bradykinin. With advancing gestation, the reactivity of the fetal pulmonary vascular bed increases (Rudolph, 1977). Reflex pulmonary vasoconstriction acting via sympathetic nerves can be elicited in fetal lambs (Dawes, 1968). However, in utero there is little resting autonomic tone, as autonomic blockade (α-adrenergic, β-adrenergic and muscarinic) has no effect on pulmonary blood flow (Lewis, Heymann & Rudolph, 1976). Furthermore, autonomic blockade does not alter the pulmonary vasoconstriction which accompanies fetal hypoxaemia (Lewis et al., 1976) or the profound vasodilatation at birth (Dawes, 1968). Angiotensin II (AII) is considered to be important in the pulmonary vasoconstrictor response to hypoxaemia in the adult lung, but blockade of AII activity in fetal lambs has no effect on resting pulmonary vascular resistance or the vasoconstriction in response to hypoxaemia (Hyman et al., 1975). Rather, AII is a dilator of the fetal pulmonary circulation (Iwamoto & Rudolph, 1981).

Fetal pulmonary vasculature is extremely reactive to oxygen, and small differences of blood PO_2 cause large changes in pulmonary blood flow (Peeters, 1978). Thus, high pulmonary vascular resistance in the fetus can be attributed predominantly to hypoxic vasoconstriction, because pulmonary vessels are exposed to low blood PO_2. With advancing gestation, vasodilatation in response to oxygen increases; near term, raising fetal blood oxygen levels in utero without ventilating the lungs can induce the entire pulmonary flow increase that normally occurs at birth (Morin et al., 1988).

At birth, the important respiratory changes that occur in the lung are gaseous expansion and clearance of fetal lung liquid from the alveoli, rhythmic pulmonary ventilation, and an increase in the oxygen tension in the environment of the pulmonary vessels. The pulmonary vascular changes are illustrated in Fig. 7.3. Within minutes of the onset of spontaneous air breathing, pulmonary vascular resistance decreases to 10% of fetal values, and pulmonary flow increases approximately tenfold (Leffler, Hessler & Green, 1984). The rapid increases in alveolar and fetal blood oxygen levels occurring at this time (Comline & Silver, 1972; Berger et al., 1991) substantially explain these changes. The powerful vasodilating effect of oxygen alone (without ventilation) in the fetal lung has been demonstrated by studies of hyperbaric oxygenation, perfusion of unventilated lungs by oxygenated blood, and lung expansion with oxygenated liquids (Dawes, 1968; Morin et al., 1988).

The decrease in pulmonary vascular resistance at birth is also explained partly by mechanical expansion of the alveoli with gas. This effect has been attributed to the creation of surface forces at the gas–liquid interface within the alveoli which lower vascular resistance by decreasing perivascular pressure and physically expanding small vessels. Also, at least part of the mechanical response appears to be mediated by dilator prostaglan-

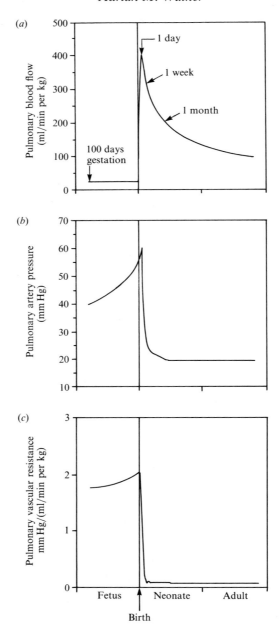

Fig. 7.3(*a*)(*b*)(*c*). Changes in the pulmonary circulation during fetal and neonatal life in lambs. For a description of the immediate changes occurring at birth see text. (Based on data from: Lewis et al., 1976; Leffler et al., 1984; Smolich, 1986; Davidson, 1987; Iwamoto et al., 1987; Smolich et al., 1991.)

dins. Expansion and rhythmic ventilation of fetal lungs (Leffler, Hessler & Terragno, 1980), and the onset of spontaneous air breathing (Leffler et al., 1984) stimulates pulmonary production of prostaglandins. Inhibition of prostaglandin synthesis by indomethacin does not prevent the rapid pulmonary vasodilatation which immediately follows the onset of air ventilation (Leffler, Tyler & Cassin, 1978), so this may be the result of physical forces. However, a slower component of the vasodilatation which develops subsequently is attenuated if prostaglandin production is blocked. Dilator prostaglandins which could play a role in the slow phase include PGI_2 and PGD_2 (Leffler et al., 1978, 1984; Cassin et al., 1981). Recently it has been proposed that bradykinin, which produces marked pulmonary vasodilatation, may be involved in each of these phases (Fineman, Soiffer & Heymann, 1991). In the rapid phase, it is envisaged that bradykinin stimulates release by the pulmonary endothelium of endothelium derived relaxing factor (EDRF), a powerful dilator of arterial smooth muscle; PGI_2 production, also stimulated by bradykinin, may be responsible for the subsequent slower fall of pulmonary vascular resistance.

Experimental studies in which gaseous ventilation and oxygenation have been studied sequentially have not succeeded in determining which of these changes at the onset of air breathing is the more important. Dawes (1968) attributed one third of the total vasodilatation caused by gaseous expansion of the lungs to each of ventilation, increasing oxygen levels and decreasing carbon dioxide levels. More recent studies have attributed almost the entire response to oxygenation alone (Morin et al., 1988) or ventilation alone (Teitel, Iwamoto & Rudolph, 1990); individual responses within a group of animals can vary between these two extremes (Teitel et al., 1990). As the lungs are liquid-filled in fetal life, and as the degree of lung inflation substantially affects pulmonary vascular resistance (Walker et al., 1988), it is possible that individual differences in lung liquid clearance and lung compliance produce varying responses in the pulmonary circulation at birth.

Changes in ventricular outputs

In the lamb fetus at term, the right ventricle ejects 300 ml/min per kg of fetal body weight, and the left ventricle ejects 150 ml/min per kg (Table 7.1). At birth, these outputs both increase to 400 ml/min per kg (Fig. 7.4); thus there is a modest increase in right ventricular output (about 30 %) and a very substantial increase of left ventricular output (more than 100 %). Studies of cardiac function at the onset of spontaneous breathing

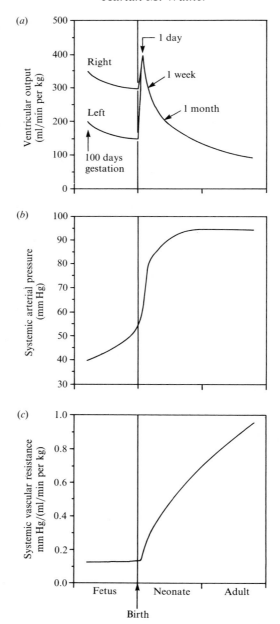

Fig. 7.4(*a*)(*b*)(*c*). Changes in the systemic circulation during fetal and neonatal life in lambs. For a description of the immediate changes occurring at birth see text. (Based on data from: Heymann et al., 1981; Lewis et al., 1976; Klopfenstein & Rudolph, 1978; Peeters, 1978; Berman and Musselman, 1979; Sidi et al., 1983; Smolich, 1986; Davidson, 1987; Iwamoto et al., 1987; Smolich et al., 1991.)

in the lamb (Smolich et al., 1991) show that both right and left ventricular output increase quite rapidly, within the first hour of birth. As functional closure of the ductus arteriosus occurs rapidly in lambs, right and left ventricular output are equal at this time. Increases of ventricular output, which closely parallel the rapid increases of heart rate and pulmonary flow, are sustained throughout the first day of life.

In full-term human infants of 2–34 h of age, ventricular outputs significantly exceed those in older children and adults (Emmanouilides et al., 1970). Due to continuing patency of the ductus arteriosus, there is a substantial left-to-right shunt of approximately 35%; thus left ventricular output (approximately 250ml/min per kg) exceeds right ventricular output (approximately 175 ml/min per kg). Cardiac outputs are greater after vaginal delivery than after elective Caesarean section delivery (Gessner et al., 1965), and (corrected for body weight) greater in healthy preterm infants than in full-term infants (Walther et al., 1985). A number of factors may contribute to the sudden and dramatic increase of ventricular outputs at birth, but the exact mechanisms are uncertain. The four cardiovascular factors that are important are heart rate, preload, afterload, and cardiac contractility (Rudolph, 1985).

High baseline levels of cardiac output in the fetus and newborn are partly explained by greater heart rate (Table 7.1). Further increases of heart rate are not effective in increasing cardiac output in the fetus as stroke volume falls (Walker et al., 1985). Nevertheless the rapid and substantial increase of heart rate that occurs at birth does contribute to the augmentation of cardiac output at this time, as stroke volume is maintained (Smolich et al., 1991). Further increments of heart rate are inefficient in the newborn and neonate, as the percentage increases of heart rate exceed the percentage increases of cardiac output (Walker et al., 1985; Sidi et al., 1983).

In adult life, the heart responds with progressively greater output as end-diastolic pressure (preload) is increased above normal – the Starling effect. At birth, left ventricular preload increases, but an increase in preload above normal resting levels has little effect on left ventricular output in the fetus (Faber et al., 1985). Decreases of end-diastolic pressure, however, are reflected by reductions in ventricular output. Thus the heart in the fetus and newborn operates at atrial pressures near the peak of the ventricular function curve (Starling curve), with essentially no reserve capacity (Rudolph, 1985). The physiological basis for this difference between fetal, newborn and adult Starling curves, as yet unexplained, may be related to the low compliance of fetal myocardium (Rudolph, 1985). As the fetal ventricle is very stiff, increases of filling pressure will have little effect in distending the ventricle and changing sarcomere length, the cellular basis of the Starling effect.

Mechanical factors associated with liquid clearance and gaseous expansion of the fetal lung at birth may also augment cardiac function via the Starling effect. Recently it has been recognised that the dimensions of the fetal heart are significantly influenced by the constraint of the surrounding tissues (rib cage, lungs and pericardium), just as in adults (Grant et al., 1988, 1991). The plateau of the fetal left ventricular function curve is largely a result of limitations imposed upon ventricular filling by thoracic tissues; when these are retracted from around the heart, the plateau is not observed and left ventricular stroke volume increases as preload is raised. In the fetus the fluid-filled lungs, as well as the amniotic fluid and maternal tissues, probably add to the constraint present in the adult thorax. At birth, the transition to air-filled lungs, together with relief of the constraint imposed by the amniotic fluid and maternal tissues, may contribute to the increase in cardiac output.

The developing heart is very sensitive to changes in afterload, presumably because of its structural immaturity. The fetal right ventricle is particularly sensitive to changes of arterial pressure (Thornburg & Morton, 1983, see Chapter 6); thus the rapid fall in pulmonary artery pressure occurring at birth probably contributes to the ability of the right ventricle to increase its output in the newborn. The fetal left ventricle is less sensitive to afterload than the right (Thornburg & Morton, 1986). Nevertheless, low afterload may enable the left ventricle to sustain high levels of output when the ductus arteriosus is patent and pulmonary vascular resistance is low; left ventricular stroke volume and output are substantially greater in infants with patent ductus arteriosus (Lindner et al., 1990).

Myocardial contractility in the first few days of life strikingly exceeds adult values (Klopfenstein & Rudolph, 1978; Berman & Musselman, 1979). This may be explained by the postnatal increase of arterial oxygen content, or by the birth-related surge in sympatho-adrenal stimulation which elevates plasma catecholamines to a life-time high level (Lagercrantz & Slotkin, 1986; Padbury & Martinez, 1988). The immediate postnatal rise of cardiac output requires the prenatal influence of thyroid hormone, as thyroidectomy prevents the normal increase (Breall, Rudolph & Heymann, 1984). Thyroid hormone might enhance cardiac function at birth by a modification of β-adrenergic receptor numbers or responsiveness, so improving the response to catecholamines.

Changes in arterial pressure

Systemic arterial pressure in the newborn lamb rises rapidly above fetal levels immediately after birth, then declines during the first day after birth (Leffler et al., 1984; Smolich et al., 1991). Similarly, arterial pressure is not substantially increased during the first day after birth in human infants (Oh, Lind & Gessner, 1966). Failure of arterial pressure to rise substantially at birth is seen after Caesarean section delivery and after vaginal delivery (Comline & Silver, 1972), although the immediate increase may be greater after vaginal delivery (Berger et al., 1990). Thus the mechanical effect of cord clamping and the elimination of the placental circulation are transient at most, in keeping with the haemodynamic studies of Guyton (1981) who demonstrated that the overshoot in systemic arterial pressure that occurs with abrupt closure of an arteriovenous shunt is transient, lasting approximately 1 minute.

The precise mechanisms which determine the level of arterial pressure immediately after birth are not known. As low arterial pressure persists after the ductus arteriosus closes (Smolich et al., 1991; Breall et al., 1984), low systemic blood flow due to left-to-right shunting is not an explanation for low levels of arterial pressure. Low vascular resistance can be partly explained by the requirement for high tissue blood flows to support increased metabolism and maintain body temperature on the day of birth. Subsequently over the first weeks of postnatal life in lambs systemic vascular resistance and arterial pressure rise toward adult values (Fig. 7.4).

Changes in regional circulations

At birth, overall systemic perfusion is not changed from fetal levels, but specific tissues do undergo quite substantial flow alterations. Myocardial blood flow changes (ml/min per 100 g tissue, Fig. 7.5(a)) reflect the perinatal changes in ventricular work and oxygen consumption (Fisher, 1984a; Smolich, 1986; Smolich et al., 1991). In the mature circulation the heart rate-arterial pressure product and the stroke volume–arterial pressure product are measures of myocardial work which correlate well with myocardial blood flow and oxygen consumption. Thus flow to the fetal right ventricular myocardium, reflecting the greater right ventricular output in the fetus, significantly exceeds that to the left in which the output is much less. The right–left flow ratio is reversed as myocardial flow to the left ventricle increases and flow to the right ventricle decreases

Adrian M. Walker

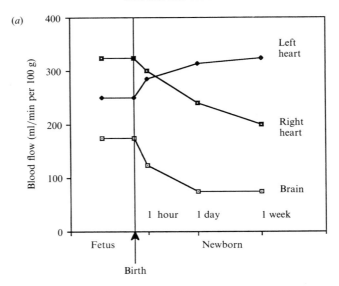

Fig. 7.5(*a*). Changes in regional blood flows in the fetal and newborn lamb at birth. (Based on data from: Jones & Traystman, 1984; Fisher, 1984*a, b*; Koehler et al., 1985; Jensen et al., 1986; Rosenberg et al., 1986; Iwamoto et al., 1987; Richardson et al., 1989*a, b*; Smolich et al., 1991.)

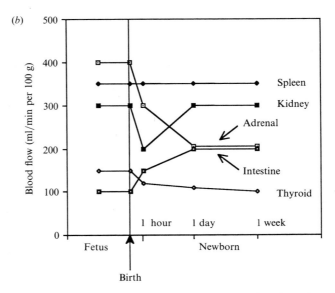

Fig. 7.5(*b*). Changes in regional blood flows in the fetal and newborn lamb at birth. (Based on data from: Aperia et al., 1977; Fisher, 1984*b*; Koehler et al., 1985; Jensen et al., 1986; Iwamoto et al., 1987; Richardson et al., 1989*b*; Smolich et al., 1991.)

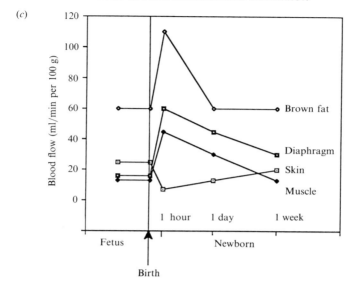

Fig. 7.5(*c*). Changes in regional blood flows in the fetal and newborn lamb at birth. (Based on data from: Fisher, 1984*b*; Koehler et al., 1985; Jensen et al., 1986; Iwamoto et al., 1987; Richardson et al., 1989*b*; Berger et al., 1991; Smolich et al., 1991.)

after birth. These myocardial flow changes are associated with the postnatal increase of aortic pressure and the decrease of pulmonary artery pressure, as well as the respective increases of ventricular outputs. The changes are gradual, much slower than the rapid changes in pulmonary artery pressure and arterial oxygenation which occur promptly with the onset of pulmonary ventilation, suggesting that there are significant alterations in myocardial oxygen metabolism in the perinatal period. Beyond 1 week of postnatal age there are continuing gradual changes of myocardial flow toward adult levels in association with substantial growth and remodelling of the myocardium (Smolich et al., 1989).

Cerebral blood flow decreases promptly and substantially after birth (Fig. 7.5(*a*)). As cerebral metabolic rate is not changed at birth (Richardson et al., 1989*a*), this change is largely in response to increasing arterial oxygen levels and possibly to decreasing arterial PCO_2, each of which are powerful vasoconstricting influences in the cerebral circulation. Regionally within the brain there is a significant redistribution of flow after birth; notably, cortical flow increases relative to brainstem and cerebellum, perhaps reflecting enhanced cortical activity in the newborn (Szymonowicz et al., 1988; Richardson et al., 1989*a*).

Kidney blood flow, presumably reflecting a perinatal continuity of renal function, is transiently depressed immediately after birth, but recovers promptly to fetal levels (Fig. 7.5(*b*)). Similarly, splenic and thyroid flows are unchanged at birth (Fig. 7.5(*b*)). Adrenal flow decreases progressively in inverse correlation to arterial oxygenation, whereas flow to the small intestine increases promptly following feeding (Fig. 7.5(*b*)). Tissues with significant thermoregulatory functions change substantially and rapidly at birth (Fig. 7.5(*c*)). Diaphragm flow, reflecting the high oxygen requirements of the newborn, and possibly increased work of breathing, increases significantly above the levels measured during fetal non-breathing periods and usually exceeds the flow measured during fetal breathing (Berger et al., 1991). Increasing flow to brown fat and skeletal muscle and decreasing skin flow are explained by the need for increased metabolic heat production and thermal insulation required to sustain body temperature in the newborn. Muscle flow may also be increased to support the postural needs of the awake lamb.

Neonatal circulation

Postnatal changes

During the first weeks of life there are substantial growth-related changes in the circulation related to changes in thermoregulatory capacity, oxygen consumption and the important haematological determinants of oxygen transport: the percentage of fetal haemoglobin, haemoglobin concentration, and oxygen affinity.

High cardiac output immediately after birth is required principally to sustain overall systemic perfusion, and only partly to support the increased oxygen metabolism required to maintain body temperature. The increased left ventricular output of the newborn results from the left ventricle taking over the perfusion of tissues that had been supplied by the right ventricle in utero. No increase of left ventricular output is required for increased perfusion of tissues, as on average these remain at fetal levels (Smolich et al., 1991). Thus, the greater oxygen requirements of the newborn immediately after birth are met by enhanced extraction of oxygen from arterial blood, not by increased blood flow. Subsequently cardiac output falls a little during the first week after birth to a level of 300 ml/min per kg. This change is due to a fall in stroke volume as the high perinatal level of heart rate is maintained throughout this period. With subsequent growth, cardiac output per kg of body weight declines quite rapidly over the first weeks of postnatal age, and then more slowly to the adult level of 100 ml/min per kg (Table 7.1). These postnatal changes in cardiac output are related to decreasing oxygen requirements for growth, which are very high in the neonatal period, and to maturing thermoregulatory ability (Sidi et al., 1983). Increasing efficiency of oxygen release in tissue because of the change from high affinity fetal haemoglobin to low affinity adult haemoglobin also reduces the requirement for high tissue flows, and hence cardiac output (Klopfenstein & Rudolph, 1978). Arterial pressure continues to rise slowly after the rapid increase during the first postnatal week due to steadily increasing peripheral vascular resistance. The associated fall in heart rate during this period is not a baroreflex adjustment, nor is it mediated by changes in basal autonomic tone, because the slower heart rate persists after autonomic blockade. Rather, the fall represents a developmental change in the intrinsic rate of the sino-atrial node (Walker, 1984).

Responses to stress

Associated with the high resting levels of cardiovascular performance, the capacity to increase cardiac output in response to stress (cardiac reserve) is extremely limited in the newborn (Rudolph, 1985). As the reserve is limited, redistribution of the available cardiac output is an important defence against stress in the newborn, just as it is in fetal life (Cohn et al., 1974).

In the newborn lamb, acute mild hypoxaemia is associated with systemic vasodilatation, tachycardia and limited, transient increases of cardiac output (Sidi et al., 1983; Fisher, 1984b; Koehler, Traystman & Jones, 1985). Blood flows to neural tissues (cerebrum, cerebellum and brain stem), the diaphragm, the myocardium, and the adrenal glands increase progressively in inverse relation to arterial oxygen content. Oxygen delivery (blood flow times arterial oxygen content) to the heart is increased and that to the brain is maintained constant by increased blood flow, at the expense of the spleen, gastrointestinal tract, skin and kidneys. These vasoconstrictor responses are much more intense in the newborn than in the adult vascular beds (Koehler et al., 1985). Vasoconstriction also occurs during hypercapnia in lambs, but not in adult sheep (Rosenberg, Jones & Koehler, 1984). With advancing age and greater structural maturity of the heart, the lamb is increasingly able to raise cardiac output and to maintain the rise in the face of longer and more severe exposures to hypoxia (Sidi et al., 1983). Thus, postnatal development of the cardiovascular response to stress is represented by a change from a primarily circulatory response (redistribution of cardiac output) in the newborn to a largely cardiac response (increasing cardiac output) in the adult.

Baroreceptor and chemoreceptor control

In adult life, arterial baroreceptors are the major sensing elements of the cardiovascular regulatory system. During fetal life, baroreceptors are functional from 0.6 gestation in lambs (Walker, 1984). With advancing gestation, baroreflex control of heart rate matures, as evidenced by an increasing proportion of positive responses to brief elevations of arterial pressure and by an increasing sensitivity of these responses, quantified by the ratio of heart rate slowing to the extent of blood pressure elevation (Shinebourne et al., 1972).

At birth, baroreceptor maturity differs between animal species according to general maturity. For example, cardiac slowing in response to elevation in arterial pressure is less well developed in the maternally dependent newborn puppy than in the more independent newborn lamb (Vatner & Manders, 1979). Nevertheless most species, including man, have a depressed baroreceptor-heart rate reflex at birth and a progressive postnatal maturation to adult levels (Dawes, Johnston & Walker, 1980). Surprisingly, the sensitivity of the baroreceptors themselves, measured by recording discharge in afferent fibres of the carotid sinus nerve or aortic nerve, is greater in the fetus and newborn than in the adult (Blanco et al., 1988; Hanson, 1988). Also, the efferent pathway is intact, as the vagus nerve can slow the heart from 0.4 gestation (Born, Dawes & Mott, 1956). Thus, the depressed baroreflex control of heart rate in fetal and newborn life appears to result from central nervous influences, as yet unidentified.

Baroreceptors are reset as blood pressure increases during fetal life and at birth (Blanco et al., 1988; Hanson, 1988). Resetting has two components. First, there is a movement to the right of the stimulus–response curve relating baroreceptor discharge to mean arterial blood pressure; this ensures that as baseline blood pressure increases basal baroreceptor discharge remains constant. Secondly, the sensitivity of the baroreceptors (the slope of the stimulus–response curve) is reduced. Resetting of fetal baroreflexes may occur promptly at birth, as resetting of adult baroreceptors upon exposure to elevated arterial pressure occurs rapidly, within 1 hour (Shepherd & Mancia, 1986).

Baroreflexes play an important role in regulating fetal blood pressure, as shown by increased blood pressure variability after arterial baroreceptor denervation (Yardley et al., 1983). In preterm infants, baroreceptors are functional from at least 25 weeks gestational age (Finley et al., 1984; Lagercrantz et al., 1990). In very preterm infants with a rapid baseline heart rate, there is little or no heart rate response to stimulating baroreceptors by postural tilting (Waldman, Krauss & Auld, 1979; Lagercrantz et al., 1990). However, peripheral vascular resistance responses serve to keep blood pressure constant. Older infants respond to tilting with changes in heart rate, signifying effective baroreflex control of the heart (Finley, Hamilton & MacKenzie, 1984).

Arterial chemoreceptors are active and sensitive to reductions of arterial oxygen levels in the fetus from at least 0.7 gestation (Hanson, 1988). These receptors respond to asphyxia in a way which is similar to adult receptors, producing bradycardia, increased arterial pressure and sympathetic vasoconstriction. At birth, chemoreceptors are silenced when oxygen levels increase, but remain sensitive to CO_2. Subsequently, over the first week of life, the chemoreceptors are slowly reset so that they become responsive within the adult range of arterial PO_2 (Kumar & Hanson, 1989). Postnatally, chemoreceptor stimulation also increases respiration which opposes the primary responses seen in fetal life, and produces secondary changes which include tachycardia and systemic vasodilatation.

Autonomic nervous system

Activation of the sympatho-adrenal system at birth has an important role in circulatory adaptation by supporting cardiac function and arterial pressure, and in several other adaptive processes including fetal lung liquid re-absorption, surfactant release, and non-shivering thermogenesis (Lagercrantz & Slotkin, 1986; Padbury & Martinez, 1988).

Autonomic control of the circulation begins during fetal life in many animal species. The parasympathetic arm of the cardiac innervation develops early in gestation, prior to the sympathetic innervation. In the human fetus , there is a progressive reduction of the baseline fetal heart rate from 15 weeks gestation to term which is due to growth in vagal inhibition which predominates over a smaller tonic sympathetic stimulation (Schifferli & Caldeyro-Barcia, 1973). During this period, the heart rate measured after autonomic blockade, the intrinsic heart rate, is constant. In the lamb, stimulation of the vagus can slow the heart from as early as 0.4 gestation, but the natural vagal slowing extends from 0.7 gestation to term (Walker, 1984). After increasing above fetal levels at birth, the heart rate declines progressively throughout neonatal life in the lamb; in human infants there is a peak in rate at about 1 month of age, and a decline thereafter throughout early childhood. The postnatal slowing is explained by a progressive fall in the intrinsic rate of the sino-atrial node; throughout this developmental phase a tonic vagal inhibition lowers the baseline heart rate below the intrinsic rate (Walker, 1984).

Sympathetic innervation in developing myocardium can be assessed using tissue concentrations of catecholamines as the heart stores of noradrenaline are located predominantly within sympathetic nerves (Friedman, 1972). Assessed in this way, myocardial innervation is incomplete at term and preterm birth because concentrations in the fetus are much less than in the adult. Adrenergic innervation is better developed in newborn animals that are relatively more independent at birth (Pappano, 1977). In the lamb, myocardial sympathetic innervation begins at 0.6 gestation and continues to develop after birth. Although sympathetic innervation is incomplete, other tissues, principally the adrenal medulla and also the paraganglia, are sources of catecholamines in the newborn (Lagercrantz & Slotkin, 1986).

Plasma catecholamine concentrations in the lamb fetus increase gradually from 0.7 gestation, then rapidly 2–3 days prior to delivery (Comline & Silver, 1966; Jones, 1980). At parturition, beginning with the onset of labour (Eliot et al., 1981), there is a marked increase of sympatho-adrenal activity. Sequential measurements in lambs before and after birth show that plasma adrenaline and noradrenaline levels increase abruptly in the immediate minutes after birth (Davidson, 1987) This period is associated with rapid falls in arterial pH and body temperature, transient falls of PO_2, and transient increases of PCO_2, all potent stimuli for activation of the sympatho-adrenal system. Umbilical cord cutting is also a potent stimulus for catecholamine release (Padbury et al., 1981). Vaginal delivery is associated with greater increases of plasma catecholamines than Caesarean section (Faxelius, Lagercrantz & Yao, 1984) and catecholamines are further increased when there is evidence of fetal distress (Bistoletti et al., 1983). Even healthy infants have higher catecholamine levels at birth than severely stressed or exercising adults (Lagercrantz & Slotkin, 1986). The preterm lamb shows a more substantial increase of plasma catecholamines at birth than the full-term lamb (Padbury et al., 1985). In contrast, the associated haemodynamic changes (increased heart rate and blood pressure) are less pronounced in the preterm lamb. These blunted physiological responses in the face of a greater catecholamine surge probably represent immature target tissue receptor–effector mechanisms in the preterm lamb (Padbury et al., 1985).

Vasoactive substances

In addition to the surge in plasma catecholamines, plasma concentrations of other vasoactive substances change significantly at birth. The renin–angiotensin system is, in utero and in the perinatal period, in a state of hyperactivity relative to that of the adult (Broughton- Pipkin & Symonds, 1984). Plasma renin activity and angiotensin II (AII) concentrations are elevated following delivery, particularly so in preterm infants, and somewhat less after Caesarean section delivery (Lumbers & Reid, 1977). Increases of AII occur in the immediate minutes after delivery (Davidson, 1987) then decline over the next hour. AII is a powerful vasoconstrictor of systemic arteries, more potent on a molecule-for-molecule basis than catecholamines (Lumbers & Reid, 1978). Resting AII production has a role in maintaining normal fetal blood pressure, since injection of the angiotensin antagonist saralasin causes systemic arterial pressure to fall (Heymann et al., 1981). In the newborn, AII may play an important role in maintaining systemic arterial pressure as lambs given an inhibitor of AII formation before birth develop hypotension after birth (Davidson, 1987). In the fetal pulmonary circulation AII markedly increases flow and decreases vascular resistance (Iwamoto & Rudolph, 1981). Thus AII may contribute to the pulmonary vasodilatation at birth, perhaps by inducing the pulmonary endothelium to release the dilator prostacyclin (PGI_2) (Omini, Vigano & Marini, 1983). Nevertheless, activity of the fetal renin–angiotensin system is not crucial at birth, as fetal lambs survive delivery following bilateral nephrectomy (Thorburn, 1974).

In the neonate, the renin–angiotensin system may contribute to cardiovascular homeostasis through blood volume regulation, as well as direct vascular effects. The last trimester fetus and the newborn have fully functional osmoreceptor and volume control systems (Robillard et al., 1979) and high renin–angiotensin activity may offset the low antidiuretic hormone concentrations in neonatal plasma (Broughton-Pipkin & Symonds, 1984).

Prostaglandin concentrations in fetal plasma and in umbilical cord blood following vaginal or Caesarean section delivery exceed maternal levels (Heymann, Iwamoto & Rudolph, 1981). After birth, prostaglandin levels decrease rapidly, reflecting the removal of the placental site of production and increased catabolism in the lung. Prostaglandin PGE_2 has important vasodilator properties in the fetal circulation, particularly in maintaining patency of the ductus arteriosus. The marked fall in PGE_2 concentrations after birth could contribute to the postnatal rise in arterial pressure via peripheral vasoconstriction (Heymann et al., 1981), but this has not yet been examined.

The endothelium plays important roles in regulating vascular resistance and blood flow by releasing several vasoactive substances. These include dilators such as PGI_2, the peptide bradykinin, and endothelium derived relaxing factor (EDRF), and constrictors, such as endothelin.

As stimuli for their release include haemodynamic forces such as increase in blood flow and endothelial stress, factors which occur in the pulmonary circulation at birth, it has been suggested that release of EDRF acts synergistically with PGI_2 to contribute to the reduction of pulmonary resistance at birth (Abman et al., 1990). Recently it has been proposed that bradykinin may act to stimulate pulmonary endothelial release of PGI_2 and EDRF (Fineman et al., 1991). In support of the suggestion, inhibition of EDRF production attenuates the rise of pulmonary flow at delivery (Abman et al., 1990). Endothelin is a newly described peptide with potent vasoconstrictor actions on the ductus arteriosus and in many vascular beds (Coceani, Armstrong & Kelsey, 1989). Thus endothelin may contribute to closure of the ductus arteriosus at birth, and as it is released from the vascular endothelium of umbilical vessels and found in high concentrations in fetal cord plasma, it may also contribute to umbilical cord constriction at birth (Haegerstrand et al., 1989; Nakamura et al., 1990). Endothelin is a dilator of the newborn pulmonary circulation, not a constrictor (Bradley, Czaja & Goldstein, 1990). Whether this action, and its actions on the ductus arteriosus and cord vessels, contribute to the circulatory transitions at birth remains speculative.

Atrial natriuretic factors (ANF) are circulating peptide hormones during fetal and postnatal life with potent diuretic, natriuretic, and vasodilator actions (Smith et al., 1989). ANF granules are present in ventricular and atrial myocytes of fetal and newborn animals, and concentrate in atrial cells as maturation progresses. In adult animals, a rise in atrial pressure causes release of ANF, a shift of fluid from the vascular to the interstitial space, an increase of urine output, and a reduction of blood volume. A potential role for ANF at birth is suggested by the high levels in fetal blood, and the increases in the first week postnatally. In addition to its volume regulatory actions, recent studies indicate that ANF may have important actions in the lung in newborn life, opposing pulmonary vasoconstriction and fluid accumulation (Baertschi & Teague, 1989). However, the exact roles of ANF in perinatal life remain to be determined.

Cardiovascular system in sleep

In man and other animal species behavioural states develop during fetal life. In utero, stable behavioural states can be recognized using real-time ultrasonic imaging of the fetus after 35 weeks gestational age. Distinct behavioural states are also recognizable in neonates with a gestational age of 35 weeks or more. Several states may be recognized based upon observation of behavioural features, supplemented by physiological recording: active sleep (also called rapid-eye movement sleep, REM); quiet sleep (also called non-REM, NREM or slow-wave sleep); indeterminate sleep; and quiet and active wakefulness. In preterm infants of less than 35 weeks gestation, cycles of rest and activity, regular and irregular breathing and other behavioural features, as seen in older infants, are present but alternate independently. When these become more coincident after 35 weeks and alternate in synchrony, they are recognized as true behavioural states (Casaer & Devlieger, 1984). At birth total sleep time, and in particular REM sleep duration, is at a lifetime maximum (Roffwarg, Muzio & Dement, 1966). With postnatal growth, distinct phases of sleep emerge: the stages 1–4 of quiet sleep; and the two phases of REM sleep, the longer-lasting more steady (tonic) phase and the brief, excitatory (phasic) phase. In newborns phasic REM is predominant, and the term active sleep is used to describe REM in early life.

Sleep state cycling has significant impact upon cardiovascular function and control throughout fetal and postnatal development. Contrasting behavioural state-related differences of heart rate, cardiac output and blood pressure show, as expected, highest values in alert wakefulness. Comparing sleep states, the most prominent feature of the cardiovascular system which is common to all species is the very great variability of heart rate and blood pressure in active sleep, explained by the specific nature of cardiorespiratory control in this state. During sleep, the control system receives excitatory inputs from central and peripheral chemoreceptors (the metabolic drive) and from other regions of the brain that control behaviour (behavioural drive) (Phillipson & Bowes, 1986). Behavioural drive dominates cardiorespiratory control during active wakefulness and active sleep. In quiet sleep, and perhaps during quiet wakefulness and the tonic phase of active sleep, when the cardiorespiratory system is under metabolic control, the cardiovascular system is more stable.

Cardiac output in lambs can be very high in active sleep, exceeding values in quiet sleep and other states of wakefulness (Sibley, Walker & Maloney, 1982). However, average cardiac output values in active sleep are comparable to quiet sleep and wakefulness at normal ambient temperatures (Berger, Horne & Walker, 1989). Cardiac output in active sleep becomes less than in other states when ambient temperature is lowered, because thermoregulatory compensations, which include increases of cardiac output and oxygen consumption, are suspended in active sleep.

Heart rate in active sleep in lambs is usually slightly lower than in other behavioural states, so that stroke volume is elevated (Walker et al., 1986); mean arterial pressure is comparable in quiet wakefulness, quiet sleep and active sleep. Human newborns have slightly faster heart rates, averaging about 4 beats/min greater, and slightly elevated blood pressure (about 5 mm Hg greater) in active sleep compared with quiet sleep (Haddad et al., 1980; Mukhtar, Cowan & Stothers, 1982). Faster heart rate in active sleep may reflect greater body movement in this state, and is also found in other newborn species, e.g. the kitten (Egbert & Katona, 1980). Heart rate differences between sleep states are minor compared to the striking developmental difference resulting from preterm birth. In preterm infants heart rate is about 35 beats/min greater in quiet and active sleep than in the same states in full-term infants (Rose, 1983).

Behavioural states may also influence the distribution of cardiac output. The most prominent changes occur in the cerebral circulation, in which blood flow increases in active sleep in several animal species, in adult man, and in newborn infants (Mancia & Zanchetti, 1980; Mukhtar et al., 1982). Even in animals that do not increase total brain flow in active sleep, there is a redistribution of flow toward the brainstem, the brain region in which active sleep is generated (Cote & Haddad, 1990). By contrast, blood flow to most skeletal muscle groups, and particularly to the intercostals and diaphragm, is lower in active sleep than in quiet sleep (Cote & Haddad, 1990).

As yet there is little information to assess reflex control of the circulation in sleep in newborn life. Baroreceptor control of heart rate is similar in quiet sleep and active sleep in lambs (Horne et al., 1989, 1991) and in full-term and preterm infants (Finley et al., 1984). Reflex control of blood pressure may be impaired in active sleep, as arterial pressure decreases more following haemorrhage in this state than during quiet sleep or quiet wakefulness (Fewell, Williams & Hill, 1984). Other reflex responses, for example heart rate acceleration in response to tactile stimulation, may differ in quiet sleep and active sleep in preterm infants (Rose, 1983).

References

Abman, S. H., Chatfield, B. A., Hall, S. L. & McMurtry, I. F. (1990). Role of endothelium-derived relaxing factor during transition of pulmonary circulation at birth. *American Journal of Physiology,* **259** (Heart & Circulatory Physiology 28), H1921–7.

Adeagbo, A. S. O., Coceani, F. & Olley, P. M. (1982). The response of the lamb ductus venosus to prostaglandins and inhibitors of prostaglandin and thromboxane synthesis. *Circulation Research,* **51**, 580–6.

Anderson, D., Faber, J., Morton, M., Parks, C., Pinson, C. & Thornburg, K. (1985). Flow through the foramen ovale of the fetal and newborn lamb. *Journal of Physiology,* **365**, 29–40.

Aperia, A., Broberger, O., Herin, P. & Joelsson, I. (1977). Renal hemodynamics in the perinatal period. A study in lambs. *Acta Physiologia Scandinavia,* **99**, 261–9.

Baertschi, A. J. & Teague, W. G. (1989). Alveolar hypoxia is a powerful stimulus for ANF release in conscious lambs. *American Journal of Physiology,* **256** (Heart & Circulatory Physiology 25), H990–8.

Behrman, R. E., Lees, M. H., Peterson, E. N., De Lannoy, C. W. & Seeds, A. E. (1970). Distribution of the circulation in the normal and asphyxiated fetal primate. *American Journal of Obstetrics and Gynecology,* **108**, 956–69.

Berger, P. J., Horne, R. S. C., Soust, M., Walker, A. M. & Maloney, J. E. (1990). Breathing at birth and the associated blood gas and pH changes in the lamb. *Respiration Physiology,* 251–66.

Berger, P. J., Horne, R. S. C. & Walker, A. M. (1989). Cardio-respiratory responses to cool differ with sleep-state in newborn lambs. *Journal of Physiology,* **412**, 351–63.

Berger, P. J., Soust, M., Smolich, J. J. & Walker, A. M. (1991). Respiratory muscle blood flow in the lamb before and after birth (In press).

Berman, W. & Musselman, J. (1979). Myocardial peformance in the newborn lamb. *American Journal of Physiology,* **237** (Heart & Circulatory Physiology 6), H66–70.

Bistoletti, P., Nylund, L., Lagercrantz, H., Hjendahl, P. & Strom, H. (1983). Fetal scalp catecholamines during labour. *American Journal of Obstetrics and Gynecology,* **1467(7)**, 785–8.

Blanco, C. E., Dawes, G. S., Hanson, M. A. & McCooke, H. B. (1988). Carotid baroreceptors in fetal and newborn sheep. *Pediatric Research,* **24**, 342–6.

Born, G. V. R., Dawes, G. S. & Mott, J. C. (1956). Oxygen lack and autonomic control of the foetal circulation in the lamb. *Journal of Physiology,* **134**, 149–66.

190 *Adrian M. Walker*

Bradley, L. M., Czaja, J. F. & Goldstein, R. E. (1990). Circulatory effects of endothelin in newborn piglets. *American Journal of Physiology,* **259** (Heart & Circulatory Physiology 28), H1613–17.

Breall, J. A., Rudolph, A. M. & Heymann, M. A. (1984). Role of thyroid hormone in postnatal circulatory and metabolic adjustments. *Journal of Clinical Investigation,* **73**, 1418–24.

Broughton-Pipkin, F. & Symonds, E. M. (1984). Renin-angiotensin system in early life. In *Fetal Physiology and Medicine*, ed. R. W. Beard & P. W. Nathanielsz. 2nd edn. Marcel-Dekker Inc, Butterworths, New York.

Casaer, P. & Devlieger, H. (1984). The behavioural state in human perinatal life. *Journal of Developmental Physiology,* **6**, 187–94.

Cassin, S., Tod, M., Philips, J., Frisinger, J., Jordan, J. & Gibbs, C. (1981). Effects of prostaglandin D2 on perinatal circulation. *American Journal of Physiology,* **240** (Heart & Circulatory Physiology 9), H755–60.

Challis, J. R. G., Dilley, S. R., Robinson, J. S. & Thorburn, G. D. (1976). Prostaglandins in the circulation of the fetal lamb. *Prostaglandins,* **11**, 1041–52.

Clyman, R. I. (1987). Ductus arteriosus: current theories of prenatal and postnatal regulation. *Seminars in Perinatology,* **11**, 64–71.

Clyman, R. I. (1990). Developmental physiology of ductus arteriosus. In *Fetal and Neonatal Cardiology,* ed. A. Walker & A. Long. pp. 64–75. Saunders, Philadelphia.

Clyman, R. I., Mauray, F., Heymann, M. A. & Roman, C. (1981). Effect of gestational age on pulmonary metabolism of prostaglandin E1 and E2. *Prostaglandins,* **21**, 505–13.

Clyman, R. I., Mauray, F., Heymann, M. & Roman, C. (1989). Influence of increased pulmonary vascular pressures on the closure of the ductus arteriosus in newborn lambs. *Pediatric Research,* **25**, 136–42.

Clyman, R. I., Roman, C., Heymann, M. & Mauray, F. (1987). How a patent ductus arteriosus effects the preterm lambs ability to handle additional volume loads. *Pediatric Research,* **22**, 531–5.

Coceani, F., Armstrong, C. & Kelsey, L. (1989). Endothelin is a potent constrictor of the lamb ductus arteriosus. *Canadian Journal of Physiology and Pharmacology,* **67**, 902–4.

Coceani, F. & Olley, P. M. (1980). Role of prostaglandins, prostacyclin and thromboxanes in the control of prenatal patency and postnatal closure of the ductus arteriosus. *Seminars in Perinatology,* **4**, 109–13.

Cohn, H. E., Sacks, E. J., Heymann, M. A. & Rudolph, A. M. (1974). Cardiovascular responses to hypoxaemia and acidaemia in fetal lambs. *American Journal of Obstetrics and Gynecology,* **120**, 817–24.

Comline, R. S. & Silver, M. (1966). Development of activity in the adrenal medulla of the foetus and newborn animals. *British Medical Bulletin,* **22**, 16–20.

Comline, R. S. & Silver, M. (1972). The composition of foetal and maternal blood during parturition in the ewe. *Journal of Physiology,* **222**, 233–56.

Cote, A. & Haddad, G. G. (1990). Effect of sleep on regional blood flow distribution in piglets. *Pediatric Research,* **28**, 218–22.

Davidson, D. (1987). Circulating vasoactive substances and hemodynamic adjustments at birth in lambs. *Journal of Applied Physiology,* **63**, 676–84.

Dawes, G. S. (1968). Foetal and neonatal Physiology. Year Book Medical Publishers, Chicago, Ill.

Dawes, G. S., Johnston, B. M. & Walker, D. W. (1980). Relationship of arterial pressure and heart rate in fetal, newborn and adult sheep. *Journal of Physiology,* **309**, 405–17.

Edelstone, D. I. (1980). Regulation of blood flow through the ductus venosus. *Journal of Developmental Physiology,* **2**, 219–38.

Edelstone, D. I. & Rudolph, A. M. (1979). Preferential streaming of ductus venosus blood to the brain and heart in fetal lambs. *American Journal of Physiology,* **237** (Heart & Circulatory Physiology 6), H724–9.

Edelstone, D. I., Rudolph, A. M. & Heymann, M. A. (1978). Liver and ductus venosus blood flows in fetal lambs in utero. *Circulation Research,* **42**, 426–33.

Egbert, J. R. & Katona, P. G. (1980). Development of autonomic heart rate control in the kitten during sleep. *American Journal of Physiology,* **238** (Heart & Circulatory Physiology 7), H829–35.

Eliot, R. J., Klein, A. H., Glatz, T. H., Nathanielsz, P. W. & Fisher, D. A. (1981). Plasma norepinephrine, epinephrine and dopamine concentrations in maternal and fetal sheep during spontaneous parturition and in premature sheep during cortisol-induced parturition. *Endocrinology,* **108**, 1678–82.

Emmanouilides, G. C., Moss, A. J., Monset-Couchard, M., Marcano, B. A. & Rzeznic, B. (1970). Cardiac output in newborn infants. *Biology of the Neonate,* **15**, 186–97.

Faber, J. J., Anderson, D. F., Morton, J. F. et al. (1985). Birth, its physiology, and the problems it creates. In *The Physiological Development of the Fetus and Newborn,* ed. C. T. Jones & P. W. Nathanielsz. part 4. pp 371–380. Academic Press Inc, London.

Faxelius, G., Lagercrantz, H. & Yao, A. (1984). Sympathoadrenal activity and peripheral blood flow after birth: comparison in infants delivered vaginally and by Caesarean section. *Journal of Pediatrics,* **105**, 144–8.

Fewell, J. E., Williams, B. J. & Hill, D. E. (1984). Behavioural state influences the cardiovascular response to hemorrhage in lambs. *Journal of Developmental Physiology,* **6**, 339–48.

Fineman, J. R., Soiffer, S. J. & Heymann, M. A. (1991). The role of pulmonary vascular endothelium in perinatal pulmonary circulatory regulation. *Seminars in Perinatology,* **15**, 58–62.

Finley, J. P., Hamilton, R. & MacKenzie, M. G. (1984). Heart rate response to tilting in newborns in quiet and active sleep. *Biology of the Neonate,* **45**, 1–10.

Fisher, D. J. (1984*a*). Oxygenation and metabolism in the developing heart. *Seminars in Perinatology,* **8(3)**, 217–25.

Fisher, D. J. (1984*b*). Cardiac output and regional blood flows during hypoxaemia in unanaesthetized newborn lambs. *Journal of Developmental Physiology,* **6**, 485–94.

Friedman, W. J. (1972). The intrinsic physiologic properties of the developing heart. In *Neonatal Heart Disease,* ed. W. F. Friedman, M. Lesch & E. H. Sonnenblick. pp. 21–49. Grune and Stratton, New York.

Gessner, I., Krovetz, L. J., Benson, R. W., Prystowsky, H., Stenger, V. & Eitzman, D. V. (1965). Hemodynamic adaptations in the newborn infant. *Pediatrics,* **36**, 752–62.

Grant, D. A., Kondo, C. S., Takahashi, Y., ter Keurs, H. E. D. J., Tyberg, J. V. & Maloney, J. E. (1988). Pericardial influences on the left ventricle of the neonatal lamb. In *Fetal and Neonatal Development*, ed. C. T. Jones. pp. 150–152. Perinatology Press, New York.

Grant, D. A., Maloney, J. E., Tyberg, J. V. & Walker, A. M. (1991). Effects of external constraint on the fetal left ventricular function curve. *Circulation* (In press).

Guyton, A. C. (1981). *The Textbook of Medical Physiology* (6th ed.). Philadelphia, PA: Saunders, pp. 277–278.

Haddad, G. G., Epstein, R. A., Epstein, M. A. F., Leistner, H. L. & Mellins, R. B. (1980). The R-R interval and R-R variability in normal infants during sleep. *Pediatric Research*, **14**, 809–11.

Haegerstrand, A., Hemsen, A., Larsson, C. O. & Lundberg, J. M. (1989). Endothelin: presence in human umbilical vessels, high levels in fetal blood and potent constrictor effect. *Acta Physiologica Scandinavica*, **137**, 541–2.

Hanson, M. A. (1988). The importance of baro- and chemoreflexes in the control of the fetal cardiovascular system. *Journal of Developmental Physiology*, **10**, 491–511.

Harvey, W. (1847). *The Works of William Harvey*. Translated from the Latin by Willis, R. The Sydenham Society, London. pp. 77–78.

Heymann, M. A. (1985). Management of the newborn circulation. In *The Physiological Development of the Fetus and Newborn*, part 7. ed. C. T. Jones & P. W. Nathanielsz. pp 721–731. Academic Press Inc, London.

Heymann, M. A., Iwamoto, H. S. & Rudolph, A. M. (1981). Factors effecting changes in the neonatal systemic circulation. *Annual Review of Physiology*, **43**, 371–83.

Horne, R. S. C., Berger, P. J., Bowes, G. B. & Walker, A. M. (1989). Acute hypotension and arousal from sleep in intact and sino-aortic denervated newborn lambs. *American Journal of Physiology*, **256** (Heart & Circulatory Physiology 25) H434–40.

Horne, R. S. C., de Preu, N. D., Berger, P. J. & Walker, A. M. (1991). Arousal responses to hypertension in lambs: effect of sino-aortic denervation. *American Journal of Physiology* (In press).

Hyman, A., Heymann, M. A., Levin, D. L. & Rudolph, A. M. (1975). Angiotensin is not the mediator of hypoxia induced pulmonary vasoconstriction in fetal lambs. *Circulation*, **52**, 11–132.

Iwamoto, H. S., Kaufman, T. et al. (1989). Responses to acute hypoxaemia in fetal sheep at 0.6–0.7 gestation. *American Journal of Physiology*, **256** (Heart & Circulatory Physiology 25), H613–20.

Iwamoto, H. S., Teitel, D. & Rudolph, A. M. (1987). Effects of birth-related events on blood flow distribution. *Pediatric Research*, **22**, 634–40.

Iwamoto, H. S. & Rudolph, A. R. (1981). Effects of angiotensin II on the blood flow and its distribution in fetal lambs. *Circulation Research*, **48**, 183–9.

Jensen, A., Bamford, O. S., Dawes, G. S., Hofmeyr, G. & Parkes, M. J. (1986). Changes in organ blood flow between high and low voltage electrocortical activity in fetal sheep. *Journal of Developmental Physiology*, **8**, 187–94.

Jones, C. T. (1980). Circulating catecholamines in the fetus, their origin, actions and significance. In *Biogenic amines in development*, ed. H. Parvez & S. Parvez. pp. 63–86. Elsevier/North Holland Biomedical Press, Amsterdam.

Jones, M. D. & Traystman, R. J. (1984). Cerebral oxygenation of the fetus, newborn and adult. *Seminars in Perinatology*, **8**, 205–16.

Klopfenstein, H. S. & Rudolph, A. M. (1978). Postnatal changes in the circulation and responses to volume loading in sheep. *Circulation Research,* **42**, 839–45.

Koehler, R. C., Traystman, R. J. & Jones, M. D. Jr. (1985). Regional blood flow and O_2 transport during hypoxic and CO hypoxia in neonatal and adult sheep. *American Journal of Physiology,* **248** (Heart & Circulatory Physiology 17), H118–24.

Kumar, P. & Hanson, M. A. (1989). Re-setting of the hypoxic sensitivity of aortic chemoreceptors in the new-born lamb. *Journal of Developmental Physiology,* **11**, 199–206.

Lagercrantz, H., Edwards, D., Henderson-Smart, D., Hertzberg, T. & Jeffery, H. (1990). Autonomic reflexes in preterm infants. *Acta Paediatrica Scandinavica,* **79**, 721–8.

Lagercrantz, H. & Slotkin, T. A. (1986). The 'stress' of being born. *Scientific American,* **254(4)**, 92–102.

Leffler, C. W., Hessler, J. R. & Green, R. S. (1984). The onset of breathing at birth stimulates pulmonary vascular prostacyclin synthesis. *Pediatric Research,* **18**, 938–42.

Leffler, C. W., Hessler, J. R. & Terragno, N. A. (1980). Ventilation induced release of prostaglandin-like material from fetal lungs. *American Journal of Physiology,* **238** (Heart & Circulatory Physiology 7), H282–6.

Leffler, C. W., Tyler, T. L. & Cassin, S. (1978). Effect of indomethacin on pulmonary vascular response to ventilation of fetal goats. *American Journal of Physiology,* **234** (Heart & Circulatory Physiology 3), H346–51.

Lewis, A. B., Heymann, M. A. & Rudolph, A. M. (1976). Gestational change in pulmonary vascular responses in fetal lambs in utero. *Circulation Research,* **39**, 536–41.

Lind, J. & Gessner, I. H. (1966). The circulatory and respiratory adaptation to early and late cord clamping in newborn infants. *Acta Paediatrica Scandinavica,* **55**, 17–22.

Lindner, W., Seidel, M., Versmold, H., Dohlemann, C. & Riegel, K. (1990). Stroke volume and ventricular output in preterm infants with patent ductus arteriosus. *Pediatric Research,* **27**, 278–81.

Longo, L. D., Wyatt, J. F., Hewitt, C. W. & Gilbert, R. D. (1978). A comparison of circulatory responses to hypoxic hypoxia and carbon monoxide hypoxia in fetal blood flow and oxygenation. In *Fetal and Newborn Cardiovascular Physiology,* ed. L. D. Longo & D. D. Reneau. pp. 257–287. Garland Press, New York.

Lumbers, E. R. & Reid, G. C. (1977). Effects of vaginal delivery and caesarian section on plasma renin activity and angiotensin II levels in human umbilical cord blood. *Biology of the Neonate,* **31**, 127–34.

Lumbers, E. R. & Reid, G. C. (1978). The actions of vasoactive compounds in the foetus and the effect of perfusion through the placenta on their biological activity. *Australian Journal of Experimental Biology and Medical Science,* **56**, 11–24.

Mancia, G. & Zanchetti, A. (1980). Cardiovascular regulation during sleep. In *Physiology in Sleep,* ed. J. Orem & C. D. Barnes. pp. 1–55. Academic Press, New York.

Meyer, W. W. & Lind, J. (1966). The ductus venosus and the mechanisms of its closure. *Archives of Disease in Childhood,* **41**, 597–605.

Morin, F. C. III, Egan, E. A., Ferguson, W. & Lundgren, C. E. G. (1988).

Development of pulmonary vascular response to oxygen. *American Journal of Physiology*, **254** (Heart & Circulatory Physiology 23), H542–6.

Mukhtar, A. I., Cowan, F. M. & Stothers, J. K. (1982). Cranial blood flow and blood pressure changes during sleep in the human neonate. *Early Human Development*, **6**, 59–64.

Nakamura, T., Kasai, K., Konuma, S., Emoto, T., Banba, N., Ishikawa, M. & Simoda, S-I. (1990). Immunoreactive endothelin concentrations in maternal and fetal blood. *Life Sciences*, **46**, 1045–50.

Oh, W., Lind, J. & Gessner, I. H. (1966). The circulatory and respiratory adaptation to early and late cord clamping in newborn infants. *Acta Paediatrica Scandinavica*, **55**, 17–22.

Omini, C., Vigano, T. & Marini, A. (1983). Angiotensin II: A releaser of PGI2 from fetal and newborn lungs. *Prostaglandins*, **25**, 901–10.

Padbury, J. F., Diakomanolis, E. S., Hobel, C. J., Perlman, A. & Fisher, D. A. (1981). Neonatal adaption: sympathoadrenal response to umbilical cord cutting. *Pediatric Research*, **15**, 1483–7.

Padbury, J. F. & Martinez, A. M. (1988). Sympathoadrenal system activity at birth: integration of postnatal adaptation. *Seminars in Perinatology*, **12**, 163–72.

Padbury, J. F., Polk, D. H., Newnham, J. P. & Lam, R. W. (1985). Neonatal adaption: greater sympathoadrenal response in preterm than full-term fetal sheep at birth. *American Journal of Physiology*, **248** (Endocrinology & Metabolism 11) E443–9.

Pappano, A. J. (1977). Ontogenetic development of autonomic neuroeffector transmission and transmitter reactivity in embryonic and fetal hearts. *Pharmacology Review*, **29**, 3–33.

Paton, J. B., Fisher, D. E., Peterson, E. N., DeLannoy, C. W. & Behrman, R. E. (1973). Cardiac output and organ blood flows in the baboon fetus. *Biology of the Neonate*, **22**, 50–7.

Peeters, L. L. H. (1978). *Fetal Blood Flow at Various Levels of Oxygen*. Leiter-Nijpels bv, Maastricht, Holland.

Peeters, L. L. H., Sheldon, R. E., Jones, M. D. Jr, Makowski, E. L. & Meschia, G. (1979). Blood flow to fetal organs as a function of arterial oxygen content. *American Journal of Obstetrics and Gynecology*, **135**, 637–46.

Phillipson, E. A. & Bowes, G. (1986). Control of breathing during sleep. In *Handbook of Physiology. The Respiratory System. Control of Breathing*, ed. M.D. Bethesda. sect. 3, vol II, pt 2, pp. 649–689. American Physiological Society.

Reuss, L. & Rudolph, (1980). Distribution and recirculation of umbilical and systemic venous blood flow in fetal lambs during hypoxia. *Journal of Developmental Physiology*, **2**, 71–84.

Richardson, B. S., Carmichael, L., Homan, J. & Gagnon, R. (1989a). Cerebral oxidative metabolism in lambs during perinatal period: relationship to electrocortical state. *American Journal of Physiology*, **257** (Regulatory Integrative Comparative Physiology 26), R1251–7.

Richardson, B. S., Carmichael, L., Homan, J., Tanswell, K. & Webster, A. C. (1989b). Regional blood flow change in the lamb during the perinatal period. *American Journal of Obstetrics and Gynecology*, **160**, 919–25.

Robillard, J. E., Weitzman, R. E., Fisher D. A. & Smith, F. G. Jr (1979). The dynamics of vasopressin release and blood volume regulation during fetal haemorrhage in the lamb fetus. *Pediatric Research*, **13**, 606–10.

Roffwarg, H. P., Muzio, J. N. & Dement, W. C. (1966). Ontegenic development of the human sleep-dream cycle. *Science,* **152**, 604–19.

Rose, S. A. (1983). Behavioural and psychophysiological sequelae of preterm birth : the neonatal period. In *Infants Born at Risk: Physiological, Perceptual and Cognitive Processes.* ed: T. Field & A. Sostek. pp. 45–67. Grune and Stratton, New York.

Rosenberg, A. A., Jones, M. D. & Koehler, R. C. (1984). Distribution of cardiac output in fetal and neonatal lambs with acute respiratory acidosis. *Pediatric Research,* **18**, 731–5.

Rosenberg, A. A., Harris, A. P., Koehler, R. C., Hudak, M. L., Traystman, R. J. & Jones, M. D. Jr (1986). Role of O2-hemoglobin affinity in the regulation of cerebral blood flow in fetal sheep. *American Journal of Physiology,* **251**, H56–62.

Rudolph, A. M. (1974). *Congenital Diseases of the Heart. Year Book,* Chicago.

Rudolph, A. M. (1977). Fetal and neonatal pulmonary circulation. *American Review of Respiratory Disease,* **115**, 11–18.

Rudolph, A. M. (1985). Organization and control of the fetal circulation. In *The Physiological Development of the Fetus and Newborn*, part 4, ed. C. T. Jones & P. W. Nathanielsz. pp. 343–353. Academic Press, London.

Rudolph, A. M., Heymann, M. A., Teramo, K. A. W., Barrett, C. T. & Raiha, N. C. R. (1971). Studies in the circulation of the previable human fetus. *Pediatric Research,* **5**, 452–65.

Schifferli, P. Y. & Caldeyro-Barcia, R. (1973). Effects of atropine and beta-adrenergic drugs on the heart rate of the human fetus. In *Fetal Pharmacology*, ed. L.O. Boreus. pp. 259–279. Raven Press, New York.

Shepherd, J. T. & Mancia, G. (1986). Reflex control of the human cardiovascular system. *Reviews of Physiology, Biochemistry and Pharmacology,* **105**, 3–99.

Shinebourne, E. A., Vapaavouri, E. K., Williams, R. L., Heymann, M. A. & Rudolph, A. M. (1972). Development of baroreflex activity in unanaesthetised foetal and newborn lambs. *Circulation Research,* **31**, 710–18.

Sibley, Y. D. L., Walker, A. M. & Maloney, J. E. (1982). The influence of behavioural state on the cardiovascular system of newborn lambs. *Journal of Developmental Physiology,* **4**, 107–19.

Sidi, D., Kuipers, J. R. G., Teitel, D., Heymann, M. A. & Rudolph, A. M. (1983). Developmental changes in oxygenation and circulatory responses to hypoxemia in lambs. *American Journal of Physiology,* **245** (Heart & Circulatory Physiology 14), H674–82.

Smith, F. G., Sato, T., Varille, V. A. & Robillard, J. E. (1989). Atrial natriuretic factor during fetal and postnatal life: A review. *Journal of Developmental Physiology,* **12**, 55–62.

Smolich, J. J. (1986). The structural and functional development of the sheep heart. PhD Thesis, Monash University.

Smolich, J. J., Soust, M., Berger, P. J. & Walker, A. M. (1991). Indirect relation between rises in oxygen consumption and left ventricular output at birth in lambs. (In press).

Smolich, J. J., Walker, A. M., Campbell, G. R. & Adamson, T. M. (1989). Left and right ventricular myocardial morphometry in fetal, neonatal and adult sheep. *American Journal of Physiology,* **257** (Heart & Circulatory Physiology 26), H1–9.

Szymonowicz, W., Walker, A. M., Cussen, L., Cannata, J. & Yu, V. Y. H.

(1988). Developmental changes in regional cerebral blood flow in fetal, term fetus and newborn lamb. *American Journal of Physiology,* **254** (Heart & Circulatory Physiology 23), H52–8.

Teitel, D. F., Iwamoto, H. S. & Rudolph, A. M. (1987). Effects of birth-related events on central blood flow patterns. *Pediatric Research,* **22**, 557–66.

Teitel, D. F. (1988). Circulatory adjustments to postnatal life. *Seminars in Perinatology,* **12**, 96–103.

Teitel, D. F., Iwamoto, H. S. & Rudolph, A. M. (1990). Changes in the pulmonary circulation during birth-related events. *Pediatric Research,* **27**, 372–8.

Thorburn, G. D. (1974). The role of the thyroid gland and the kidneys in fetal growth. Ciba Foundation Symposium 27, 185–200.

Thornburg, K. L. & Morton, M. J. (1983). Filling and arterial pressures as determinants of RV stroke volume in the sheep fetus. *American Journal of Physiology,* **244** (Heart & Circulatory Physiology 13), H656–63.

Thornburg, K. L. & Morton, M. J. (1986). Filling and arterial pressures as determinants of LV stroke volume in fetal lambs. *American Journal of Physiology,* **251** (Heart & Circulatory Physiology 20), H961–8.

Vatner, S. F. & Manders, W. T. (1979). Depressed responsiveness of the carotid sinus reflex in conscious newborn animals. *American Journal of Physiology,* **237** (Heart & Circulatory Physiology 6), H40–3.

Waldman, S., Krauss, A. N. & Auld, P. A. M. (1979). Baroreceptors in preterm infants. Their relationship to maturity and disease. *Developmental Medicine and Child Neurology,* **21**, 714–22.

Walker, A. M. (1984). Physiological control of the fetal cardiovascular system. In *Fetal Physiology and Medicine. The Basis of Perinatology,* 2nd edn. ed. R. W. Beard & P. W. Nathanielsz. pp. 287–317. Marcel Dekker Inc, New York.

Walker, A. M., Cannata, J. P., Ritchie, B. C. & Maloney, J. E. (1985). Different patterns of reflex heart rate control during stress in fetal and neonatal lambs: implications for ventricular function. In *The Physiological Development of the Fetus and Newborn,* ed. C. T. Jones & P. W. Nathanielsz. pp. 395–399. Academic Press, London.

Walker, A. M., Horne, R. S. C., Bowes, G. & Berger, P. (1986). The circulation in sleep in newborn lambs. *Australian Paediatric Journal* (suppl.), 71–4.

Walker, A. M., Ritchie, B. C., Adamson, T. M. & Maloney, J. E. (1988). Effect of changing lung liquid volume on the pulmonary circulation of fetal lambs. *Journal of Applied Physiology,* **64**, 61–7.

Walsh, S. Z., Myer, W. W. & Lind, J. (1974). *The Human Fetal and Neonatal Circulation.* Charles C Thomas, Springfield, Illinois.

Walther, F. J., Siassi, B., Ramadan, N., Ananda, A. K. & Wu, P. Y. K. (1985). Pulsed doppler determinations of cardiac output in neonates: normal standards for clinical use. *Pediatrics,* **76**, 829–33.

Yardley, R. W., Bowes, G., Wilkinson, M., Cannata, J. P., Maloney, J. E., Ritchie, B. C. & Walker, A. M. (1983). Increased arterial pressure variability after arterial baroreceptor denervation in fetal lambs. *Circulation Research,* **52**, 580–8.

Zink, J. & Van Petten, G. R. (1980). Time course of closure of the ductus venosus in the newborn lamb. *Pediatric Research,* **14**, 1–3.

Pathophysiology

8

Cardiovascular effects of acute fetal hypoxia and asphyxia

HARRIET S. IWAMOTO

Introduction

Acute reductions in the nutrients and oxygen supplied by the mother challenge fetal homeostatic responses. While the fetus reduces its rate of growth and utilizes proteins and carbohydrates derived from tissue reservoirs during brief periods of starvation, oxygen is not stored and the fetus remains wholly dependent upon a steady supply. Several methods have been used to characterize fetal cardiovascular responses to acute reductions in oxygen delivery and to define the mechanisms responsible for maintaining adequate oxygen delivery to fetal tissues. The most common method has involved a reduction in oxygen availability to the mother. This produces maternal and fetal hypoxaemia but usually does not affect fetal pH or carbon dioxide tension. Other methods produce fetal hypercapnia and acidaemia in addition to hypoxaemia and results from these studies differ from those that produce hypoxaemia alone because increases in H^+ and CO_2 concentrations affect chemoreceptor responses, vascular tone and neurohormonal mechanisms directly and have indirect effects on tissue oxygen delivery as a result of shifting the oxygen–haemoglobin dissociation curve (Jones & Robinson, 1975; Cohen, Piasecki & Jackson, 1982; Faucher et al., 1987; Wood & Chen, 1989).

Experimental approaches

Recent advances such as cordocentesis and ultrasound allow clinicians to obtain information from the human fetus in utero. While some important information has been obtained by applying these techniques, physiological studies of normal human fetuses are severely restricted due to ethical restraints. Thus, much current understanding of fetal cardiovascular

Table 8.1. *Comparison of the effects of an acute 50% reduction in oxygen delivery produced by several methods on umbilical venous oxygen content and umbilical blood flow*

	Hypoxic hypoxaemia[a]	Uterine artery compression[b]	Umbilical cord compression[c]	Haemoglobin exchange[d]	Fetal anaemia[e]
Umbilical venous O_2 content	↓40–50%	↓50%	⇔	↓46%	↓50%
Umbilical blood flow	⇔	⇔	↓51%	↓33%	⇔
O_2 delivery	↓40–50%	↓50%	↓54%	↓64%	↓50%

Note: Values are expressed as a percentage of the control value after 5–30 minutes of reduction in oxygen delivery.
O_2 delivery = oxygen delivery to the fetus, umbilical blood flow × umbilical venous oxygen content.

[a] Data derived from Cohn et al., 1974; Peeters et al., 1979; Reuss et al., 1982; Edelstone et al., 1980.
[b] Data derived from Jensen et al., 1991; Gu et al., 1985; Yaffe et al., 1987.
[c] Data derived from Edelstone et al., 1980; Itskovitz et al., 1987; Rudolph et al., 1989.
[d] Data derived from Itskovitz et al., 1984.
[e] Data derived from Fumia et al., 1984.

development is derived from experimental studies in animals. The fetal sheep is a widely used preparation for the study of cardiovascular development particularly because it is amenable to extensive chronic instrumentation and is sufficiently large to accommodate sequential measurements of haemodynamic and hormonal variables.

Fetal cardiovascular responses have been examined following a reduction in the inspired oxygen delivered to the ewe (hypoxic hypoxaemia) (Cohn et al., 1974; Peeters et al., 1979; Sheldon et al., 1979; Edelstone & Holzman, 1982; Reuss et al., 1982; Jones & Robinson, 1983; Court et al., 1984; Block et al., 1990), partial occlusion of the uterine artery (Gu, Jones & Parer, 1985; Yaffe et al., 1987; Jensen, Roman & Rudolph, 1991), compression of the umbilical cord (Dawes et al., 1968; Lewis, Wolf & Sischo, 1984; Itskovitz, LaGamma & Rudolph, 1987), decreases in haemoglobin concentration (Fumia, Edelstone & Holzman, 1984) and decreases in haemoglobin affinity for oxygen produced by exchanging adult for fetal haemoglobin (Battaglia et al., 1969; Itskovitz et al., 1984). To compare the changes produced by each acute stress, responses to a 50% reduction in oxygen delivery to the fetus, defined as the product of umbilical–placental blood flow and umbilical venous oxygen content, are included in Table 8.1. Hypoxic hypoxaemia and uterine artery compression reduce oxygen delivery to the fetus by reducing umbilical venous oxygen content but not umbilical–placental blood flow (Peeters et al., 1979; Sheldon et al., 1979; Reuss & Rudolph, 1980; Cohn et al., 1985; Jensen et al., 1986; Yaffe et al., 1987). Similar changes are produced with acute fetal and maternal anaemia (Paulone, Edelstone & Shedd, 1987; Fumia, Edelstone & Holzman, 1984). In contrast, umbilical cord compression reduces umbilical blood flow (Itskovitz et al., 1987; Rudolph, Roman & Rudolph, 1989) and reduces central blood volume in the fetus secondary to an increase in umbilical venous resistance. Haemoglobin exchange reduces umbilical–placental blood flow and umbilical venous oxygen content significantly; complete exchange of adult for fetal haemoglobin is associated with a 64% decrease in fetal oxygen delivery acutely (Itskovitz et al., 1984).

Effects on arterial pH and blood gases, heart rate and blood pressure

The changes in arterial blood pH, gases, and oxygen content produced by different acute stresses differ even though oxygen delivery is decreased by similar amounts (Table 8.2). Hypoxic hypoxaemia decreases PO_2 and oxygen content although acidaemia may develop (Cohn et al., 1974).

Table 8.2. *Comparison of the effect of an acute 50% reduction in oxygen delivery produced by several methods on arterial pH and blood gases*

	Control	Hypoxaemia[a]	Hypoxaemia + acidaemia[b]	Uterine artery compression[c]	Umbilical cord compression[d]	Haemoglobin exchange[e]	Fetal anaemia[f]
Ascending aorta							
pH	7.37–7.40	7.33–7.36	7.28*	7.25*	7.36	NA	NA
PO_2 (torr)	21–24	12–14*	12*	16*	18*	NA	20
PCO_2 (torr)	41–47	41–50	43	60*	46	NA	NA
O_2 content (mM)	3.3–3.5	1.5–2.0*	NA	1.7*	2.4*	NA	NA
Descending aorta							
pH	7.34–7.40	7.3–7.36	7.26*	7.25*, 7.32	7.31*–7.34*	7.23*	7.36
PO_2 (torr)	19–24	11–15*	12*	13*–15*	16*–17*	21	17
PCO_2 (torr)	40–54	41–42	43	61*, 47	47, 59*	44	46
O_2 content (mM)	2.8–3.0	1.2*	NA	1.5*	1.9–2.3*	1.1*	1.552*

Note: NA = data not available.   * Indicates a significant change from the corresponding control value in the original study.

[a] Data derived from Cohn et al., 1974; Reuss et al., 1982; Edelstone et al., 1980; Block et al., 1990.
[b] Data derived from Cohn et al., 1974; Block et al., 1990.
[c] Data derived from Jensen et al., 1991; Yaffe et al., 1987; Espinoza et al., 1989.
[d] Data derived from Itskovitz et al., 1984; Itskovitz et al., 1987; Rudolph et al., 1989.
[e] Data derived from Itskovitz et al., 1984.
[f] Data derived from Fumia et al., 1984.

Changes in $PaCO_2$ are usually prevented by increasing the PCO_2 of gas provided to the ewe. Compression of the uterine artery or umbilical cord produces hypoxaemia, acidaemia and hypercapnia. Uterine artery compression produces more marked changes primarily because it has a major effect on the composition of umbilical venous blood (Edelstone, 1984; Itskovitz et al., 1987; Yaffe et al., 1987; Jensen, Roman & Rudolph, 1991). Haemoglobin exchange produces acidaemia and reduces arterial O_2 content but does not alter PaO_2 significantly (Itskovitz et al., 1984). Acute fetal anaemia decreases arterial O_2 content but does not alter PaO_2, PCO_2 or pH significantly (Fumia et al., 1984).

It was appreciated by Sir Joseph Barcroft that PO_2 in the ascending aorta was intermediate between that in the umbilical vein, where it is greatest, and that in the descending aorta (Barcroft, 1946). It was subsequently determined that gradients for O_2 content, PCO_2, pH and nutrient concentrations exist as well (Sheldon et al., 1979; Charlton & Johengen, 1984). These gradients are maintained to different degrees when oxygen delivery is reduced by different methods (Table 8.2). Hypoxic hypoxaemia decreases the gradient more than other acute stresses; when acidaemia develops, the gradient is abolished (Cohn et al., 1974; Sheldon et al., 1979). The effects of uterine artery and umbilical cord compression are less marked, and the decreases in pH and PaO_2 in the ascending aorta are smaller than in the descending aorta.

Differences in the composition of blood in the upper and lower portions of the fetal circulation are best understood through a consideration of the pattern of blood flow shunts. Normally about half of umbilical venous return perfuses the hepatic circulation and half traverses the ductus venosus to enter the inferior vena cava, of which a major portion is preferentially distributed to perfuse upper body organs (Edelstone, Rudolph & Heymann, 1978; Edelstone & Rudolph, 1979). The proportion of umbilical venous blood flow that traverses the ductus venosus increases and hepatic blood flow falls when oxygen delivery is reduced by hypoxic hypoxaemia, uterine artery compression or umbilical cord compression (Table 8.3). More umbilical venous blood returns directly to the heart and crosses the foramen ovale so that oxygen delivery to the upper body organs from blood derived from the umbilical vein increases (Reuss & Rudolph, 1980; Itskovitz et al., 1987; Jensen et al., 1991). The degree of umbilical venous blood shunting across the ductus venosus and foramen ovale is greatest during umbilical cord compression and least during hypoxic hypoxaemia. The resulting differences in oxygenation of fetal arterial blood are certain to produce different degrees of

Table 8.3. *Comparison of the effects of an acute 50% reduction in oxygen delivery produced by several methods on umbilical, ductus venosus and hepatic blood flows in the fetus*

	Hypoxic hypoxemia[a]	Uterine artery compression[b]	Umbilical cord compression[c]
Umbilical blood flow	⇔	⇔	⇓50%*
Ductus venosus blood flow as a fraction of umbilical blood flow	⇑14%*	⇑18%*	⇑22–64%*
Liver flow	⇓23%*	⇓20%	⇓40–82%*

Note: Values are expressed as a percentage of the corresponding control values of the original study.
    * Indicates a significant change from the corresponding control value in the original study.
[a] Data derived from Reuss et al., 1982; Edelstone et al., 1980.
[b] Data derived from Jensen et al., 1991; Cohn et al., 1985.
[c] Data derived from Edelstone et al., 1980; Itskovitz et al., 1987; Rudolph et al., 1989.

chemoreceptor stimulation, recognizing that the peripheral chemorecep-
tors are sensitive to changes in oxygen tension, as well as differences in
activation of local and hormonal mechanisms that regulate vascular tone
(Jones & Robinson, 1975; Cohen et al., 1982; Faucher et al., 1987; Lewis
& Sadeghi, 1987; Hanson, 1988; Wood & Chen, 1989; Wood, Chen &
Bell, 1989).

The effects of acute reductions in fetal oxygen delivery on fetal heart
rate and arterial blood pressure have been reviewed recently in detail
(Hanson, 1988) and are discussed in Chapter 1 of this volume. Bradycardia and hypertension usually develop in response to a decrease in oxygen
delivery in late gestation fetuses (Edelstone, Rudolph & Heymann, 1980;
Reuss & Rudolph, 1980; Cohn et al., 1985; Lewis & Sadeghi, 1987; Yaffe
et al., 1987; Block et al., 1990). Bradycardia results from chemoreceptor
and baroreceptor activation, is mediated by the vagus and may last only a
few minutes due to an increase in plasma catecholamines that exert a
positive chronotropic effect (Jones & Robinson, 1983). Hypertension
depends upon the degree of peripheral vasoconstriction mediated by the
sympathetic nervous system and increases in plasma vasopressin (Jones
& Ritchie, 1983; Reuss et al., 1982; Court et al., 1984; Schuijers et al.,
1986; Jensen, Kunzel & Kastendieck, 1987*b*; Jones et al., 1988; Iwamoto,
Stucky & Roman, 1991) and catecholamines and the degree of modulation by endogenous opioids (Espinoza et al., 1989) and prostaglandins
(Millard, Baig & Vatner, 1979). Severe degrees of hypoxaemia and
acidaemia are associated with profound decreases in fetal heart rate
which precede fetal demise (Block et al., 1990). The magnitude of the
heart rate and blood pressure responses depends upon the extent to
which arterial pH and blood gases change. When PaO_2 is not altered, as
in haemoglobin exchange, fetal anaemia and carboxyhaemoglobinaemia,
mean arterial pressure and heart rate do not change significantly (Longo
et al., 1978; Fumia et al., 1984; Itskovitz et al., 1984; Edelstone et al.,
1989). Heart rate and blood pressure responses also depend on fetal
maturity. Heart rate increases rather than decreases and mean arterial
blood pressure does not change in response to hypoxic hypoxaemia or
umbilical cord compression prior to the last third of gestation in the sheep
(Boddy et al., 1974; Iwamoto et al., 1989; Iwamoto, Stucky & Roman,
1991). This reflects the relative maturity of neurohormonal mechanisms
and the incomplete development of parasympathetic regulation of heart
rate at that stage of gestation (Walker et al., 1978, 1979).

Table 8.4. *Comparison of the effects of an acute 50% reduction in oxygen delivery produced by several methods on combined ventricular output and organ blood flow*

	Hypoxic hypoxaemia[a]	Hypoxaemia + acidaemia[b]	Uterine artery compression[c]	Umbilical cord compression[d]	Haemoglobin exchange[e]	Fetal anaemia[f]
Combined ventricular output	↓5–18	↓20–23*	↓12	↓18*	↓18	⇕
Umbilical–placenta	⇕	⇕	⇕	↓51*	↓33*	⇕
Fetal body	↓16	↓41*	↓22	⇕	⇕	⇕
Organ						
Brain	↑75*	↑54*	↑77*	↑43*	↑17	↑93
Heart	↑151*	↑161*	↑126*	↑41	↑130*	↑114
Adrenal	↑206*	↑183*	↑278*	↑101*	↑50*	↑92
Lungs	↓55	↓44*	↓35	↓50*	↓68*	NA
GI tract	↓21	↓57*	↓33	↑22	↑17	↑35
Kidneys	↓22*	↓50*	↓30	↑13	↓8	⇕
Periphery	↓30	↓70*	↓40*	↓26*	↓23*	⇕

Note: Values are expressed as a percentage of the corresponding control value in the original study. NA = data not available.
* Indicates a significant change from the corresponding control value in the original study. Periphery is the skin, muscle, and skeleton of the fetus; Fetal Body = Combined ventricular output–umbilical–placental blood flow.

[a] Data derived from Cohn et al., 1974; Peeters et al., 1979; Block et al., 1990; Fisher et al., 1982; Boyle et al., 1990; Iwamoto & Rudolf, 1985; Reuss et al., 1982; Edelstone et al., 1980.
[b] Data derived from Cohn et al., 1974; Block et al., 1990.
[c] Data derived from Jensen et al., 1991; Yaffe et al., 1987; Espinoza et al., 1989.
[d] Data derived from Itskovitz et al., 1987; Rudolph et al., 1989; Edelstone et al., 1980.
[e] Data derived from Itskovitz et al., 1984.
[f] Data derived from Fumia et al., 1984.

Combined ventricular output and patterns of blood flow distribution

Combined ventricular output, the sum of right and left ventricular outputs in the fetus, is maintained or decreases slightly when oxygen delivery is reduced by 50% by a variety of methods (Table 8.4). When oxygen delivery is reduced by more than 50%, or when acidaemia develops, combined ventricular output falls as a consequence of brady-cardia and a decrease in stroke volume (Cohn et al., 1974; Jensen, Hohmann & Kunzel, 1987*a*; Yaffe et al., 1987; Block et al., 1990) and hypotension (Block et al., 1990). Different acute stresses have different effects on the distribution of combined ventricular output to either the fetal body or the umbilical circulation. Blood flow in the umbilical circulation is generally maintained during hypoxic hypoxaemia, hypoxae-mia and acidaemia, and uterine artery compression (Cohn et al., 1974; Peeters et al., 1979; Yaffe et al., 1987; Jensen et al., 1991; Table 8.4). In these instances, heart rate decreases and arterial blood pressure in-creases. These two factors, which can directly influence umbilical blood flow (Rudolph, 1976), oppose each other and blood flow does not change significantly. Umbilical blood flow falls during umbilical cord compres-sion secondary to the increase in umbilical venous resistance. In other studies, factors other than perfusion pressure and heart rate appear to regulate umbilical blood flow. Haemoglobin exchange does not change arterial blood pressure, heart rate, or perfusion pressure significantly, but umbilical blood flow falls acutely by 33% (Itskovitz et al., 1984), though the decrease is not maintained for 24–48 h (Edelstone et al., 1989). The mechanism of this response is not known. In fetal sheep, prior to the last third of gestation, acute hypoxaemia and acidaemia decrease umbilical blood flow markedly even though mean arterial blood pressure does not change and heart rate increases (Iwamoto et al., 1989). This may be a direct effect of hypoxia on placental blood vessels because hypoxia has been shown to decrease blood flow in isolated perfused cotyledons (Howard, Hosokawa & Maguire, 1987). Chemoreceptors may be in-volved because acute hypoxaemia decreases umbilical blood flow in fetal sheep when afferents from the aortic and carotid chemoreceptors are cut (Jansen et al., 1989). Vasopressin may also be involved because inhi-bition of V1 pressor receptors increases umbilical blood flow in hypoxae-mic fetal sheep even though it decreases arterial blood pressure (Peréz et al., 1989). Recently direct vasoconstrictor actions of angiotension II and norepinephrine on extraplacental umbilical vessels have been demon-strated in intact fetal sheep (Adamson et al., 1989). Sympathetic and renin–angiotension systems are activated in the hypoxaemic fetus, but it is not known to what extent these extraplacental vascular responses are activated.

Blood flow to the fetal brain, heart and adrenals increases when oxygen delivery to the fetus decreases (Table 8.4). Blood flow to these vascular beds is preserved relative to other areas of the fetal circulation, particularly when the degree of hypoxaemia or asphyxia becomes severe (Johnson et al., 1979; Jensen et al., 1987*b*; Yaffe et al., 1987; Block et al., 1990). Failure to maintain blood flow to the brain and adrenals during an acute asphyxic period portends fetal demise (Block et al., 1984; Jensen et al., 1987*b*; Yaffe et al., 1987). These responses mature early and are present prior to the last third of gestation in the sheep (Iwamoto et al., 1989, 1991). These organs serve important functions for the fetus and depend largely upon aerobic metabolism to meet energy requirements. Thus, preservation of oxygen delivery to these organs during acute stress is an important adaptive response.

Blood flow to the brain, heart and adrenals varies with metabolic rate. Cerebral oxygen and glucose consumption in the fetal sheep is greater during low voltage than high voltage electrocortical activity, and blood flow to most areas of the fetal brain is greater during low voltage electrocortical activity (Abrams et al., 1984; Richardson, Patrick & Abduljabbar, 1985; Jensen et al., 1986; Rankin et al., 1987). When fetuses are made hypoxaemic, electrocortical activity switches from low to high voltage activity, perhaps to reduce fetal oxygen requirements and protect the brain from hypoxic damage (Boddy et al., 1974; Rankin et al., 1987). In the myocardium, blood flow to the right ventricular free wall (Fisher, Heymann & Rudolph, 1982) and right ventricular output is twice that of the left ventricle. Blood flow to the adrenals increases in response to acute stress, when catecholamine and steroid hormone secretion from them is increased and, presumably, when the oxygen requirements and metabolic rate of the glands are also increased (Cohen et al., 1984; Jackson et al., 1989).

It is not clear which factors mediate metabolic regulation of blood flow in the fetal brain, heart, and adrenal. Several investigators have demonstrated that blood flow varies as an inverse function of arterial oxygen content so that oxygen delivery is maintained at a stable level (Jones et al., 1977, 1978; Peeters et al., 1979; Ashwal, Dale & Longo, 1984). Thus, by comparison with the data shown in Tables 8.2 and 8.4, hypoxic hypoxaemia (Cohn et al., 1974; Jones et al., 1977; Peeters et al., 1979;

Fisher, Heymann & Rudolph, 1982; Block et al., 1990), hypoxaemia and acidaemia (Cohn et al., 1974; Block et al., 1990), and uterine artery compression (Jensen et al., 1991; Yaffe et al., 1987) produce the largest decreases in PaO_2 content and the largest increases, expressed as a percentage of the control value, in blood flow to the heart, brain and adrenal. Umbilical cord compression produces a smaller decrease in PaO_2 content and smaller increase in blood flow to the brain, heart and adrenal. A close relationship between O_2 content and blood flow is not always observed but PO_2 may be an important regulator (Szymonicz et al., 1988). Complete haemoglobin exchange produces the largest decrease in PaO_2 content and the smallest increase in blood flow. This may be because PaO_2 does not change. Similarly, during haemorrhage, blood flow to the brain, heart and adrenal does not change even though arterial O_2 content decreases significantly (Toubas et al., 1981; Itskovitz, Goetzman & Rudolph, 1982). Again, PO_2 may be the important regulator as it does not change significantly with haemorrhage (Toubas et al., 1981; Itskovitz et al., 1982). Recently, a revised hypothesis was proposed that relates the fetal cerebral blood flow response to O_2 deficit to the baseline of ratio of O_2 demand/O_2 supply rather than arterial O_2 content (Hudak et al., 1988). Clearly, additional studies are needed to test this hypothesis.

Pulmonary vascular resistance in the fetus is normally high and pulmonary blood flow constitutes only 5–7% of combined ventricular output in late gestation (Rudolph & Heymann, 1970). When O_2 delivery to the fetus is reduced by a number of methods, pulmonary vascular resistance increases and blood flow falls to about 50% of the control value (Table 8.4). This hypoxaemic vasoconstrictor response in the lungs serves to shunt blood flow away from the lungs through the ductus arteriosus and primarily to the placenta, the site of gas exchange in the fetus. This adaptive response develops early and the pulmonary circulation vasoconstricts in response to hypoxaemia and umbilical cord compression prior to the last third of gestation (Iwamoto et al., 1989, 1991). In the pulmonary vascular bed, local vascular responses to hypoxia appear to be important regulatory factors in the fetus as they are in the adult (Grover et al., 1983). A potentiating effect of increases in H^+ concentration on the pulmonary response to hypoxaemia has not been directly examined in the fetus as it has in the postnatal animal (Rudolph & Yuan, 1966). The important regulatory mechanisms of pulmonary blood flow appear to be local vascular responses because sympathectomy and α-adrenergic antag-

onists do not affect the pulmonary vasoconstrictor response to hypoxaemia (Reuss et al., 1982; Iwamoto et al., 1983). Locally produced regulators of pulmonary blood flow are discussed in detail in Chapter 12.

Blood flow to the gastrointestinal, renal, and peripheral (cutaneous
and musculoskeletal) vascular beds has been reported to decrease or not
change in response to decreases in O_2 delivery to the fetus (Cohn et al.,
1974; Edelstone & Holzman, 1982; Iwamoto & Rudolph, 1985; Yaffe et
al., 1987; Jansen et al., 1989; Block et al., 1990; Boyle et al., 1990). As
fetal O_2 delivery decreases from normal to half-normal values, blood flow
through these vascular beds remains constant (Sheldon et al., 1979;
Edelstone & Holzman, 1982; Boyle et al., 1990). When O_2 delivery to the
fetus falls below half normal values and aterial O_2 content is less than 1.5–
2 mM, blood flow to these organs decreases markedly (Boyle et al., 1990;
Edelstone & Holzman, 1982; Sheldon et al., 1979). These vascular beds
can survive on anaerobic metabolism for at least short periods of time,
and in the fetus their continuous function is not essential for survival.

As evident from the data in Table 8.4, different methods used to reduce
fetal O_2 delivery produce different degrees of vasoconstriction in the
gastrointestinal, renal and peripheral vascular beds. The vasoconstrictor
responses are not a result of local vascular responses to hypoxaemia,
acidaemia and hypercarbia, which would cause vasodilation. This indicates that local regulatory mechanisms play a minor role in regulating
blood flow in these areas of the circulation. In support of this concept is
the observation that vasoconstrictor responses in these vascular beds are
not present in fetuses prior to the last third of gestation (Iwamoto et al.,
1989, 1991), a time when neurohormonal response mechanisms are not
fully mature. In late-gestation fetuses, neural and hormonal mechanisms
that are activated by hypoxaemia and acidaemia are important regulators
of blood flow to the gastrointestinal, renal and peripheral vascular beds.
The vasoconstrictor response to hypoxaemia or asphyxia is reduced by
peripheral denervation (Dawes et al., 1968), chemoreceptor denervation
(Jansen et al., 1989), sympathectomy (Lewis, Donovan & Platzker, 1980;
Iwamoto et al., 1983; Jones & Ritchie, 1983; Schuijers et al., 1986), α-
adrenergic blockade (Reuss et al., 1982), and vasopressin blockade
(Peréz et al., 1989). Endogenous opioids counteract vasoconstriction in
the periphery and kidneys and reduce the hypertensive response (Espinoza, 1989) and prostaglandins modulate the renal vasoconstrictor response (Millard et al., 1979; Robillard, Nakamura & DiBona, 1986). The
degree to which neurohormonal mechanisms are activated depends upon
the magnitude of changes in pH and blood gases (Jensen et al., 1987*a,b*;

Lewis & Sadeghi, 1987; Wood & Chen, 1989; Wood et al., 1989). It is concluded that differences in the activation of neurohormonal mechanisms are responsible for the different degrees of vasoconstriction observed during acute hypoxaemia and asphyxia.

One apparent exception is the study by Itskovitz et al. (1987) where occlusion of the umbilical cord for 5 min resulted in an increase in blood flow to the periphery even though secretion of catecholamines and other vasoactive substances probably increased (Lewis, Wolf & Sischo, 1984). The vasodilatory response in the periphery was not confirmed in a subsequent study from the same laboratory after 15–30 min of cord compression (Rudolph et al., 1989), and it was concluded that the vasoconstrictor response in the periphery required more than 5 min to develop fully.

Conclusions

Acute reductions in O_2 delivery to the fetus alter the distribution of blood flow to fetal organs in a manner that is directly related to the degree of hypoxaemia or acidaemia produced. Organs that are crucial to fetal survival, the brain, heart and adrenals, respond directly to local changes in PO_2 or O_2 content such that O_2 delivery to these areas is maintained at the expense of delivery to other areas of the body. Blood flow to other fetal organs, such as the kidneys, gastrointestinal tract, skin, muscle and bone, decreases secondary to increases in the activity of sympathetic, adrenergic, and vasopressin mechanisms stimulated by hypoxaemia and acidaemia. Other locally produced and neuroendocrine factors are most likely involved, though their roles remain to be clarified.

References

Abrams, R. M., Ito, M., Frisinger, J. E., Patlak, C. S., Pettigrew, K. D. & Kennedy, C. (1984). Local cerebral glucose utilization in fetal and neonatal sheep. *American Journal of Physiology,* **246**, 608–18.

Adamson, S. L., Morrow, R. J., Bull, S. B. & Langille, B. L. (1989). Vasomotor responses of the umbilical circulation in fetal sheep. *American Journal of Physiology,* **256**, 1056–62

Ashwal, S., Dale, P. S. & Longo, L. D. (1984). Regional cerebral blood flow: studies in the fetal lamb during hypoxia, hypercapnia, acidosis and hypotension. *Pediatric Research,* **18**, 1309–16.

Barcroft, J. (1946). *Researches on Prenatal Life.* pp. 197–210. Blackwell Scientific Publications, Oxford.

Battaglia, F. C., Bowes, W., McGaughey, H. R., Makowski, E. L. & Meschia,

G. (1969). The effect of fetal exchange transfusions with adult blood upon fetal oxygenation. *Pediatric Research,* **2**, 60–5.

Block, B. S., Schlafer, D. H., Wentworth, R. A., Kreitzer, L. A. & Nathanielsz, P. W. (1990). Intrauterine asphyxia and the breakdown of physiologic circulatory compensation in fetal sheep. *American Journal of Obstetrics and Gynecology,* **162**, 1325–31.

Boddy, K., Dawes, G. S., Fisher, R., Pinter, S. & Robinson, J. S. (1974). Foetal respiratory movements, electrocortical and cardiovascular responses to hypoxaemia and hypercapnia in sheep. *Journal of Physiology (London),* **243**, 599–618.

Boyle, D. W., Hirst, K., Zerbe, G. O., Meschia, G. & Wilkening, R. B. (1990). Fetal hind limb oxygen consumption and blood flow during acute graded hypoxia. *Pediatric Research,* **28**, 94–100.

Charlton, V. & Johengen, M. (1984). Nutrient and waste product concentration differences in upper and lower body arteries of fetal sheep. *Journal of Developmental Physiology,* **6**, 431–7.

Cohen, W. R., Piasecki, G. J., Cohn, H. E., Young, J. B. & Jackson, B. T. (1984). Adrenal secretion of catecholamines during hypoxemia in fetal lambs. *Endocrinology,* **114**, 383–90.

Cohen, W. R., Piasecki, G. J. & Jackson, B. T. (1982). Plasma catecholamines during hypoxemia in fetal lamb. *American Journal of Physiology,* **243**, 520–5.

Cohn, H. E., Jackson, B. T., Piasecki, G. J., Cohen, W. R. & Novy, M. J. (1985). Fetal cardiovascular responses to asphyxia induced by decreased uterine perfusion. *Journal of Developmental Physiology,* **7**, 289–97.

Cohn, H. E., Sacks, E. J., Heymann, M. A. & Rudolph, A. M. (1974). Cardiovascular responses to hypoxemia and acidemia in fetal lambs. *American Journal of Obstetrics and Gynecology,* **120**, 817–24.

Court, D. J., Parer, J. T., Block, B. S. B. & Llanos, A. J. (1984). Effects of beta-adrenergic blockade on blood flow distribution during hypoxaemia in fetal sheep. *Journal of Developmental Physiology,* **6**, 349–58.

Dawes, G. S., Lewis, B. V., Milligan, J. E., Roach, M. R. & Talner, N. S. (1968). Vasomotor responses in the hindlimbs of foetal and new-born lambs to asphyxia and aortic chemoreceptor stimulation. *Journal of Physiology (London),* **195**, 55–81.

Edelstone, D. I. (1984). Fetal compensatory responses to reduced oxygen delivery. *Seminars in Perinatology,* **8**, 184–91.

Edelstone, D. I., Darby, M. J., Bass, K., & Miller, K. (1989). Effects of reductions in hemoglobin-oxygen affinity and hematocrit level on oxygen consumption and acid-base state in fetal lambs. *American Journal of Obstetrics and Gynecology,* **160**, 820–8.

Edelstone, D. I. & Holzman, I. R. (1982). Fetal intestinal oxygen consumption at various levels of oxygenation. *American Journal of Physiology,* **242**, H50–4.

Edelstone, D. I., Rudolph, A. M. & Heymann, M. A. (1978). Liver and ductus venosus blood flows in fetal lambs in utero. *Circulation Research,* **42**, 426–33.

Edelstone, D. I., Rudolph, A. M. & Heymann, M. A. (1980). Effects of hypoxemia and decreasing umbilical flow liver and ductus venosus blood flows in fetal lambs. *American Journal of Physiology,* **238**, 656–63.

Edelstone, D. I. & Rudolph, A. M. (1979). Preferential streaming of ductus venosus blood to the brain and heart in fetal lambs. *American Journal of Physiology*, **237**, 724–9.

Espinoza, M., Riquelme, R., Germain, A. M., Tevah, J., Parer, J. T. & Llanos, A. J. (1989). Role of endogenous opioids in the cardiovascular responses to asphyxia in fetal sheep. *American Journal of Physiology*, **256**, 1063–8.

Faucher, D. J., Lowe, T. W., Magness, R. R., Laptook, A. R., Porter, J. C. & Rosenfeld, C. R. (1987). Vasopressin and catecholamine secretion during metabolic acidemia in the ovine fetus. *Pediatric Research*, **21**, 38–43.

Fisher, D. J., Heymann, M. A. & Rudolph, A. M. (1982). Fetal myocardial oxygen and carbohydrate consumption during acutely induced hypoxemia. *American Journal of Physiology*, **242**, 657–61.

Fisher, D. J., Heymann, M. A. & Rudolph, A. M. (1982). Regional myocardial blood flow and oxygen delivery in fetal, newborn and adult sheep. *American Journal of Physiology*, **243**, 729–31.

Fumia, F. D., Edelstone, D. I. & Holzman, I. R. (1984). Blood flow and oxygen delivery to fetal organs as functions of fetal hematocrit. *American Journal of Obstetrics and Gynecology*, **150**, 274–82.

Grover, R. F., Wagner, W. W. Jr, McMurty, I. F. & Reeves, J. T. (1983). Pulmonary circulation. In *Handbook of Physiology, Section 2: The Cardiovascular System, Volume III, Peripheral Circulation and Organ Blood Flow, Part 1*, ed. J. T. Shepherd & F. M. Abboud. pp. 103–136. American Physiological Society, Bethesda, MD.

Gu, W., Jones, C. T. & Parer, J. T. (1985). Metabolic and cardiovascular effects on fetal sheep of sustained reduction in uterine blood flow. *Journal of Physiology (London)* **368**, 109–29.

Hanson, M. A. (1988). The importance of baro- and chemoreflexes in the control of the fetal cardiovascular system. *Journal of Developmental Physiology*, **10**, 491–511.

Howard, R. B., Hosokawa, T. & Maguire, M. H. (1987). Hypoxia-induced fetoplacental vasoconstriction in perfused human placental cotyledons. *American Journal of Obstetrics and Gynecology*, **157**, 1261–6.

Hudak, M. L., Tang, Y. L., Massik, J., Koehler, R. C., Traystman, R. J. & Jones, M. D. Jr (1988). Base-line O_2 extraction influences cerebral blood flow response to hematocrit. *American Journal of Physiology*, **254**, 156–62.

Itskovitz, J., Goetzmann, B. W., Roman, C. & Rudolph, A. M. (1984). Effects of fetal–maternal exchange transfusion on fetal oxygenation and blood flow distribution. *American Journal of Physiology*, **247**, 655–60.

Itskovitz, J., Goetzman, B. W. & Rudolph, A. M. (1982). Effects of hemorrhage on umbilical venous return and oxygen delivery in fetal lambs. *American Journal of Physiology*, **242**, 543–8.

Itskovitz, J., LaGamma, E. F. & Rudolph, A. M. (1987). Effects of cord compression on fetal blood flow distribution and O_2 delivery. *American Journal of Physiology*, **252**, 100–9.

Iwamoto, H. S., Kaufman, T., Keil, L. C. & Rudolph, A. M. (1989). Responses to acute hypoxemia in fetal sheep at 0.6–0.7 gestation. *American Journal of Physiology*, **256**, 613–20.

Iwamoto, H. S. & Rudolph, A. M. (1985). Metabolic responses of the kidney in fetal sheep. Effect of acute and spontaneous hypoxemia. *American Journal of Physiology*, **249**, 836–41.

Iwamoto, H. S., Rudolph, A. M., Mirkin, B. L. & Keil, L. C. (1983).

Circulatory and humoral responses of sympathectomized fetal sheep to hypoxemia. *American Journal of Physiology,* **245**, 767–72.

Iwamoto, H. S., Stucky, E. & Roman, C. (1991). Effects of graded umbilical cord compression in fetal sheep at 0.6–0.7 gestation. *American Journal of Physiology,* **261**, H1268–74.

Jackson, B. T., Morrison, S. H., Cohn, H. E. & Piasecki, G. J. (1989). Adrenal secretion of glucocorticoids during hypoxemia in fetal sheep. *Endocrinology,* **125**, 2751–7.

Jansen, A. H., Belik, J., Ioffe, S. & Chernick, V. (1989). Control of organ blood flow in fetal sheep during normoxia and hypoxia. *American Journal of Physiology,* **257**, 1132–9.

Jensen, A., Bamford, O. S., Dawes, G. S., Hofmeyr, G. & Parkes, M. J. (1986). Changes in organ blood flow between high and low voltage electrocortical activity in fetal sheep. *Journal of Developmental Physiology,* **8**, 187–94.

Jensen, A., Hohmann, M. & Kunzel, W. (1987*a*). Dynamic changes in organ blood flow and oxygen consumption during acute asphyxia in fetal sheep. *Journal of Developmental Physiology,* **9**, 543–59.

Jensen, A., Kunzel, W. & Kastendieck, E. (1987*b*). Fetal sympathetic activity, transcutaneous PO_2, and skin blood flow during repeated asphyxia in sheep. *Journal of Developmental Physiology,* **9**, 337–46.

Jensen, A., Roman, C. & Rudolph, A. M. (1991) Effects of reducing uterine blood flow distribution and oxygen delivery. *Journal of Developmental Physiology,* **15**, 309–23.

Johnson, G. N., Palahniuk, R. J., Tweed, W. A., Jones, M. V. & Wade, J. G. (1979). Regional cerebral blood flow changes during severe fetal asphyxia produced by slow partial umbilical cord compression. *American Journal of Obstetrics and Gynecology,* **135**, 48–52.

Jones, C. T. & Ritchie, J. W. K. (1983). The effects of adrenergic blockade on fetal response to hypoxia. *Journal of Developmental Physiology,* **5**, 211–22.

Jones, C. T. & Robinson, J. S. (1983). Studies on experimental growth retardation in sheep. Plasma catecholamines in fetuses with small placenta. *Journal of Developmental Physiology,* **5**, 77–87.

Jones, C. T. & Robinson, R. O. (1975). Plasma catecholamines in foetal and adult sheep. *Journal of Physiology (London),* **248**, 15–33.

Jones, C. T., Roebuck, M. M., Walker, D. W. & Johnston, B. M. (1988). The role of the adrenal medulla and peripheral sympathetic nerves in the physiological responses of the fetal sheep to hypoxia. *Journal of Developmental Physiology,* **10**, 17–36.

Jones, M. D. Jr, Sheldon, R. E., Peeters, L. L., Makowski, E. L. & Meschia, G. (1978). Regulation of cerebral blood flow in the ovine fetus. *American Journal of Physiology,* **235**, 162–66.

Jones, M. D. Jr, Sheldon, R. E., Peeters, L. L., Meschia, G., Battaglia, F. C. & Makowski, E. L. (1977). Fetal cerebral oxygen consumption at different levels of oxygenation. *Journal of Applied Physiology,* **43**, 1080–4.

Lewis, A. B., Donovan, M. & Platzker, A. C. G. (1980). Cardiovascular responses to autonomic blockade in hypoxemic fetal lambs. *Biology of the Neonate,* **37**, 233–42.

Lewis, A. B. & Sadeghi, M. (1987). Acidemia potentiates the plasma catecholamine response to hypoxemia in fetal sheep. *Biology of the Neonate,* **52**, 285–91.

Lewis, A. B., Wolf, W. J. & Sischo, W. (1984). Cardiovascular and catecholamine responses to successive episodes of hypoxemia in the fetus. *Biology of the Neonate*, **45**, 105–11.

Longo, L. D., Wyatt, J. F., Hewitt, C. W. & Gilbert, R. D. (1978). A comparison of circulatory responses to hypoxic hypoxia and carbon monoxide hypoxia in fetal blood flow and oxygenation. In *Fetal and Newborn Cardiovascular Physiology*, ed. L. D. Longo & D. D. Reneau. pp. 259–287. Garland STPM Press, New York.

Millard, R. W., Baig, H. & Vatner, S. F. (1979). Prostaglandin control of the renal circulation in response to hypoxemia in the fetal lamb in utero. *Circulation Research*, **45**, 172–9.

Paulone, M. E., Edelstone, D. I. & Shedd, A. (1987). Effects of maternal anemia on uteroplacental and fetal oxidative metabolism in sheep. *American Journal of Obstetrics and Gynecology*, **156**, 230–6.

Peeters, L. L. H., Sheldon, R. E., Jones, M. D. Jr, Makowski, E. L. & Meschia, G. (1979). Blood flow to fetal organs as a function of arterial oxygen content. *American Journal of Obstetrics and Gynecology*, **135**, 637–46.

Peréz, R., Espinoza, M., Riquelme, R., Parer, J. T. & Llanos, A. J. (1989). Arginine vasopressin mediates cardiovascular responses to hypoxemia in fetal sheep. *American Journal of Physiology*, **256**, 1011–18.

Rankin, J. H. G., Landauer, M., Tian, Q. & Phernetton, T. M. (1987). Ovine fetal electrocortical activity and regional cerebral blood flow. *Journal of Developmental Physiology*, **9**, 537–42.

Reuss, M. L., Parer, J. T., Harris, J. L. & Krueger, T. R. (1982). Hemodynamic effects of alpha-adrenergic blockade during hypoxia in fetal sheep. *American Journal of Obstetrics and Gynecology*, **142**, 410–15.

Reuss, M. L. & Rudolph, A. M. (1980). Distribution and recirculation of umbilical and systemic venous blood flow in fetal lambs during hypoxia. *Journal of Developmental Physiology*, **2**, 71–84.

Richardson, B. S., Patrick, J. E. & Abduljabbar, H. (1985). Cerebral oxidative metabolism in the fetal lamb: relationship to electrocortical state. *American Journal of Obstetrics and Gynecology*, **153**, 426–31.

Robillard, J. E., Nakamura, K. T. & DiBona, G. F. (1986). Effects of renal denervation on renal responses to hypoxemia in fetal lambs. *American Journal of Physiology*, **250**, 294–301.

Rudolph, A. M. (1976). Factors affecting umbilical blood flow in the lamb in utero. *5th European Congress of Perinatal Medicine*, 159–72.

Rudolph, A. M. & Heymann, M. A. (1970). Circulatory changes during growth in the fetal lamb. *Circulation Research*, **26**, 289–99.

Rudolph, A. M. & Yuan, S. (1966). Response of the pulmonary vasculature to hypoxia and H^+ ion concentration changes. *Journal of Clinical Investigation*, **45**, 399–411.

Rudolph, C. R., Roman, C. & Rudolph, A. M. (1989). Effect of acute umbilical cord compression on hepatic carbohydrate metabolism in the fetal lamb. *Pediatric Research*, **25**, 228–33.

Schuijers, J. A., Walker, D. W., Browne, C. A. & Thorburn, G. D. (1986). Effect of hypoxemia on plasma catecholamines in intact and immunosympathectomized fetal lambs. *American Journal of Physiology*, **251**, 893–900.

Sheldon, R. E., Peeters, L. L. H., Jones, M. D. Jr, Makowski, E. L. & Meschia, G. (1979). Redistribution of cardiac output and oxygen delivery in the hypoxemic fetal lamb. *American Journal of Obstetrics and Gynecology,* **135**, 1071–8.

Szymonowicz, W., Walker, A. M., Cussen, L., Cannata, J. & Yu, V. Y. H. (1988). Developmental changes in regional cerebral blood flow in fetal and newborn lambs. *American Journal of Physiology,* **254**, 52–8.

Toubas, P. L., Silverman, N. H., Heymann, M. A. & Rudolph, A. M. (1981). Cardiovascular effects of acute hemorrhage in fetal lambs. *American Journal of Physiology,* **240**, 45–8.

Walker, A. M., Cannata, J., Dowling, M. H., Ritchie, B. & Maloney, J. E. (1978). Sympathetic and parasympathetic control of heart rate in unanesthetized fetal and newborn lambs. *Biology of the Neonate* **33**, 135–43.

Walker, A. M., Cannata, J. P., Dowling, M. H., Ritchie, B. C. & Maloney, J. E. (1979). Age-dependent pattern of autonomic heart rate control during hypoxia in fetal and newborn lambs. *Biology of the Neonate,* **35**, 198–208.

Wood, C. E. & Chen, H. G. (1989). Acidemia stimulates ACTH, vasopressin, and heart rate responses in fetal sheep. *American Journal of Physiology,* **257**, 344–9.

Wood, C. E., Chen, H. G. & Bell, M. E. (1989). Role of vagosympathetic fibers in the control of adrenocorticotropic hormone, vasopressin, and renin responses to hemorrhage in fetal sheep. *Circulation Research,* **64**, 515–23.

Yaffe, H., Parer, J. T., Block, B. S. & Llanos, A. J. (1987). Cardiorespiratory responses to graded reductions of uterine blood flow in the sheep fetus. *Journal of Developmental Physiology,* **9**, 325–36.

9

Effects of chronic hypoxaemia on circulatory control

ALAN D. BOCKING

Introduction

The effects of hypoxaemia on the developing fetus are of great interest to both physiologists and clinicians. Much attention has been devoted to the effects of acute hypoxaemia produced by a variety of means, such as decreasing maternal inspired oxygen fraction, reducing uterine blood flow and compressing the umbilical cord. Some of the information gained from these studies has been utilized in developing strategies to assess fetal health in clinical practice (Manning, Platt & Sipos, 1980). It is only recently that attention has been directed towards determining the effects of more prolonged periods of hypoxaemia on fetal development. This chapter will review some of the information which has been obtained recently from experiments conducted in chronically catheterized fetal sheep regarding the effects of long-term (i.e. more than a few hours) hypoxaemia on fetal behaviour and circulatory control.

Fetal behaviour

It has been recognized since the early 1970s that acute hypoxaemia in fetal sheep during the latter third of gestation gives rise to a profound inhibition of fetal breathing movements (for review see Dawes, 1984). This inhibition of FBM is now known to be mediated through the activation of neural networks which either arise from, or pass through, the upper lateral pons (Dawes, Gardner, Johnston & Walker, 1983; Gluckman & Johnston, 1987).

It has been recognized recently that more prolonged hypoxaemia, in the absence of acidaemia, is associated with an initial inhibition of FBM followed by a return to the normal incidence of FBM within 12–16 h (Fig. 9.1). This behavioural adaptation of the sheep fetus has been observed in

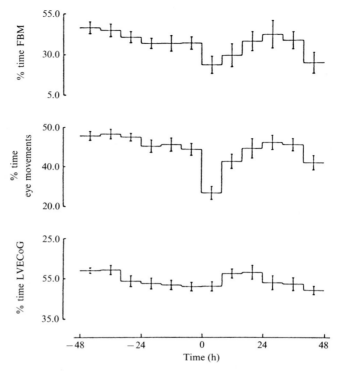

Fig. 9.1. Mean (±SEM) percentage of time spent making fetal breathing movements (FBM), making eye movements, and spent in low-voltage electrocortical activity (LVECoG) in 8 h epochs for 48 h before and 48 h during restricted uterine blood flow ($n = 10$).

fetuses made hypoxaemic either through the restriction of uterine blood flow (Bocking et al., 1988a; Hooper & Harding, 1990) or by a reduction in maternal inspired oxygen fraction (Koos et al., 1988). A similar inhibition followed by a return to normal incidence has been observed for eye movements during prolonged restrictions in uterine blood flow, although there is no change in the incidence of low-voltage electrocortical activity (Bocking et al., 1988a). Sustained hypoxaemia in association with progressive acidaemia results in continued inhibition of both FBM and eye movements (Patrick et al., 1987).

The mechanism(s) whereby the incidence of FBM return to normal during prolonged hypoxaemia in the absence of acidaemia is unknown. The initial inhibition of FBM with hypoxaemia is thought to be a way in which the fetus can conserve oxygen for more vital functions (Rurak & Gruber, 1983). In the long term, however, FBM are known to be important for normal lung growth (Wigglesworth & Desai, 1979; Liggins et al., 1981) and it would therefore appear to be in the best interest of the fetus for FBM to be resumed. It is of note that, although the incidence of FBM is normal during prolonged hypoxaemia, the normal outward flow of lung liquid with FBM is reversed under conditions of restricted uterine blood flow (Hooper & Harding, 1990). This suggests that there may be differences in the characteristics of FBM under conditions of hypoxaemia compared to normoxaemic FBM: these are yet to be determined.

One method of producing growth restriction in the sheep fetus is to remove a proportion of the uterine caruncles which make up the placenta. Such fetuses make FBM, although their incidence is slightly less than that of the appropriately grown sheep fetus (Worthington, Piercy & Smith, 1981). Quite clearly, then, despite the acute inhibitory effect of hypoxaemia on FBM and eye movements, the sheep fetus is able to adapt behaviourally to a prolonged reduction in oxygen delivery as long as progressive acidaemia does not occur. The importance of these observations in fetal sheep to the use of FBM as an indicator of fetal health in the human remains to be determined.

Heart rate

The effect of acute hypoxia and/or asphyxia on fetal heart rate (FHR) has been described in Chapters 1 and 8 of this volume. More prolonged hypoxaemia in the absence of acidaemia secondary to a restriction in uterine blood flow leads to an initial bradycardia followed by a tachycardia lasting for up to 24 h (Fig. 9.2). It is possible that this prolonged increase in FHR is related to a sustained release of catecholamines (Bocking et al., 1988b). In addition to these changes in mean FHR, there is an initial increase in the number of FHR accelerations and decelerations during the first 12–16 h of hypoxaemia, following which FHR variability is unchanged from that of the normoxaemic sheep fetus (Bocking et al., 1989). It is of interest that acute hypoxaemia in the sheep fetus also gives rise to an increase in short-term FHR variability and it is only with severe acidosis that this variability decreases (Dalton, Dawes & Patrick, 1977).

Mean FHR normally decreases with advancing gestation during the latter stages of ovine pregnancy. This normal progression is unchanged in fetal sheep exposed to a 10 mm Hg decrease in PaO_2 for up to 28 days through the reduction of maternal inspired oxygen in an environmental chamber (Kitanaka et al., 1989). It is of interest that these fetuses compensated by increasing haemoglobin synthesis such that for the

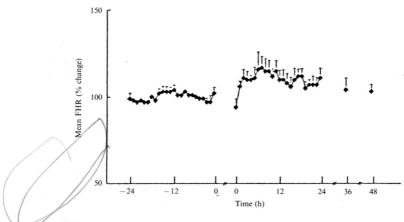

Fig. 9.2. Mean (±SEM) hourly fetal heart rate (FHR) shown as per cent of control (mean FHR over 24 hours) for 24 h before and 48 h during hypoxaemia produced by restriction of uterine blood flow ($n = 10$).

majority of the study period, fetal O_2 content was unchanged from control and there was no effect on fetal body weight at term. Similarly, minimal changes were observed in mean FHR in fetal sheep made hypoxaemic for a 2-week period by infusing nitrogen into a maternal tracheal catheter (Alonso et al., 1989). Prolonged hypoxaemia with progressive acidaemia does not result in significant alterations in mean FHR (Rurak et al., 1990a). Mean FHR is only slightly higher in the chronically hypoxaemic growth-restricted sheep fetus compared to fetuses which are appropriately grown (Robinson, Jones & Kingston, 1983). There appears to be very little effect, therefore, of prolonged or chronic hypoxaemia on mean FHR in sheep.

Arterial pressure

Fetal arterial pressure is initially increased with acute hypoxaemia as described in Chapters 1 and 8. This occurs when fetal hypoxaemia is induced either by restricting uterine blood flow (Bocking, Harding & Wickham, 1986) or by reducing maternal inspired oxygen (Boddy et al., 1974). Following this initial pressor response, if hypoxaemia is maintained, fetal blood pressure returns to normal both in the presence or absence of acidaemia (Bocking et al., 1988b; Rurak et al., 1990a).

Under normal conditions, as FHR decreases during the last 30 days of ovine pregnancy, fetal blood pressure increases. A similar rise in fetal blood pressure is observed in those fetuses made hypoxaemic for 3–4 weeks by reducing maternal inspired oxygen (Kitanaka et al., 1989). Blood pressure in the chronically hypoxaemic, growth-restricted sheep fetus is not different from that of the appropriately grown fetus (Robinson, Jones & Kingston, 1983). Chronic hypoxaemia therefore has very little effect on fetal blood pressure under resting conditions.

Distribution of cardiac output

In contrast to the minimal changes in fetal heart rate and blood pressure, the redistribution of cardiac output known to occur with acute hypoxaemia in fetal sheep is maintained with prolonged hypoxaemia. When uterine blood flow is reduced sufficient to decrease fetal arterial O_2 content by approximately 40% in the absence of progressive acidaemia, there is a significant increase in blood flow to the brain, heart and adrenal glands which is maintained for up to 48 h (Bocking et al., 1988*b*). Umbilical blood flow is increased at 1 h, which is a time when mean FHR is also elevated, but by 24 h umbilical blood flow has returned to control, as has mean FHR (Fig. 9.3).

The increase in cerebral blood flow is maximal at 1 h when fetal arterial PCO_2 is increased and pH is decreased, both of which will augment cerebral blood flow. At 24 and 48 h, when fetal blood gases have returned to normal except for the sustained decrease in fetal PO_2, blood flow to the brain remains elevated (Fig. 9.4). The observed increase in cerebral

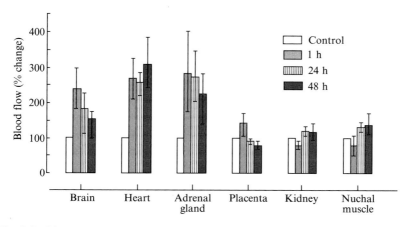

Fig. 9.3. Change from control in fetal blood flow to various organs at 1, 24 and 48 h of hypoxaemia secondary to the restriction of uterine blood flow ($n = 9$).

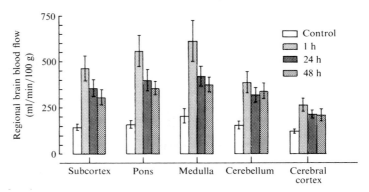

Fig. 9.4. Mean (±SEM) brain blood flow to various regions before (control) and at 1, 24 and 48 h of hypoxaemia secondary to the restriction of uterine blood flow ($n = 9$).

blood flow with prolonged hypoxaemia is greatest to subcortical and brain stem structures as is seen with acute hypoxaemia (Ashwal, Dale & Longo, 1984).

Fetal plasma cortisol concentration is elevated during prolonged hypoxaemia in the absence of progressive acidaemia, in keeping with the sustained increase in adrenal blood flow (Challis et al., 1989). It is of interest that, although fetal ACTH concentration increases markedly with an acute reduction in uterine blood flow, there is a subsequent fall in immunoreactive ACTH, such that by 16 h it is only slightly greater than control (Fig. 9.5). Plasma concentrations of arginine vasopressin follow a similar pattern to that of ACTH and therefore cannot solely be responsible for the redistribution of cardiac output which is observed with prolonged hypoxaemia (Hooper et al., 1990). It is of interest that noradrenaline concentration remains elevated for 24 h of hypoxaemia whereas adrenaline concentration which rises initially with acute hypoxaemia, has returned to control values by 12 h. Fetal plasma PGE_2 concentration rises progressively with restriction of uterine blood flow, reaching a plateau at 10 h and remaining elevated for up to 24 h. The importance of these endocrine alterations in regulating the distribution of cardiac output with prolonged hypoxaemia is yet to be determined.

Prolonged hypoxaemia secondary to a reduction in maternal inspired oxygen fraction gives rise to an initial fall in right ventricular function at 3 days but this is unchanged from control by 7 days. These changes appear to parallel changes in fetal arterial oxygen content secondary to a progressive rise in haemoglobin concentration (Alonso et al., 1989).

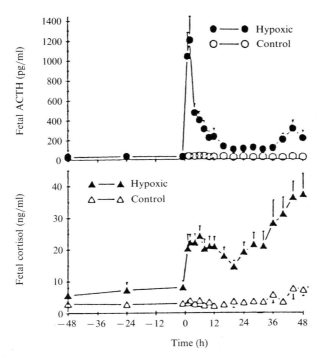

Fig. 9.5. Mean (±SEM) concentrations of immunoreactive ACTH and cortisol in arterial plasma of control fetuses (open symbols, *n* = 4) and in hypoxaemic fetuses (closed symbols, *n* = 8) before and during the restriction of uterine blood flow.

Blood flow to the brain, heart and adrenal gland is also increased with· fetal hypoxaemia and progressive acidaemia secondary to reduced maternal inspired oxygen fraction which is maintained even with severe acidosis (pH of 6.9). Under these conditions, blood flow to brown fat is also increased and flow to the spleen and kidney is decreased (Rurak et al., 1990*b*).

Oxygen consumption by the fetus is maintained with sustained maternal (and therefore fetal) hypoxaemia until severe acidosis has developed at approximately 7 h (Rurak et al., 1990*a*). In contrast, there is no change in overall fetal oxygen consumption for up to 24 h of prolonged hypoxaemia in the absence of progressive acidaemia (Bocking et al., 1991). This is of interest since, by 24 h of prolonged hypoxaemia secondary to the restriction of uterine blood flow, there are already significant reductions in the synthesis of DNA in the fetal lung, skeletal

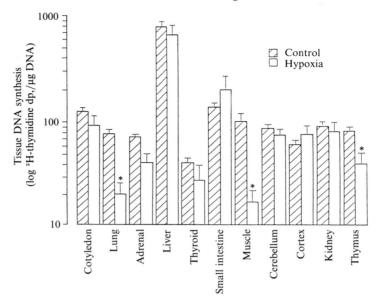

Fig. 9.6. Tissue DNA synthesis rate (DPM of ^{3}H-thymidine/μg of DNA), plotted on a logarithmic scale in sheep fetuses exposed to 24 h of hypoxaemia secondary to the restriction of uterine blood flow ($n = 6$) and control fetuses ($n = 6$). * = significantly different from control.

muscle and thymus gland (Hooper et al., 1991). It is possible that the selective effect of prolonged hypoxaemia on fetal growth may be related in some cases to the redistribution of cardiac output which is maintained under these conditions (Fig. 9.6).

The sheep fetus, therefore, is quite capable of maintaining the redistribution of cardiac output seen with acute hypoxaemia for prolonged periods of time. This is in agreement with the previous observations from growth-restricted sheep fetuses exposed to the daily embolization of the maternal side of the placenta with 15 μm micro-spheres (Creasy et al., 1973). It is through this redistribution of cardiac output that the fetus is able to sustain the necessary growth and metabolism of vital organs such as the brain, heart and adrenal glands.

References

Alonso, J. G., Okal, T., Longo, L. D. & Gilbert, R. D. (1989). Cardiac function during long-term hypoxemia in fetal sheep. *American Journal of Physiology,* **257**, H581–9.

Ashwal, S., Dale, P. S. & Longo, L. D. (1984). Regional cerebral blood flow: studies in the fetal lamb during hypoxia, hypercapnia, acidosis and hypertension. *Pediatric Research,* **18**, 1309–16.

Bocking, A. D., Harding, R. & Wickham, P. J. D. (1986). Effects of reduced uterine blood flow on accelerations and decelerations in heart rate of fetal sheep. *American Journal of Obstetrics and Gynecology,* **154**, 329–35.

Bocking, A. D., Gagnon, R., Milne, K. M. & White, S. E. (1988*a*). Behavioral activity during prolonged hypoxemia in fetal sheep. *Journal of Applied Physiology,* **65**, 2420–6.

Bocking, A. D., Gagnon, R., White, S. E., Homan, J., Milne, K. M. & Richardson, B. (1988*b*). Circulatory responses to prolonged hypoxemia in fetal sheep. *American Journal of Obstetrics and Gynecology,* **159**, 1418–24.

Bocking, A. D., White, S. E., Gagnon, R. & Hansford, H. (1989). Effect of prolonged hypoxemia on fetal heart rate accelerations and decelerations in sheep. *American Journal of Obstetrics and Gynecology,* **161**, 722–7.

Bocking, A. D., White, S. E., Homan, J. & Richardson, B. S. (1991). Effect of prolonged hypoxemia in the absence of acidemia on oxygen consumption in fetal sheep. *Proceedings of the Society for Gynecologic Investigation,* Abstract 576.

Boddy, K., Dawes, G. S., Fisher, R., Pinter, S. & Robinson, J. S. (1974). Foetal respiratory movements, electrocortical and cardiovascular responses to hypoxemia and hypercapnia in sheep. *Journal of Physiology,* **243**, 599–618.

Challis, J. R. G., Fraher, L., Oosterhuis, J., White, S. E. & Bocking, A. D. (1989). Fetal and maternal endocrine responses to prolonged reductions in uterine blood flow in pregnant sheep. *American Journal of Obstetrics and Gynecology,* **160**, 926–32.

Creasy, R. K., de Swiet, M., Kahanpaa, K. V., Young, W. P. & Rudolph, A. M. (1973). Pathophysiological changes in the foetal lambs with growth retardation. In *Foetal and Neonatal Physiology,* ed. R. S. Comline, K. W. Cross, G. S. Dawes & P. W. Nathanielz. pp. 398–402. Cambridge University Press.

Dalton, K. J., Dawes, G. S. & Patrick, J. E. (1977). Diurnal, respiratory and other rhythms of fetal heart rate in lambs. *American Journal of Obstetrics and Gynecology,* **127**, 414–24.

Dawes, G. S. (1984). The central control of fetal breathing and skeletal muscle movements. *Journal of Physiology,* **346**, 1–18.

Dawes, G. S., Gardner, W. N., Johnston, B. M. & Walker, D. W. (1983). Breathing in fetal lambs: the effects of brainstem section. *Journal of Physiology,* **335**, 535–53.

Gluckman, P. D. & Johnston, B. M. (1987). Lesions in the upper lateral pons abolish the hypoxic depression of breathing in unanaesthetized fetal lambs in utero. *Journal of Physiology,* **382**, 373–83.

Hooper, S. B., Coulter, C. L., Deayton, J. M., Harding, R. & Thorburn, G. D. (1990). Fetal endocrine responses to prolonged hypoxemia in sheep. *American Journal of Physiology,* **259**, R703–8.

Hooper, S. B. & Harding, R. (1990). Changes in lung liquid dynamics induced by prolonged fetal hypoxemia. *Journal of Applied Physiology,* **69**, 127–35.

Hooper, S. B., Bocking, A. D., White, S. E., Challis, J. R. G. & Han, V. K. M. (1991). DNA synthesis is reduced in selected fetal tissues during prolonged hypoxemia. *American Journal of Physiology,* **261**, R508–14.

Kitanaka, T., Alonso, J. G., Gilbert, R. D., Benjamin, L. S., Clemons, G. K.

& Longo, L. D. (1989). Fetal responses to long-term hypoxemia in sheep. *American Journal of Physiology*, **256**, R1348–54.

Koos, B. J., Kitanaka, T., Matsuda, K., Gilbert, R. D. & Longo, L. D. (1988). Fetal breathing adaptation to prolonged hypoxemia in sheep. *Journal of Developmental Physiology*, **10**, 161–6.

Liggins, G. C., Vilos, G. A., Campos, G. A., Kitterman, J. A. & Lee, C. H. (1981). The effect of spinal cord transection on lung development in fetal sheep. *Journal of Developmental Physiology*, **3**, 267–74.

Manning, F. A., Platt, L. D. & Sipos, L. (1980). Antepartum fetal evaluation: Development of a fetal biophysical profile. *American Journal of Obstetrics and Gynecology*, **136**, 787–95.

Patrick, J., Richardson, B. S., Rurak, D., Carmichael, L. & Homan, J. (1987). Biophysical variables during sustained hypoxemia in fetal sheep. *Proceedings of the Society for Gynecologic Investigation,* Abstract 8.

Robinson, J. S., Jones, C. T. & Kingston, E. J. (1983). Studies on experimental growth retardation in sheep. The effects of maternal hypoxemia. *Journal of Developmental Physiology*, **5**, 89–100.

Rurak, D. W. & Gruber, N. C. (1983). Increased oxygen consumption associated with breathing activity in fetal lambs. *Journal of Applied Physiology*, **54**, 701–7.

Rurak, D. W., Richardson, B. S., Patrick, J. E., Carmichael, L. & Homan, J. (1990a). Oxygen consumption in the fetal lamb during sustained hypoxemia with progressive acidemia. *American Journal of Physiology*, **258**, R1108–15.

Rurak, D. W., Richardson, B. S., Patrick, J. E., Carmichael, L. & Homan, J. (1990b). Blood flow and oxygen delivery to fetal organs and tissues during sustained hypoxemia. *American Journal of Physiology*, **258**, R1116–22.

Wigglesworth, J. S. & Desai, R. (1979). Effects on lung growth of cervical cord section in the rabbit fetus. *Early Human Development*, **3**, 51–65.

Worthington, D., Piercy, W. N. & Smith, B. T. (1981). Effects of reduction of placental size in sheep. *Obstetrics and Gynecology*, **58**, 215–21.

10

Persistent pulmonary hypertension of the newborn

SCOTT J. SOIFER AND MICHAEL A. HEYMANN

Introduction

In the syndrome of persistent pulmonary hypertension of the newborn (PPHN), pulmonary vascular resistance does not decrease with the initiation of ventilation and oxygenation at birth. Consequently, pulmonary blood flow does not increase. There is persistent pulmonary hypertension, with right-to-left shunting of blood through the foramen ovale, the ductus arteriosus or both resulting in hypoxaemia. In addition, these newborns often have increased systemic vascular resistance, right ventricular dysfunction with tricuspid insufficiency and right ventricular failure, and/or left ventricular dysfunction with mitral insufficiency, hypotension, and cardiogenic shock (Emmanouilides & Baylen, 1979; Graves, Redmond & Arensman, 1988). Newborns with the syndrome of PPHN account for approximately 1% of all admissions to newborn intensive care units (Goetzman & Riemenschneider, 1980; Graves et al., 1988; Spitzer et al., 1988). Their treatment is supportive and consists of the administration of supplemental oxygen, mechanical hyperventilation or alkalosis, correction of metabolic abnormalities, the infusion of nonspecific vasodilators to lower pulmonary arterial pressure, the infusion of cardiotonic agents to improve cardiac function and, most recently, the use of extracorporeal membrane oxygenation (ECMO). Despite treatment, the clinical course is variable and the mortality rate may be 20–50% (Drummond, Peckham & Fox, 1977; Emmanouilides & Baylen, 1979; Goetzman & Riemenschneider, 1980; Graves et al., 1988; Spitzer et al., 1988). Many anatomical and physiological factors are responsible for the control of pulmonary vascular resistance in the fetus and for its normal decrease after birth. PPHN occurs when there are alterations in, or failure of, one or more of these factors.

The normal pulmonary circulation

Morphological development

In the fetus and newborn, pulmonary arteries (regardless of size) have a thicker medial smooth muscle coat relative to the external diameter of the artery than do similar pulmonary arteries in the adult (Hislop & Reid, 1972; Reid, 1977, 1979). This greater muscularity is responsible, in part, for the higher pulmonary vascular resistance and greater pulmonary vascular reactivity in the near term fetus. In fetal lamb lungs, fixed by perfusion at fetal arterial pressure, the medial smooth muscle coat was thickest in the 20–50 μm external diameter arteries (Levin et al., 1976*b*). During the first few weeks after birth there is thinning of the medial smooth muscle coat of the small pulmonary arteries (Hislop & Reid, 1973; Rendas, Branthwaite & Reid, 1978). Similar observations have been made in human fetal lungs (Hislop & Reid, 1972, 1973; Reid, 1979).

Small pulmonary arteries may be identified by their relationship to airways. Pre-acinar pulmonary arteries are proximal to, or course with, the terminal bronchioli. Intra-acinar pulmonary arteries course with the respiratory bronchioli and alveolar ducts, or are within the alveolar walls (Hislop & Reid, 1972). In the late gestation fetus, only about 50% of the pulmonary arteries associated with respiratory bronchioli are partially or completely muscularized, and the pulmonary arteries within alveolar walls are non-muscularized (Hislop & Reid, 1972). The partially muscularized and non-muscularized pulmonary arteries contain pericytes and intermediate cells (intermediate in position & structure between pericytes and mature smooth muscle cells) (Meyrick & Reid, 1979). These cells are precursors of smooth muscle cells and, under certain conditions such as hypoxia, they may rapidly differentiate into mature smooth muscle cells (Meyrick & Reid, 1978). In the adult, smooth muscle extends peripherally along the intra-acinar arteries so that the majority of small pulmonary arteries within alveolar walls are completely muscularized (Hislop & Reid, 1973; Reid, 1977, 1979).

Physiology

In the fetus, normal gas exchange occurs in the placenta. Pulmonary blood flow is low, supplying the lungs with nutritional requirements for growth and serving metabolic functions (Rudolph & Heymann, 1967; Rudolph, 1979; Heymann & Hoffman, 1986). Pulmonary blood flow in the near term fetal lamb is about 100 ml/100 g wet lung weight which is 8 to 10% of the combined left and right ventricular output (400–450 ml/kg/min) (Rudolph & Heymann, 1967, 1970; Heymann, Creasy & Rudolph, 1973). Fetal pulmonary arterial pressure increases progressively with gestation. At term, mean pulmonary arterial pressure is about 50 mm Hg, generally exceeding mean descending aortic pressure by 1 to 2 mm Hg (Lewis, Heymann & Rudolph, 1976). Early in gestation, pulmonary vascular resistance is much higher than in the infant or adult, due to the small number of pulmonary arteries present (Rudolph, 1979). Pulmonary vascular resistance decreases during fetal life (Rudolph & Heymann, 1970; Rudolph, 1979) with the growth of new pulmonary arteries and the increase in total cross sectional area of the pulmonary vascular bed (Levin et al., 1976b). Near term, however, pulmonary vascular resistance was still much higher than after birth (Rudolph et al., 1961; Rudolph, 1979).

Many factors regulate the tone of the fetal pulmonary circulation. In the fetus, the high pulmonary vascular resistance is associated with the low PO_2 in systemic and pulmonary arteries (pulmonary arterial PO_2 is 17 to 20 mm Hg) (Rudolph & Heymann, 1970; Rudolph, 1979; Heymann & Hoffman, 1986). Pulmonary vascular resistance was increased by decreasing the oxygen tension (Lewis, Heymann & Rudolph, 1976) and was decreased by increasing the PO_2 (Cassin et al., 1964; Heymann et al., 1969; Iwamoto, Teitel & Rudolph, 1987) or by infusion of acetylcholine (Lewis, Heymann & Rudolph, 1976), bradykinin (Campbell et al., 1968; Heymann et al., 1969), or prostaglandins (PG) E_2, PGI_2 and PGD_2 (Cassin, Tyler & Wallis, 1975; Tyler, Leffler & Cassin, 1977; Leffler & Hessler, 1979; Cassin, 1980; Tripp et al., 1980; Cassin et al., 1981a,b).

Prostaglandins, cyclo-oxygenase products of arachidonic acid metabolism, are produced by the fetal vasculature (Terragno & Terragno, 1979; Cassin, 1980; Clyman & Heymann, 1981). Pulmonary vascular resistance is high despite the presence of these endogenous vasodilators, indicating active vasoconstriction. Leukotrienes (LT) C_4 and D_4, lipoxygenase products of arachidonic acid metabolism, are potent pulmonary vasoconstrictors (Schreiber, Heymann & Soifer, 1987) and may be responsible, at least in part, for maintaining the high pulmonary vascular resistance in the fetus. In fetal lambs, leukotriene receptor antagonists or synthesis inhibitors (Soifer et al., 1985; Le Bidois et al., 1987) increased pulmonary blood flow eight-fold similar to the increase which occurs with ventilation and oxygenation after birth. Leukotrienes have also been isolated from the tracheal fluid of fetal lambs (Velvis et al., 1990) and from lung lavage fluid of newborns with PPHN (Stenmark et al., 1983) suggesting a role for them in regulating the high pulmonary vascular resistance in the fetus.

Other vasoactive substances, such as platelet activating factor or endo-thelin, may also play a role in maintaining the high pulmonary vascular resistance in the fetus.

After birth and initiation of oxygenation and ventilation by the lungs, pulmonary vascular resistance decreases and pulmonary blood flow increased by eight-to-tenfold (Cassin et al., 1964; Rudolph, 1979; Leffler, Hessler & Green, 1984*a, b*; Heymann & Hoffman, 1986; Iwamoto et al., 1987). The large increase in pulmonary blood flow increases pulmonary venous return to the left atrium, increasing left atrial pressure. Then the valve of the foramen ovale closes, preventing any significant right-to-left shunting of blood (Rudolph et al., 1961; Cassin et al., 1964; Iwamoto et al., 1987). In addition, the ductus arteriosus constricts and closes func-tionally within several h after birth (Moss, Emmanouilides & Duffie, 1963; Clyman & Heymann, 1981), effectively separating the pulmonary and systemic circulations. Mean pulmonary arterial pressure decreases and, by 24 h of age, it is approximately 50% of mean systemic arterial pressure (Rudolph et al., 1961; Moss et al., 1963; Heymann & Hoffman, 1986). Adult values are reached by 2–6 weeks after birth (Rudolph et al., 1961; Krovetz & Goldbloom, 1972).

The decrease in pulmonary vascular resistance with ventilation and oxygenation at birth is the result of many factors. Physical expansion of the lung without oxygenation (Cassin et al., 1964; Enhorning, Adams & Norman, 1966; Tyler et al., 1977; Iwamoto et al., 1987), an increase in alveolar PO_2 (during ventilation) or arterial PO_2 (following exposure to hyperbaric oxygen without ventilation) all increased fetal pulmonary blood flow (Enhorning et al., 1966; Tyler et al., 1977; Leffler et al., 1984*a,b*; Iwamoto et al., 1987; Graves et al., 1988). Physical expansion of the lung decreased pulmonary vascular resistance by replacing the fluid in the alveoli with gas which allowed the unkinking of the small pulmonary arteries (Enhorning et al., 1966). Physical expansion of the lung also caused the release of PGI_2 (Edmonds, Berry & Wyllie, 1969; Tyler et al., 1977; Gryglewski, Korbut & Ocetkiewicz, 1978; Gryglewski, 1980; Leffler & Hessler, 1979; Leffler et al., 1984) which is known to decrease pulmonary vascular resistance in the fetal goat and lamb (Tyler et al., 1977; Leffler & Hessler, 1979; Cassin, 1980; Cassin et al., 1981*a*). In addition, it has been shown that inhibitors of prostaglandin synthesis attenuate the initial decrease in pulmonary vascular resistance that occurs with ventilation (Leffler, Tyler & Cassin, 1978) and block the decrease in pulmonary vascular resistance that occurs with physical expansion of the lung but not the decrease that occurs with oxygenation (Tyler et al., 1977).

The increase in alveolar or arterial PO_2 may decrease pulmonary vascular resistance either directly, by dilating the small pulmonary arteries, or indirectly by stimulating the production of vasodilator substances (Cassin et al., 1964; Rudolph, 1979; Heymann & Hoffman, 1986). In the fetal lamb, bradykinin production was increased by ventilation at birth (Campbell et al., 1968) and by hyperbaric oxygenation (Heymann et al., 1969). Bradykinin stimulates PGI_2 production and release from endothelial cells (McIntyre et al., 1985) which may cause vasodilatation. In addition, bradykinin stimulated the production of endothelium-derived relaxing factor (EDRF) by endothelial cells (Ignarro, 1991). Once released, EDRF diffuses into vascular smooth muscle cells, stimulates guanylate cyclase and increases the concentration of cyclic 3', 5' guanosine monophosphate, which initiates a cascade that results in smooth muscle relaxation and vasodilatation (Ignarro, 1991). In the fetal lamb, inhibition of EDRF production by N^w nitro-L-arginine increased pulmonary vascular resistance and attenuated the decrease in pulmonary vascular resistance produced by ventilation with 100% oxygen (Fineman, Heymann & Soifer, 1991; Moore et al., 1991). N^w nitro-L-arginine did not block the initial decrease in pulmonary vascular resistance but prevented the successful transition to extrauterine life.

Control of the perinatal pulmonary circulation, therefore, probably reflects a balance between factors producing pulmonary vasoconstriction (low PO_2, leukotrienes and other substances) and those producing pulmonary vasodilatation (high PO_2, PGI2, EDRF, & other vasoactive substances). The dramatic increase in pulmonary blood flow with the initiation of ventilation and oxygenation at birth is the result of a shift from active pulmonary vasoconstriction to active pulmonary vasodilatation.

The abnormal pulmonary circulation

Morphological development

The pathophysiological mechanisms preventing the normal fall in pulmonary vascular resistance which therefore result in the increased systemic vascular resistance and cardiac dysfunction in newborns with PPHN are not well understood. There may be increased concentration of, or responsiveness to, vasoconstrictor substances and/or decreased concentration of, or responsiveness to, vasodilator substances. In new-borns who died with PPHN (Haworth & Reid, 1976; Levin et al., 1978; McKenzie & Haworth, 1981; Murphy et al., 1981) there is an increase in the thickness of the medial smooth muscle coat of the small pulmonary arteries and muscularization of otherwise partially muscularized pulmon-ary arteries becomes complete, with extension of this muscle coat to the arteries within the alveolar wall (generally muscularized only in adults). In some patients, microvascular thrombi further decrease the cross sectional area of the pulmonary vascular bed (Lewis et al., 1976). There is also proliferation of adventitial tissue (Murphy et al., 1981). Infarction of the papillary muscles of the tricuspid and mitral valves and necrosis of the ventricular septum occurs (Emmanouilides & Baylen, 1979). These structural changes take time to develop, indicating that in utero events have altered the pulmonary circulation and may account for the altered response to vasodilator and to vasoconstrictor stimuli seen. The abnor-malities of the systemic vasculature and cardiac function suggest a more generalized effect on the fetal circulation.

Chronic stress in utero induces anatomical and physiological changes in the pulmonary circulation similar to newborns with PPHN. Pregnant rats exposed to hypoxic gas mixtures produce offspring with an increased medial smooth muscle coat in the small pulmonary arteries (Fox & Duara, 1983). After birth, the ratio of the medial smooth muscle coat to the external diameter of these arteries decreased at a slower rate than controls. Newborn calves also develop severe pulmonary vascular changes, including smooth muscle thickening, cellular proliferation and extra-matrix deposition, after being placed in a hypobaric oxygen chamber (Stenmark et al., 1987, 1988; Prosser et al., 1989). Similar vascular changes develop in newborn pigs (Allen & Haworth, 1986) and adult rats (Meyrick & Reid, 1978) exposed to hypoxia. However, other studies, using pregnant rats or guinea pigs in a hypobaric chamber to produce maternal hypoxia and fetal hypoxaemia have failed to reproduce these changes (Geggel, Aronovitz & Reid, 1986; Murphy, Aronovitz & Reid, 1986). There was a significant decrease in cardiac output in the guinea pigs suggesting that chronic in utero hypoxaemia produced cardiac dysfunction. The estimated pulmonary vascular resistance (mean pulmonary arterial pressure/cardiac output) was also increased. In the pregnant ewe, embolization of the maternal utero-placental circulation with microspheres produced fetal hypoxaemia, haematocrit elevation, growth retardation, and a decrease in pulmonary blood flow in the fetal lamb (Creasy et al., 1972, 1973; Drummond & Bissonnette, 1978). With the initiation of ventilation and oxygenation at birth these lambs had an increased pulmonary arterial pressure (Drummond & Bissonnette, 1978).

Umbilical cord compression is a common cause of fetal distress and may result in heart rate decelerations (Itskovitz, LaGamma & Rudolph, 1983). In fetal lambs, short periods of umbilical cord compression decreased umbilical blood flow and fetal PaO_2. Systemic arterial pressure increased and heart rate decreased (Itskovitz, La Gamma & Rudolph, 1983, 1987) even after the compression was released, suggesting that hormonal release may mediate these changes (Daniel et al., 1975, 1978). After prolonged periods of severe umbilical cord compression the decrease in combined ventricular output and pulmonary blood flow were more pronounced (Itskovitz et al., 1987). In the fetal lamb, chronic umbilical cord compression for 10 to 15 days decreased PaO_2 (Soifer et al., 1987). At birth, these lambs had increased pulmonary vascular resistance and pulmonary arterial pressure, and an exaggerated response to alveolar hypoxia. In addition, they had excessive muscularization of the small pulmonary arteries, similar to newborns with PPHN. These studies suggest that chronic in utero hypoxaemia induces both anatomical and physiological changes in the pulmonary circulation as well as cardiac dysfunction.

Fetal systemic hypertension is transmitted to the pulmonary arteries if the ductus arteriosus is widely patent (Rudolph, 1979; Heymann & Hoffman, 1986). In the fetal lamb, systemic hypertension produced by constriction of a renal or umbilical artery for 6 to 14 days, or pulmonary hypertension produced by mechanical constriction of the ductus arteriosus for 8 days, increased the ratio of the medial smooth muscle coat to the external diameter of the small pulmonary arteries (Levin et al., 1978).

Pharmacological constriction of the ductus arteriosus by administration of indomethacin to the pregnant ewe for 2 to 4 days, or ligation or compression of the ductus arteriosus in the fetal sheep produced persistent pulmonary hypertension after birth which was unresponsive to oxygenation, hyperventilation and non-specific vasodilators, and was accompanied by an exaggerated response to alveolar hypoxia, structural changes in the pulmonary arteries and infarction of the papillary muscles of the tricuspid valve (Agarwal, Paltoo & Palmer, 1970; Ruiz et al., 1972; Levin, Mills & Weinberg, 1979; Levin, 1980; Abman, Shanley & Accurso, 1989; Morin, 1989; Wild, Nickerson & Morin, 1989). Administration of indomethacin to the pregnant rat (Harker et al., 1981), although not to the guinea pig (Demello et al., 1987), produced similar changes. Use of this and other inhibitors of prostaglandin synthesis, during pregnancy has been linked to the development of PPHN (Manchester, Margolis & Sheldon, 1976; Csaba, Sulyok & Ertl, 1978; Levin et al., 1978*a*, *b*; Wilkinson, Aynsley-Green & Mitchell, 1979), but an association is not clearly established. These studies suggest that chronic in utero systemic and/or pulmonary hypertension produces a generalized circulatory effect on the fetus, inducing anatomical changes in the pulmonary circulation and heart.

To summarize, newborns with PPHN demonstrate failure of normal pulmonary vasodilatation with the initiation of ventilation and oxygenation at birth. There is also an exaggerated response to pulmonary vasoconstrictor stimuli, increased systemic vascular resistance and cardiac dysfunction. These changes may be caused by the increased muscularization of the small pulmonary arteries, increased concentration of, or responsiveness to vasoconstrictor substances, or decreased concentration of, or responsiveness to, vasodilator substances. The effects of potentially specific pulmonary vasodilator agents have been studied extensively in the normal fetal lamb and goat to determine whether they are responsible for the decrease in pulmonary vascular resistance and the increase in pulmonary blood flow with the initiation of ventilation and oxygenation at birth. The results of these studies have been applied to the treatment of newborns with PPHN with little success. Chronic in utero stress (chronic hypoxaemia, systemic and/or pulmonary hypertension, or umbilical cord compression) produces similar anatomical and physiological changes in the pulmonary and systemic circulations and the heart. A better understanding of the mechanisms responsible for the pulmonary and systemic vascular and myocardial changes in newborns with PPHN is required before improved treatment is likely.

Physiology

The pathophysiological feature common to all newborns with PPHN is the failure of the pulmonary vascular resistance to fall normally with the initiation of ventilation and oxygenation at birth. As a result, pulmonary blood flow remains low, and pulmonary arterial pressure remains elevated. Right-to-left shunting of blood occurs through the ductus arteriosus (which often remains patent). Right ventricular end-diastolic and right atrial pressures remain elevated resulting in right-to-left shunting of blood across the foramen ovale (Levin et al., 1976a; Drummond et al., 1977; Fox et al., 1977; Emmanouilides & Baylen, 1979; Goetzman &

Riemenschneider, 1980; Fox & Duara, 1983; Heymann & Hoffman, 1986; Graves et al., 1988; Spitzer et al., 1988). The presence of tricuspid valve insufficiency often accentuates this shunting. All newborns with PPHN have decreased systemic PaO_2 and hypoxaemia. The higher the pulmonary vascular resistance the lower the PaO_2.

Pulmonary vascular resistance is related to several factors and can be estimated by applying the hydraulic equivalent of Ohm's law and the Poiseuille–Hagen relationship (Prandtl & Tietjens, 1957; Roos, 1962; Caro, 1966). The hydraulic equivalent of Ohm's law states that resistance to flow between two points along a tube equals the pressure drop between the two points divided by flow. For the pulmonary vascular bed where R is resistance and Q is pulmonary blood flow, the pressure drop occurs from the pulmonary artery (Ppa) to the pulmonary vein (Ppv). Thus:

$$R = (Ppa - Ppv)/Q \qquad (1)$$

An increase in pulmonary artery pressure caused by pulmonary vasoconstriction secondary to alveolar hypoxia or other noxious stimuli, increases pulmonary vascular resistance. To maintain the driving pressure across the lungs an increase in pulmonary venous pressure also increases pulmonary arterial pressure and pulmonary vascular resistance (Caro, 1966). This results in delayed clearance of fetal lung liquid and increased fluid in the interstitial spaces, alveolar hypoxia, and further pulmonary vasoconstriction (Iliff, Greene & Hughes, 1972). Pulmonary venous pressure is also increased by left ventricular myocardial dysfunction (secondary to asphyxia or electrolyte imbalance, such as hypocalcaemia, or hypoglycaemia) which increases left ventricular end-diastolic pressure producing left atrial and pulmonary venous hypertension. Therefore, depression of myocardial performance would worsen pulmonary hypertension in newborns with PPHN.

Other factors that affect pulmonary vascular resistance can be defined by the Poiseuille–Hagen relationship (Roos, 1962; Caro, 1966) which describes the resistance to flow of a Newtonian fluid through a straight glass tube of circular cross section:

$$\text{Resistance} = (8l\eta)/(\pi r^4) \qquad (2)$$

where l is the length of the tube, r is its internal radius, and η is the viscosity of the fluid. However, there are differences between physical and biological systems. First, blood is not a Newtonian fluid; the viscosity of blood increases with haematocrits greater than 55% (Argawal, Paltoo & Palmer, 1970; Benis, Usami & Chien, 1970). Secondly, blood flow through the pulmonary circulation is pulsatile rather than laminar and the small pulmonary arteries are branched, curved, and tapered rather than smooth (Roos, 1962). In addition, the small pulmonary arteries are in parallel and the radii of these arteries may differ in different lung zones. However, the effects of these factors on pulmonary vascular resistance are minimal (Caro, 1966; Whitmore, 1968). Despite these differences from physical systems, changes in viscosity or radius affect pulmonary vascular resistance. Increasing the viscosity of blood perfusing the lungs or decreasing the radius or cross sectional area of the pulmonary vascular bed (r^4) increases pulmonary vascular resistance (Roos, 1962; Caro, 1966).

Blood viscosity is related to red cell number, fibrinogen concentration, and red cell deformability. An increased haematocrit (after twin to twin, or maternal to fetal blood transfusion, or delayed clamping of the umbilical cord) will increase viscosity (Whitmore, 1968; Argawal et al., 1970). Pulmonary vascular resistance increases logarithmically with increasing haematocrit (Argawal et al., 1970). Chronic intrauterine hypoxaemia increases haematocrit and fibrinogen concentration (Pickart, Creasy & Thaler, 1976), and is associated with PPHN. In the newborn, red blood cells are less deformable than in the adult. This is accentuated by acidaemia which may increase pulmonary vascular resistance.

The cross sectional area of the pulmonary vascular bed is reduced in newborns with PPHN because of an increased thickness of the medial smooth muscle coat of the small pulmonary arteries, failure of the fetal pulmonary circulation to undergo normal postnatal vasodilatation, or under-development of the pulmonary circulation resulting in a decreased number of small pulmonary arteries. Chronic in utero stress can induce these pulmonary vascular changes, although why some stressed fetuses develop pulmonary hypertension whereas many others, equally stressed, do not, is unclear.

There is not only increased thickness of the medial smooth coat of the small pulmonary arteries in newborns with PPHN, there is also an accelerated distribution of the smooth muscle to arteries that are normally partially or non-muscularized. These abnormal small pulmonary arteries have an exaggerated constrictor response to alveolar hypoxia (Soifer et al., 1987; Morin, 1989) and an abnormal response to vasoactive substances. For example, PGD_2 decreased pulmonary arterial pressure and increased cardiac output without changing systemic arterial pressure in newborn lambs with hypoxia induced pulmonary hypertension (Soifer, Morin & Heymann, 1982; Soifer et al., 1983), while it increased pulmonary arterial pressure in older lambs (Soifer et al., 1983). In newborns with PPHN, PGD_2 also increased pulmonary arterial pressure, suggesting that there had been a functional as well as structural alteration of the pulmonary vascular bed (Soifer, Clyman & Heymann, 1988). Other mechanisms involved in normal regulation of perinatal pulmonary vascular resistance may also be altered resulting in the inability to sustain pulmonary vasodilation during the transition to extra-uterine life.

Clinical syndrome

Persistent pulmonary hypertension of the newborn is characterized by the onset of cyanosis and tachypnoea, often with moderate, or even severe, respiratory distress within 4–8 h of birth. It occurs most commonly in full and post-term newborns and very rarely in the preterm newborn (Gersony, 1973; Levin et al., 1976*a*; Drummond et al., 1977; Fox et al., 1977; Emmanouilides & Baylen, 1979; Goetzman & Riemenschneider, 1980; Fox & Duara, 1983; Graves et al., 1988; Spitzer et al., 1988). The clinical presentation may be indistinguishable from certain types of congenital heart disease (such as total anomalous pulmonary venous return), or pneumonia or sepsis (caused by group B *β*-haemolytic *Streptococcus* or *Escherichia coli*). In addition, some newborns with diaphragmatic hernia or chest wall abnormalities have hypoplastic lungs, an underdeveloped pulmonary vascular bed, and pulmonary hypertension after birth. Newborns with PPHN can be divided into two groups. The first group have intrinsic pulmonary disease secondary to the aspiration of meconium or blood. The second group have no intrinsic pulmonary disease. The mortality rate is higher in those newborns with aspiration syndromes (Fox et al., 1977; Fox & Duara, 1983).

In newborns with PPHN there is often a history of a difficult or abnormal labour and delivery, or perinatal asphyxia. The Apgar scores are low and there is meconium staining of the amniotic fluid, even without evidence of aspiration. Numerous physical signs and symptoms are present. Most newborns have cyanosis and tachypnoea. In addition, intercostal retraction, nasal flaring, rales, rhonchi and wheezing are associated with increased airway resistance and respiratory distress. In many newborns with PPHN, a systolic murmur is heard along the lower left sternal border. This is due either to myocardial dysfunction or to an increase in afterload, which causes dilatation of the right and/or the left ventricle and secondary tricuspid (more commonly) and/or mitral insufficiency (Heymann & Hoffman, 1986). Because of the cyanosis and heart murmur, congenital heart disease must be excluded early in the management of newborns suspected of having PPHN (Emmanouilides & Baylen, 1979).

Laboratory tests are often abnormal. Hypoglycaemia, hypocalcaemia, increased haematocrit, and acidaemia are commonly found. Thrombocytopenia may occur after several days of illness in newborns who are the most severely ill (Segall, Goetzman & Schick, 1980), secondary to the development of micro-thromboembolism of the small pulmonary arteries (Levin, Weinberg & Perkin, 1983). The chest X-ray in newborns with aspiration syndrome shows parenchymal lung changes while the chest X-ray in those without aspiration syndrome shows clear lung fields and decreased pulmonary vascular markings. However, the radiographic appearance of the lungs is quite variable. Often the severity of the hypoxaemia does not correlate with the chest X-ray findings (Heymann & Hoffman, 1986). The chest X-ray will help in the diagnosis of other conditions which cause cyanosis and respiratory distress, including hyaline membrane disease, diaphragmatic hernia and congenital heart disease. Cardiomegaly is present in half of the newborns (Drummond et al., 1977; Emmanouilides & Baylen, 1979). The ECG may be normal or may show nonspecific changes. Because pulmonary hypertension does not allow the normal regression of the right ventricular free wall mass, the electrocardiogram may show an increased right ventricular contribution (Heymann & Hoffman, 1986). Right atrial enlargement, and ST segment and T wave abnormalities, suggestive of myocardial ischaemia may be present. Ultrasound examination (M-mode, two-dimensional, Doppler, & colour Doppler) is useful in newborns for the diagnosis of PPHN (Emmanouilides & Baylen, 1979; Henry, 1984). An echocardiogram can differentiate newborns with PPHN from those with congenital heart disease. It is also useful in the assessment of cardiac function. Right-to-left atrial shunting is confirmed by Doppler examination or by contrast two-dimensional echocardiography, performed by injecting saline into a vein and observing the microcavitations entering the left atrium across the atrial septum. The pulmonary arterial pressure may also be estimated using the ratio (increased in newborns with PPHN) of the pre-ejection period to the ejection time (PEP/ET) measured from the M-mode echocardiogram (Henry, 1984), or by the Doppler measurement of right ventricular pressure if tricuspid insufficiency is present. In some newborns, cardiac catheterization may be necessary to exclude congenital heart disease (Levin et al., 1976a). The hyperoxia–hyperventilation test will also differentiate between newborns with PPHN and those with congenital heart disease. In this test, the newborn is hyperventilated manually using an anaesthesia bag connected to the endotracheal tube (Fox & Duara, 1983). When the pH reaches a 'critical value' (generally greater than 7.55) pulmonary vascular resistance decreases (Schreiber, Heymann & Soifer, 1986), right-to-left shunting of blood decreases and PaO_2 increases (Drummond et al., 1981). If, after 5 min of hyperventilation, PaO_2 is greater than 100 mm Hg, the newborn has PPHN and not congenital heart disease.

Decreased systemic arterial oxygen tension and hypoxaemia are always present with PPHN. Systemic arterial hypercarbia and acidosis develop with time. Hypoxaemia, measured as a lower than normal PaO_2 or haemoglobin oxygen saturation or as a decrease in saturation (arterial pulse oximetry) or transcutaneous PO_2 measurement, is secondary to right-to-left shunting of blood across a patent foramen ovale or through the lungs (intrapulmonary shunt). An additional right-to-left shunt through the ductus arteriosus was evidenced by a difference in PaO_2 of greater than 5 mm Hg between blood samples drawn simultaneously from an artery arising from the ascending aorta (right radial artery) and from the descending aorta (usually via an indwelling umbilical arterial catheter) or by differences in pulse oximetry or transcutaneous measurements (Fox & Duara, 1983; Heymann & Hoffman, 1986). These differences often correlate with the degree of pulmonary hypertension. This PaO_2 difference may be more easily demonstrated when the newborn is ventilated with 100% oxygen.

Management

General management

Management of the newborn with PPHN begins prior to birth. Obstetric management attempts to identify the chronically stressed fetus so as to minimize further stress and prevent perinatal asphyxia. At the time of delivery, care is taken to prevent the newborn from aspirating meconium (before the first breath) by suctioning the mouth with a bulb syringe and the airway with deep endotracheal suction. Rapid resuscitation may be necessary to minimize the effects of hypoxaemia and asphyxia.

After birth, if cyanosis or respiratory distress has developed, other causes must be excluded. PPHN is a diagnosis of exclusion. Serum glucose and calcium concentrations should be measured and any electrolyte abnormalities should be corrected. Sepsis or pneumonia may mimic

238   *Scott J. Soifer and Michael A. Heymann*

PPHN; after blood and urine cultures are obtained, appropriate broad spectrum antibiotics should be started. The clinical presentation of PPHN may be indistinguishable from congenital heart disease. To exclude congenital heart disease, a chest X-ray, electrocardiogram, echocardiogram, or cardiac catheterization, should be performed as necessary. If the haematocrit is greater than 55% it should be lowered by performing a partial exchange transfusion (Argawal et al., 1970). This may lower pulmonary vascular resistance and increase PaO_2. Because hypoxaemia limits O_2 delivery in newborns with PPHN, O_2 consumption should be minimized by maintaining the newborn in a neutral thermal environment.

Ventilatory management

The goal of ventilatory management is to maintain the PaO_2 (obtained from blood withdrawn from an umbilical arterial catheter) between 60 and 80 mm Hg, $PaCO_2$ between 35 and 45 mm Hg and the arterial pH between 7.45 and 7.55 (Dworetz et al., 1989). Initially, this may be achieved by administering supplemental O_2 to the spontaneously breathing newborn. If hypoxaemia, hypercarbia, or acidosis develops then the newborn is intubated and mechanical ventilation started. Sedation (Nembutal, 1–5 mg/kg or Versed, 0.1 mg/kg), analgesia (morphine sulfate, 0.05–0.2 mg/kg), and muscle relaxation (vecuronium, 0.1 mg/kg) may be necessary to prevent the newborn from 'struggling' against the mechanical ventilator. Inflation pressures (peak inspiratory pressure and positive end-expiratory pressure) should be minimized to prevent the development of a pneumothorax, barotrauma and bronchopulmonary dysplasia (Fox et al., 1977; Graves et al., 1988; Dworetz et al., 1989).

Changes in arterial pH affect pulmonary vascular resistance (Rudolph & Yuan, 1966; Drummond et al., 1981; Schreiber, Heymann & Soifer, 1986). Acidosis increases pulmonary vascular resistance while alkalosis decreases pulmonary vascular resistance. Newborns with PPHN demonstrated a 'critical pH' associated with increasing PaO_2 (Rudolph & Yuan, 1966; Fox et al., 1977; Peckham & Fox, 1978; Drummond et al., 1981; Schreiber, Heymann & Soifer, 1986). Previously, the increased PaO_2 was achieved by hyperventilation which resulted in increased morbidity and mortality secondary to barotrauma and bronchopulmonary dysplasia (Dworetz et al., 1989). In the newborn lamb with hypoxia-induced pulmonary hypertension, alkalosis (arterial pH between 7.55 and 7.65), produced by the infusion of sodium bicarbonate or by hyperventilation decreased pulmonary arterial pressure and resistance equally (Schreiber, Heymann & Soifer, 1986). The infusion of sodium bicarbonate allows the maintenance of the desired pH without resorting to hyperventilation.

In newborns with PPHN the PaO_2 decreases in response to tactile stimuli. Therefore, handling these newborns should be kept to a minimum. Endotracheal suction is necessary to clear the airway of meconium or blood and to maintain the patency of the endotracheal tube. However, this treatment often results in profound hypoxaemia unresponsive to increased oxygenation or hyperventilation. This is an exaggerated response to alveolar hypoxia. Endotracheal suction should be performed when clinically indicated, not as a routine. Once stability of arterial blood gases has been achieved, changes in ventilation should be made very slowly. Peak inspiratory pressure should be reduced in 1 cm H_2O decrements. Next, the inspired oxygen concentration should be reduced in 1 to 2% decrements. Ventilatory rate should also be decreased slowly (Heymann & Hoffman, 1986).

High frequency jet ventilators have been developed to deliver small volumes of gas at high frequencies to achieve adequate gas exchange at lower mean airway pressures (Spitzer et al., 1988). This is to decrease barotrauma and the incidence of bronchopulmonary dysplasia. High frequency jet ventilation has been associated with an increased incidence of tracheal injury and intracranial haemorrhage in premature infants. Despite these complications, it has been used successfully in the treatment of newborns with PPHN who have failed to maintain adequate arterial blood gases with conventional ventilation (Spitzer et al., 1988).

Pharmacological therapy

If there is no response to mechanical ventilation then administration of vasodilating drugs is the next step in management. No drug specifically dilates the pulmonary circulation; all are general vasodilators with systemic effects. The goal of pharmacological therapy is a sustained increase in PaO_2 without a significant decrease in systemic arterial pressure.

The most commonly used vasodilator is tolazoline, an α-adrenergic antagonist with histamine-like action (Fox et al., 1977; Emmanouilides & Baylen, 1979; Goetzman & Riemenschneider, 1980; Drummond et al., 1981; Graves et al., 1988). The dose of tolazoline is 0.25 to 1.0 mg/kg, injected intravenously over 15 min followed by a 1.0 mg/kg per h continuous infusion. Tolazoline is effective in 10 to 50% of newborns with

PPHN (Drummond et al., 1977; Fox et al., 1977; Drummond et al., 1981; Heymann & Hoffman, 1986). Factors predicting success are unknown. The complication rate of tolazoline is at least 70%, the most common complications being systemic hypotension, gastrointestinal bleeding, and renal failure (Fox et al., 1977). Fluid resuscitation with colloid or crystalloid, or the infusion of dopamine, are often necessary to maintain systemic arterial pressure.

Prostaglandins have been used in the treatment of newborns with PPHN. PGI_2 markedly decreased pulmonary arterial pressure in fetal animals (Leffler & Hessler, 1979; Cassin, 1980; Cassin et al., 1981a). It is likely to be that PGI_2 is involved in the decrease in pulmonary vascular resistance occurring with the initiation of ventilation and oxygenation at birth (Leffler et al., 1978; Leffler & Hessler, 1979; Leffler, Hessler & Green, 1984a, b; Velvis et al., 1990). However, PGI_2 has resulted in severe hypotension and death in newborns with PPHN. PGE_1 (0.05 to 0.2 μg/kg/min) is used to prevent the closure of the ductus arteriosus in newborns with congenital heart disease (Clyman & Heymann, 1981). PGE_1 decreased pulmonary arterial pressure in fetal and newborn lambs (less than PGI_2), but the effect appears to be nonspecific (Tripp et al., 1980). PGE_1 is not useful in the treatment of newborns with PPHN. Finally, PGD_2, a selective pulmonary vasodilator in fetal and newborn lambs (Cassin, 1980; Soifer et al., 1982, 1983), did not improve oxygenation or lower pulmonary arterial pressure in newborns with PPHN (Soifer et al., 1988).

Other drugs are also used in the treatment of newborns with PPHN. Isoprenaline, a β-adrenergic agonist, stimulates adenylate cyclase to increase the concentration of cyclic 3', 5' adenosine monophosphate which relaxes vascular smooth muscle, and increases heart rate and myocardial contractility (Crowley, Fineman & Soifer, 1991). In the newborn lamb with pulmonary hypertension, isoprenaline (0.01 to 0.05 μg/kg per min) selectively decreased pulmonary arterial pressure and increased cardiac output, while higher doses (1.0 to 2.0 μg/kg per min) also decreased systemic arterial pressure (Crowley et al., 1991). Dobutamine (5 to 20 μg/kg per min), another β-adrenergic agonist, also decreased pulmonary arterial pressure and increased cardiac output although to a lesser degree than isoprenaline (Crowley et al., 1991). Amrinone, a putative cyclic AMP phosphodiesterase inhibitor, increases the concentration of cyclic 3', 5' adenosine monophosphate in vascular smooth muscle cells and the heart. This results in vasodilation and increased myocardial contractility. Amrinone (1 to 5 mg/kg bolus injection, followed by 5 to 10 μg/kg per min continuous infusion) decreases pulmonary arterial pressure and increases cardiac output in newborn lambs with pulmonary hypertension (Crowley, Fineman & Soifer, 1990). In infants and older children, amrinone has been used in the treatment of pulmonary hypertension after cardiac surgery. Nitroprusside (0.05 to 10 μg/kg per min) and other nitrovasodilators donate nitric oxide (biologically identical to endothelium-derived relaxing factor) within the vascular smooth muscle cell, where it stimulates guanylate cyclase and increases the concentration of cyclic guanosine 3', 5' monophosphate (Fineman et al., 1991; Ignarro, 1991). This second messenger initiates a cascade that results in smooth muscle dilatation. These effects are non-specific. Nitroprusside has been used to treat newborns with PPHN (Rhine, Benitz & Stevenson, 1988). Combination therapy with drugs that have different mechanisms of action should be administered to newborns with PPHN so that lower doses can be used with fewer side effects.

Monitoring

Monitoring of haemodynamic variables and arterial blood gases is necessary for the successful treatment of newborns with pulmonary hypertension. The haemodynamic and arterial blood gas responses to ventilation and pharmacological agents are rapid and they require continuous assessment (Fox et al., 1977; Peckham & Fox, 1978; Heymann & Hoffman, 1986). Indwelling umbilical arterial catheters are used to measure systemic arterial pressure continuously and to obtain blood samples for arterial blood gases and pH. If the umbilical artery cannot be cannulated then another artery (radial, posterior tibial, dorsalis pedis, or axillary) may be used. Central venous pressure is measured by placing a catheter at the right atrial-vena caval junction from either the umbilical, jugular, subclavian, or femoral veins. Central venous pressure measurements help in the assessment of the preload (or filling pressures) of the heart. Catheters placed in the central circulation are also useful when large volumes of fluid are administered rapidly.

It is assumed that in newborns with PPHN, systemic PaO_2 correlates with the degree of right-to-left shunting of blood and with pulmonary arterial pressure. However, some newborns have clinical and echocardiographic evidence of PPHN with normal pulmonary arterial pressures (Soifer et al., 1988). Pulmonary arterial pressure can be measured directly by 'floating' a balloon-tipped flow directed catheter into the pulmonary artery (under pressure guidance) from either the jugular, subclavian, or femoral veins (Peckham & Fox, 1978; Drummond et al., 1981; Soifer et al., 1988). Echo-cardiography or fluoroscopy may be helpful in catheter placement. However, use of such catheters is not routine (Peckham & Fox, 1978; Heymann & Hoffman, 1986) even though they provide additional information about the relationship of pulmonary to systemic arterial pressure and allow for changes in therapy before blood gas deteriorates. These catheters (if they are positioned distal to the ductus arteriosus) also allow the infusion of vasoactive drugs directly into the pulmonary circulation.

Systemic arterial oxygen tension is measured continuously by using either transcutaneous PO_2 monitoring or pulse oximetry. Electrodes or probes are placed on the right upper and lower body to obtain pre- and postductus arteriosus measurements. Reduction in the differences between these measurements indicates a reduction in the right-to-left shunting of blood through the ductus arteriosus and a decrease in pulmonary vascular resistance.

Extracorporeal membrane oxygenation

Despite improvements in the care of the critically ill newborn and advances in therapy for newborns with PPHN, the mortality rate is 20–50%. Extracorporeal membrane oxygenation (ECMO) has been used in the treatment of newborns with respiratory failure since 1976 (Bartlett et al., 1985; Graves et al., 1988; Fugate & Ryan, 1989; O'Rourke et al., 1989). ECMO is a method of cardiopulmonary bypass that provides normal blood oxygenation, cardiac output, and oxygen delivery, providing relief from pulmonary ventilation. The ECMO circuit consists of tubing, the membrane oxygenator, a heat exchanger, and a roller pump (Fugate & Ryan, 1989). To place a newborn on ECMO, the right internal jugular vein and right common carotid artery are surgically exposed. Cannulae are inserted and advanced into the right atrium (venous) and ascending aorta (arterial). Blood is removed from the venous cannula by gravity, oxygenated by the extracorporeal circuit, and pumped back by a roller pump via the arterial cannula. During ECMO, ventilation is minimized to rest the lungs and to prevent further lung injury. Once stable on ECMO, the newborn is assessed for organ dysfunction and treatment is begun. Adequate nutrition, sedation, and diuresis are necessary. Once improvement in lung (improved PaO_2) and heart function (by echocardiography) have been documented the newborn is weaned from ECMO, the cannulae are clamped and removed after a few hours, and the blood vessels repaired (Fugate & Ryan, 1989).

There are significant complications associated with ECMO. Since the mid 1970's over 3,500 newborns have been placed on ECMO with an overall survival of 80%. The survival rate is higher for newborns with PPHN or aspiration syndromes (Neonatal ELSO Registry Report, October, 1990). Mechanical complications have been reported with all parts of the 'circuit'. They include accidental decannulation, rupture of tubing, and malfunction of the oxygenator and heat exchanger (Fugate & Ryan, 1989). Intracranial haemorrhage occurs in 10 to 30% of newborns treated with ECMO and is associated with a 50% mortality rate (Taylor et al., 1989). It is secondary to heparinization, necessary to prevent the circuit from clotting, and to the thrombocytopenia that often develops. Frequent cranial ultrasound scans are necessary for any newborn on ECMO. Bleeding can also occur from other areas including cannulation sites, chest tubes or other deep punctures (Fugate & Ryan, 1989). Long-term neurological follow-up of newborns treated with ECMO has been satisfactory (Taylor et al., 1989). Some newborns have also developed bronchopulmonary dysplasia.

As more and more centres establish ECMO programmes, the question of who needs ECMO becomes important. Most centres have developed criteria to predict which patients would (in their experience) have an 80% chance of dying. It is important that each centre develops its own criteria and does not rely on published information. The 80% mortality criteria of Bartlett et al., 1985 are:

1. $PaO_2 < 40$ mm Hg or pH < 7.15 for 2 h, or
2. 2 of the following for 3 h – $PaO_2 < 55$ mm Hg, pH < 7.40, or hypotension, or
3. indicators of severe barotrauma;

The 80% mortality criteria of Short (Dworetz et al., 1989; Taylor et al., 1989) are

1. $AaDO_2 \geq 610$ for 8 h of maximal medical therapy, or
2. $AaDO_2 \geq 605$ with a peak inspiratory pressure ≥ 38 cm H_2O for 4 h of maximal medical therapy;

When these were applied retrospectively to other newborns (who did not receive ECMO), 90% of these newborns survived (Benis et al., 1970). More research is needed, including a large multicentre randomized clinical trial (vs today's conventional therapy) before ECMO is used on newborns who are likely to survive without it. In addition, more research is needed on the physiology of ECMO, different cannulation techniques, and heparin bonded circuits, etc. so that the morbidity and mortality of this potentially valuable technique can be reduced.

Conclusion

Persistent pulmonary hypertension of the newborn is characterized by increased pulmonary vascular resistance, right-to-left shunting of blood through the foramen ovale and ductus arteriosus, and hypoxaemia. Although the pathophysiological mechanisms producing PPHN are unknown, chronic in utero stress and perinatal asphyxia play a role. There are structural changes in the pulmonary circulation of newborns dying secondary to PPHN suggesting that there is accelerated maturation and abnormal development of the medial smooth muscle coat of the small pulmonary arteries. Current management is largely supportive because the mechanisms producing pulmonary vasodilatation at birth are not completely understood. Extracorporeal membrane oxygenation is used to treat the most critically ill newborns with PPHN. The development of animal models will help our understanding of the pathophysiological mechanisms producing PPHN and may lead to specific therapies or prevention.

References

Abman, S. H. & Accurso, F. J. (1989). Acute effects of partial compression of ductus arteriosus on fetal pulmonary circulation. *American Journal of Physiology*, **257**, H626–34.

Abman, S. H., Shanley, P. F. & Accurso, F. J. (1989). Failure of postnatal adaptation of the pulmonary circulation after chronic intrauterine pulmonary hypertension in fetal lambs. *Journal of Clinical Investigation*, **83**, 1849–58.

Agarwal, J. B., Paltoo, R. & Palmer, W. H. (1970). Relative viscosity of blood at varying hematocrits in pulmonary circulation. *Journal of Applied Physiology*, **29**, 866–71.

Allen, K. & Haworth, S. G. (1986). Impaired adaptation of intrapulmonary arteries to extrauterine life in the newborn pigs exposed to hypoxia: an ultrastructural study. *Journal of Pathology*, **150**, 205–12.

Bartlett, R. H., Roloff, D. W., Cornell, R. G., Andrews, A. F., Dillon, P. W. & Zwischenberger, J. B. (1985). Extracorporeal circulation in neonatal respiratory failure: a prospective randomized study. *Pediatrics*, **76**, 479–87.

Benis, A. M., Usami, S. & Chien, S. (1970). Effect of hematocrit and inertial losses on pressure flow relations in the isolated hind paw of the dog. *Circulation Research,* **27**, 1047–68.

Campbell, A. G. M., Dawes, G. S., Fishman, A. P., Hyman, A. I. & Perks, A. M. (1968). The release of a bradykinin-line pulmonary vasodilator substance in foetal and newborn lambs. *Journal of Physiology,* **195**, 83–96.

Caro, C. G. (1966). Mechanics of the pulmonary circulation. In *Advances in Respiratory Physiology*, ed. C. G. Caro. pp. 255–296. Edwin Arnold, London.

Cassin, S. (1980). Role of prostaglandins and thromboxanes in the control of the pulmonary circulation in the fetus and newborn. *Seminars in Perinatology,* **4**, 101–7.

Cassin, S., Dawes, G. S., Mott, J. C., Ross, B. B. & Strang, L. B. (1964). The vascular resistance of the foetal and newly ventilated lung of the lamb. *Journal of Physiology,* **171**, 61–79.

Cassin, S., Tod, M., Philips, J., Frisinger, J., Jordan, J. & Gibbs, C. (1981*a*). Effects of prostaglandin D_2 in perinatal circulation. *American Journal of Physiology,* **240**, H755–60.

Cassin, S., Tyler, T. L. & Wallis, R. (1975). The effects of prostaglandin E_1 on fetal pulmonary vascular resistance. *Proceedings of the Society for Experimental Biology and Medicine,* **148**, 584–7.

Cassin, S., Winikor, I., Tod, M., Philips, J., Frisinger, S., Jordan, J. & Gibbs, C. (1981*b*) Effects of prostacyclin on the fetal pulmonary circulation. *Pediatriatric Pharmacology,* **1**, 197–207.

Clyman, R. I. & Heymann, M. A. (1981). Pharmacology of the ductus arteriosus. *Pediatric Clinics of North America,* **28**, 77–93.

Creasy, R. K., Barrett, C. T., DeSwiet, M., Kahanpaa, K. V. & Rudolph, A. M. (1972). Experimental intrauterine growth retardation in the sheep. *American Journal of Obstetrics and Gynecology,* **112**, 566–73.

Creasy, R. K., DeSwiet, M., Kahanpaa, K. V., Young, W. P. & Rudolph, A. M. (1973). Pathophysiological changes in the foetal lamb with growth retardation. In *Foetal and Neonatal Physiology. Proceedings of the Sir Joseph Barcroft Centenary Symposium*, ed. K. S. Comline, K. W. Cross, G. S. Dawes & P. W. Nathanielsz. pp. 398–402. Cambridge University Press, Cambridge.

Crowley, M. R., Fineman, J. R. & Soifer, S. J. (1991). Effects of vasoactive drugs on thromboxane A_2 mimetic-induced pulmonary hypertension in newborn lambs. *Pediatric Research,* 29, 167–72.

Crowley, M. R., Fineman, J. R. & Soifer, S. J. (1990). Amrinone causes pulmonary vasodilatation during thromboxane-mimetic-induced pulmonary hypertension. *Pediatric Research,* **27**, 298A.

Csaba, I. F., Sulyok, E. & Ertl, T. (1978). Relationship of maternal treatment with indomethacin to persistence of fetal circulation syndrome. *Journal of Pediatrics,* **92**, 484–8.

Daniel, S. S., Husain, M. K., Milliez, J., Yeh, M. N. & James, L. S. (1978). Renal response of fetal lamb to complete occlusion of umbilical cord. *American Journal of Obstetrics and Gynecology,* **131**, 514–19.

Daniel, S. S., Yeh, M. N., Bowe, E. T., Fukunaga, A. & James, L. S. (1975). Renal response of the lamb fetus to partial occlusion of the umbilical cord. *Journal of Pediatrics,* **87**, 788–94.

Demello, D. E., Murphy, J. D., Aronovitz, M. J., Davies, P. & Reid, L. M.

(1987). Effects of indomethacin in utero on the pulmonary vasculature of the newborn guinea pig. *Pediatric Research,* **22**, 693–7.

Drummond, W. H. & Bissonnette, J. M. (1978). Persistent pulmonary hypertension in the neonate: development of an animal model. *American Journal of Obstetrics and Gynecology,* **131**, 761–3.

Drummond, W. H., Gregory, G. A., Heymann, M. A. & Phibbs, R. A. (1981). The independent effects of hyperventilation, tolazoline, and dopamine on infants with persistent pulmonary hyertension. *Journal of Pediatrics,* **98**, 603–11.

Drummond, W. H., Peckham, G. J. & Fox, W. W. (1977). The clinical profile of the newborn with persistent pulmonary hypertension. *Clinical Pediatrics,* **16**, 335–41.

Dworetz, A. R., Moya, F. R., Sabo, B., Gladstone, I. & Gross, I. (1989). Survival of infants with persistent pulmonary hypertension without extracorporeal membrane oxygenation. *Pediatrics,* **84**, 1–6.

Edmonds, J. F., Berry, E. & Wyllie, J. H. (1969). Release of prostaglandins by distension of the lungs. *British Journal of Surgery,* **56**, 622–3.

Emmanouilides, G. C. & Baylen, B. G. (1979). Neonatal cardiopulmonary distress without congenital heart disease. *Current Problems in Pediatrics,* **IX** (7), 1–38.

Enhorning, G., Adams, F. H. & Norman, A. (1966). Effect of lung expansion on the fetal lamb circulation. *Acta Paediatrica Scandinavica,* **55**, 441–51.

Fineman, J. R., Heymann, M. A. & Soifer, S. J. (1991). N^w-nitro-L-arginine attenuates endothelium-dependent pulmonary vasodilation in lambs. *American Journal of Physiology,* **260**, H1299–306.

Fox, W. W., Gewitz, M. H., Dinwiddie, R., Drummond, W. H., Peckham, G. J. (1977). Pulmonary hypertension in the perinatal aspiration syndromes. *Pediatrics,* **59**, 205–11.

Fox, W. W. & Duara, S. (1983). Persistent pulmonary hypertension in the neonate: diagnosis and management. *Journal of Pediatrics,* **103**, 505–14.

Fox, W. W., Gewitz, M. H., Dinwiddie, R., Drummond, W. H. & Peckham, G. J. (1989). Pulmonary hypertension in the perinatal aspiration syndromes. *Pediatrics,* **59**, 205–11.

Fugate, J. H. & Ryan, D. P. (1989). Extracorporeal membrane oxygenation. *Problems in Anesthesia,* **3**, 271–87.

Geggel, R. L., Aronovitz, B. S. & Reid, L. M. (1986). Effects of chronic in utero hypoxemia on rat neonatal pulmonary arterial structure. *Journal of Pediatrics,* **108**, 756–9.

Gersony, W. M. (1973). Persistence of the fetal circulation: a commentary. *Journal of Pediatrics,*, **82**, 1103–6.

Goetzman, B. W. & Riemenschneider, T. A. (1980). Persistence of the fetal circulation. *Pediatrics in Review,* **2**, 37–40.

Goldberg, S. J., Levy, R. A., Siassi, B. & Betten, J. (1971) . The effects of maternal hypoxia and hyperoxia upon the neonatal pulmonary vasculature. *Pediatrics,* **48**, 528–33.

Graves, E. D., Redmond, C. R. & Arensman, R. M. (1988). Persistent pulmonary hypertension in the neonate. *Chest,* **93**, 638–41.

Gryglewski, R. J. (1980). The lung as a generator of prostacyclin. *Ciba Foundation Symposium,* **78**, 147–64.

Gryglewski, R. J., Korbut, R. & Ocetkiewicz, A. (1978). Generation of prostacyclin by lungs in vivo and its release into the arterial circulation. *Nature,* **273**, 765–7.

Harker, L. C., Kirkpatrick, S. E., Friedman, W. F. & Bloor, C. M. (1981). Effects of indomethacin on fetal rat lungs: a possible cause of persistent fetal circulation (PFC). *Pediatric Research*, **15**, 147–51.

Haworth, S. G. & Reid, L. (1976). Persistent fetal circulation: newly recognized structural features. *Journal of Pediatrics*, **88**, 614–20.

Henry, G. W. (1984). Noninvasive assessment of cardiac function and pulmonary hypertension in persistent pulmonary hypertension of the newborn. *Clinics in Perinatology*, **11**, 627–40.

Heymann, M. A., Creasy, R. K. & Rudolph, A. M. (1973). Quantitation of blood flow patterns in the foetal lamb in utero. In *Proceedings of the Sir Joseph Barcroft Centenary Symposium. Foetal and Neonatal Physiology.* pp. 129–135, Cambridge University Press, Cambridge.

Heymann, M. A. & Hoffman, J. I. E. (1986). Pulmonary circulation in the perinatal period. In *Neonatal Pulmonary Care,* ed. D. W. Thibeault & G. A. Gregory. pp. 149–174. Appleton-Century-Crofts, Norwalk, Connecticut.

Heymann, M. A., Rudolph, A. M., Nies, A. S. & Melmon, K. L. (1969). Bradykinin production associated with oxygenation of the fetal lamb. *Circulation Research*, **25**, 521–34.

Hislop, A. & Reid, L. M. (1972). Intra-pulmonary arterial development during fetal life-branching pattern and structure. *Journal of Anatomy*, **113**, 35–48.

Hislop, A. & Reid, L. M. (1973) . Pulmonary arterial development during childhood: branching pattern and structure. *Thorax*, **28**, 129–35.

Ignarro, L. J. (1991).Pharmacology of endotheliun-derived nitric oxide and nitro-vasodilators. *Western Journal of Medicine*, **154**, 51–62.

Iliff, L. D., Greene, R. E. & Hughes, J. M. B. (1972). Effect of interstitial edema on distribution of ventilation and perfusion in isolated lung. *Journal of Applied Physiology*, **33**, 462–7.

Itskovitz, J., LaGamma, E. F. & Rudolph, A. M. (1983). The effect of reducing umbilical blood flow on fetal oxygenation. *American Journal of Obstetrics and Gynecology*, **145**, 813–18.

Itskovitz, J., LaGamma, E. F. & Rudolph, A. M. (1987). Effects of cord compression on fetal blood flow distribution and oxygen delivery. *American Journal of Physiology*, **21**, H100–9.

Iwamoto, H. S., Teitel, D. & Rudolph, A. M. (1987). Effects of birth-related events on blood flow distribution. *Pediatric Research*, **22**, 634–40.

Krovetz, L. J. & Goldbloom, J. (1972). Normal standards for cardiovascular data. II. Pressure and vascular resistances. *Johns Hopkins Medical Journal*, **130**, 187–95.

Le Bidois, J., Soifer, S.J., Clyman, R. I. & Heymann, M. A. (1987). Piriprost: a putative leukotriene synthesis inhibitor increases pulmonary blood flow in fetal lambs. *Pediatric Research*, **22**, 350–4.

Leffler, C. W. & Hessler, J. R. (1979). Pulmonary and systemic vascular effects of exogenous prostaglandin I$_2$ in fetal lambs. *European Journal of Pharmacology*, **54**, 37–42.

Leffler, C. W., Hessler, J. R. & Green, R. S. (1984a). Mechanism of stimulation of pulmonary prostaglandin synthesis at birth. *Prostaglandins*, **28**, 877–87.

Leffler, C. W., Hessler, J. R. & Green, R. S. (1984b). The onset of breathing at birth stimulates pulmonary vascular prostacyclin synthesis. *Pediatric Research*, **18**, 938–42.

Leffler, C. W., Tyler, T. L. & Cassin, S. (1978). Effect of indomethacin on pulmonary vascular response to ventilation of fetal goats. *American Journal of Physiology,* **234**, H346–51.

Levin, D. L. (1980). Effects of inhibition of prostaglandin synthesis on fetal development, oxygenation and the fetal circulation. *Seminars in Perinatology,* **4**, 35–44.

Levin, D. L., Fixler, D. E., Morriss, F. C. & Tyson, J. (1978). Morphologic analysis of the pulmonary vascular bed in infants exposed in utero to prostaglandin synthetase inhibitors. *Journal of Pediatrics,* **92**, 478–83.

Levin, D. L., Heymann, M. A., Kitterman, J. A., Gregory, G. A., Phibbs, R. H. & Rudolph, A. M. (1976a). Persistent pulmonary hypertension of the newborn infant. *Journal of Pediatrics,* **89**, 626–30.

Levin, D. L., Hyman, A. I., Heymann, M. A. & Rudolph, A. M. (1978). Fetal hypertension and the development of increased pulmonary vascular smooth muscle: a possible mechanism for persistent pulmonary hypertension of the newborn infant. *Journal of Pediatrics,* **92**, 265–9.

Levin, D. L., Mills, L. J. & Weinberg, A. G. (1979). Hemodynamic, pulmonary, vascular, and myocardial abnormalities secondary to pharmacologic constriction of the fetal ductus arteriosus. *Circulation,* **60**, 360–4.

Levin, D. L., Rudolph, A. M., Heymann, M. A. & Phibbs, R. H. (1976b). Morphological development of the pulmonary vascular bed in fetal lambs. *Circulation,* **53**, 144–51.

Levin, D. L., Weinberg, A. G. & Perkin, R. M. (1983). Pulmonary microthrombi syndrome in newborn infants with unresponsive persistent pulmonary hypertension. *Journal of Pediatrics,* **102**, 299–302.

Lewis, A. B., Heymann, M. A. & Rudolph, A. M. (1976). Gestational changes in pulmonary vascular responses in fetal lambs in utero. *Circulation Research,* **39**, 536–41.

Manchester, D., Margolis, H. S. & Sheldon, R. E. (1976). Possible association between maternal indomethacin therapy and primary pulmonary hypertension of the newborn. *American Journal of Obstetrics and Gynecology,* **126**, 467–9.

McIntyre, T. M., Zimmerman, G. A., Satoh, K. & Prescott, S. M. (1985). Cultured endothelial cells synthesize both platelet-activating factor and prostacyclin in response to histamine, bradykinin, and adenosine triphosphate. *Journal of Clinical Investigation,* **76**, 271–80.

McKenzie, S. & Haworth, S. G. (1981). Occlusion of peripheral pulmonary vascular bed in a baby with idiopathic persistent fetal circulation. *British Heart Journal,* **46**, 675–8.

McMurtry, I. F., Rodman, D. M., Yamaguchi, T. & O'Brien, R. F. (1988). Pulmonary vascular reactivity. *Chest,* **93**, 88S–91S.

Meyrick, B. & Reid, L. (1978). The effect of continued hypoxia on rat pulmonary arterial circulation: an ultrastructural study. *Laboratory Investigation,* **38**, 188–200.

Meyrick, B. & Reid, L. (1979). Ultrastructural features of the distended pulmonary arteries of the normal rat. *Anatomical Record,* **193**, 71–97.

Moore, P., Velvis, H., Soifer, S. J. & Heymann, M. A. (1991). EDRF inhibition blocks the pulmonary vasodilatory response to ventilation with oxygen in fetal lambs. *Pediatric Research,* **29**, 245A.

Morin, F. C. (1989). Ligating the ductus arteriosus before birth causes persistent pulmonary hypertension in the newborn lamb. *Pediatric Research,* **25**, 245–50.

Moss, A. J., Emmanouilides, G. & Duffie, E. R. Jr (1963). Closure of the ductus arteriosus in the newborn infant. *Pediatrics,* **32**, 25–30.

Murphy, J. D., Aronovitz, M. J. & Reid, L. M. (1986). Effects of chronic in utero hypoxia on the pulmonary vasculature of the newborn guinea pig. *Pediatric Research,* **20**, 292–5.

Murphy, J. D., Rabinovitch, M., Goldstein, J. D. & Reid, L. M. (1981). The structural basis of persistent pulmonary hypertension of the newborn infant. *Journal of Pediatrics,* **98**, 962–7.

Omini, C., Vigano, T., Marini, A., Pasargiklian, R., Fano, M. & Maselli, M. A. (1983). Angiotensin II: a releaser of PGI_2 from fetal and newborn rabbit lungs. *Prostaglandins,* **25**, 901–10.

O'Rourke, P. P., Crone, R. K., Vacanti, J. P., Ware, J. H., Lillehei, C. W., Parad, R. B. & Epstein, M. F. (1989). Extracorporeal membrane oxygenation and conventional medical therapy in neonates with persistent pulmonary hypertension of the newborn: a prospective randomized study. *Pediatrics,* **84**, 957–63.

Peckham, G. J. & Fox, W. W. (1978). Physiologic factors affecting pulmonary artery pressure in infants with persistent pulmonary hypertension. *Journal of Pediatrics,* **93**, 1005–10.

Pickart, L. R., Creasy, R. K. & Thaler, M. M. (1976). Polycythemia and hyperfibrinogenemia as factors in experimental intrauterine growth retardation. *American Journal of Obstetrics and Gynecology,* **124**, 268–71.

Prandtl, L. & Tietjens, O. G. (1957). *Applied Hydro- and Aeromechanics.* pp. 14–57, Dover Publications, Inc., New York.

Prosser, I. W., Stenmark, K. R., Suthar, M., Crouch, E. D., Mecham, R. P. & Parks, W. C. (1989). Regional heterogeneity of elastin and collagen gene expression in intralobar arteries in response to hypoxic pulmonary hypertension as demonstrated by in situ hybridization. *American Journal of Pathology,* **135**, 1073–88.

Reid, L. M. (1977). The lung: its growth and remodelling in health and disease. *American Journal of Roentgenology,* **129**, 777–88.

Reid, L. M. (1979). The pulmonary circulation: remodelling in growth and disease. *American Review of Respiratory Disease,* **119**, 531–46.

Rendas, A., Branthwaite, M. & Reid, L. (1978). Growth of the pulmonary circulation in normal pig: structural analysis and aspects of cardiopulmonary function. *Journal of Applied Physiology,* **45**, 806–17.

Rhine, W. D., Benitz, W. E. & Stevenson, D. K. (1988). Nitroprusside for severe respiratory distress syndrome. *American Journal of Perinatology,* **5**, 381A.

Roos, A. (1962). Poiseuille's law and its limitations in vascular systems. *Medicina Thoracalis,* **19**, 224–38.

Rudolph, A. M. (1979). Fetal and neonatal pulmonary circulation. *Annual Review of Physiology,* **41**, 383–95.

Rudolph, A. M., Auld, P. A. M., Golinko, R. J. & Paul, M. H. (1961). Pulmonary vascular adjustments in the neonatal period. *Pediatrics,* **28**, 28–34.

Rudolph, A. M. & Heymann, M. A. (1967). The circulation of the fetus in utero. Methods for studying distribution of blood flow, cardiac output and organ blood flow. *Circulation Research,* **21**, 163–84.

Rudolph, A. M. & Heymann, M. A. (1970). Circulatory changes during growth in the fetal lamb. *Circulation Research,* **26**, 289–99.

Rudolph, A. M. & Yuan, S. (1966). Response of the pulmonary vasculature to hypoxia and H^+ ion concentration changes. *Journal of Clinical Investigation*, **45**, 399–411.

Ruiz, U., Piasecki, G. J., Balogh, K., Polansky, B. J. & Jackson, B. T. (1972). An experimental model for fetal pulmonary hypertension. *American Journal of Surgery*, **123**, 468–71.

Schreiber, M. D., Heymann, M. A. & Soifer, S. J. (1986). Increased arterial pH, not decreased $PaCO_2$, attenuates hypoxia-induced pulmonary vasoconstriction in newborn lambs. *Pediatric Research*, **20**, 113–17.

Schreiber, M. D., Heymann, M. A. & Soifer, S. J. (1987). The differential effects of leukotriene C_4 and D_4 on the pulmonary and systemic circulations in newborn lambs. *Pediatric Research*, **21**, 176–82.

Segall, M. L., Goetzman, B. W. & Schick, J. B. (1980). Thrombocytopenia and pulmonary hypertension in the perinatal aspiration syndromes. *Journal of Pediatrics*, **96**, 727–30.

Soifer, S. J., Clyman, R. I. & Heymann, M. A. (1988). Effects of prostaglandin D_2 on pulmonary arterial pressure and oxygenation in newborn infants with persistent pulmonary hypertension. *Journal of Pediatrics*, **112**, 774–7.

Soifer, S. J., Kaslow, D., Roman, C. & Heymann, M. A. (1987). Umbilical cord compression produces pulmonary hypertension in newborn lambs: a model to study the pathophysiology of persistent pulmonary hypertension in the newborn. *Journal of Developmental Physiology*, **9**, 239–52.

Soifer, S. J., Loitz, R. D., Roman, C. & Heymann, M. A. (1985). Leukotriene end organ antagonists increase pulmonary blood flow in fetal lambs. *American Journal of Physiology*, **249**, H570–6.

Soifer, S. J., Morin, F. C. III & Heymann, M. A. (1982). Prostaglandin D_2 reverses induced pulmonary hypertension in the newborn lamb. *Journal of Pediatrics*, **100**, 458–63.

Soifer, S. J., Morin, F. C. III, Kaslow, D. C. & Heymann, M. A. (1983). The developmental effects of prostaglandin D_2 on the pulmonary and systemic circulations in the newborn lamb. *Journal of Developmental Physiology*, **5**, 237–50.

Spitzer, A. R., Davis, J., Clarke, W. T., Bernbaum, J. & Fox, W. W. (1988). Pulmonary hypertension and persistent fetal circulation in the newborn. *Clinics in Perinatology*, **15**, 389–410.

Stenmark, K. R., Fasules, J., Hyde, D. M., Voelkel, N. F., Henson, J., Tucker, A., Wilson, H. & Reeves, J. T. (1987). Severe pulmonary hypertension and arterial adventitial changes in newborn calves at 4,300 m. *Journal of Applied Physiology*, **62**, 821–30.

Stenmark, K. R., James, S. L., Voekel, N. F., Toews, W. H., Reeves, J. T. & Murphy, R. C. (1983). Leokotriene C4 and D4 in neonates with hypoxemia and pulmonary hypertension. *New England Journal of Medicine*, **309**, 77–80.

Stenmark, K. R., Orton, E. C., Reeves, J. T., Voelkel, N. F., Crouch, E. C., Parks, W. C. & Mecham, R. P. (1988). Vascular remodeling in neonatal pulmonary hypertension: role of the smooth muscle cell. *Chest*, **93**, 127S–33S.

Taylor, G. A., Fitz, C. R., Glass, P. & Short, B. L. (1989). CT of cerebrovascular injury after neonatal extracorporeal membrane oxygenation: implications for neurodevelopmental outcome. *American Journal of Roentgenology*, **153**, 121–6.

Terragno, N. A. & Terragno, A. (1979). Prostaglandin metabolism in the fetal and maternal vasculature. *Federation Proceedings*, **38**, 75–7.

Tripp, M. E., Drummond, W. H., Heymann, M. A. & Rudolph, A. M. (1980). Hemodynamic effects of pulmonary arterial infusion of vasodilators in newborn lambs. *Pediatric Research*, **14**, 1311–15.

Tyler, T. L., Leffler, C. W. & Cassin, S. (1977). Effects of prostaglandin precursors, prostaglandins, and prostaglandin metabolites on pulmonary circulation in perinatal goats. *Chest*, **71**, 271S–3S.

Velvis, H., Krusell, J., Roman, C., Soifer, S. J., Riemer, R. K. & Heymann, M. A. (1990). Leukotrienes in fetal lamb tracheal fluid: further suggestive evidence for their regulation of fetal pulmonary vascular tone. *Journal of Developmental Physiology*, **14**, 37–41.

Velvis, H., Moore, P. & Heymann, M. A. (1991). Prostaglandin inhibition prevents the fall in pulmonary vascular resistance due to rhythmic distension of the lungs in fetal lambs. *Pediatric Research*, **30**, 62–8.

Whitmore, R. L. (1968). *Rheology of the Circulation*. Pergamon Press, London.

Wild, L. M., Nickerson, P. A. & Morin, F. C. (1989). Ligating the ductus arteriosus before birth remodels the pulmonary vasculature of the lamb. *Pediatric Research*, **25**, 251–7.

Wilkinson, A. R., Aynsley-Green, A. & Mitchell, M. D. (1979). Persistent pulmonary hypertension and abnormal PGE levels in preterm infants after maternal treatment with naproxen. *Archives of Disease in Childhood*, **54**, 942–5.

11

Birthweight and blood pressure in childhood and adult life

CATHERINE M. LAW AND
DAVID J. P. BARKER

Introduction

Hypertension increases the risk of stroke and ischaemic heart disease, which together account for nearly half of all deaths in England and Wales (HMSO, 1991). This risk is a continuum, a rise in cardiovascular mortality being associated with each unit increase in population mean blood pressure (MacMahon et al., 1990). The determinants of hypertension remain largely unexplained. Factors related to adult lifestyle, such as salt consumption, do not account for much of the variation in adult blood pressure. Nor does considerable reduction in salt intake result in much fall in blood pressure. A recent analysis of 45 trials of salt reduction concluded that lowering of the daily intake of sodium by 50 mmol resulted in a 5 to 7 mm Hg fall in systolic blood pressure, depending on blood pressure level before the dietary changes (Law, Frost & Wald, 1991*b*).

There is now considerable evidence that adult blood pressure is closely related to fetal size at birth. This chapter will describe that evidence, and discuss the implications for future research.

Birthweight and blood pressure

Three studies have shown that adult blood pressure is inversely related to birthweight. The Medical Research Council's national survey of health and development is a follow-up study from birth of 5362 people born in one week of March, 1946: it comprises all single, legitimate births to the wives of non-manual and agricultural workers and a randomly selected one-in-four sample of single, legitimate births to manual workers. When the study population was aged 36 years, blood pressure, height and weight were measured in 3259 men and women (Barker et al., 1989). Table 11.1 shows the relation of systolic pressure to birthweight and

Table 11.1. *Mean systolic blood pressures (mm Hg) of 1625 men and 1634 women at age 36 by thirds of weight and birthweights*

	Men Current weight (kg)				Women Current weight (kg)			
Birthweight*	<71.1	71.1–80.0	>80.0	All men	<56.6	56.6–64.5	>65.5	All women
Lowest	123.2	124.2	124.6	124.0	118.7	117.3	120.2	118.6
Middle	122.2	121.2	125.5	122.8	117.5	115.0	117.1	116.7
Highest	121.3	119.8	123.2	121.5	116.8	115.3	118.6	116.7
All	122.4	122.0	124.4	122.9	117.8	116.1	118.6	117.4

* Men: Lower tertiles of birthweight 3180, 3200, and 3410 g; upper tertiles 3520, 3770, and 3750 g. Women: Lower tertiles of birthweight 3070, 3180, and 3180 g; upper tertiles 3410, 3520, and 3640 g. Numbers of subjects in each cell within table ranged from 121 to 236; standard errors ranged from 0.96 to 1.38.

Table 11.2. *Mean systolic pressure (mm Hg) in men aged 59–70 years*

Body mass index (kg/m²)	Birthweight (pounds)			
	−7.25	−8.25	8.25+	Total
−25.2	161	159	156	156 (269)
−25.2–27.9	167	168	165	167 (255)
>27.9	172	163	164	167 (261)
Total	167 (243)	163 (268)	162 (274)	164 (785)

Note: Number of men in parentheses.

weight at 36 years. Mean systolic pressure was 2 mm Hg higher in the group with the lowest third of birthweights compared with the group with the heaviest third in men. The difference was 1.8 mm Hg in women. These differences were similar in magnitude to those found with present body weight, higher pressure also being found in the higher weight groups.

Birthweight was also and more strongly related to adult blood pressure in a study of older men born in Hertfordshire, England. Since 1911, every baby born in the county has been weighed at birth. These records have been preserved and 785 men born and still resident in the county have been visited at home at around the age of 64 and had their blood pressure measured. As in the 1946 cohort, blood pressure was inversely related to birthweight: it ranged from a mean of 169 mm Hg in those who had weighed 5.5 pounds or less at birth, to 162 mm Hg in those who had birthweights in excess of 9.5 pounds (Barker, 1991). This relation was independent of current body mass index and statistically significant (Table 11.2). Furthermore, after allowing for birthweight, blood pressure was not related to weight at one year, suggesting that differences in fetal rather than infant growth underpin the relation. A similarly strong inverse relation between birthweight and blood pressure was found in 50 year-old men and women in Preston (Barker et al., 1990): this study is described in more detail later in the chapter.

The inverse relationship between birthweight and subsequent blood pressure has also been noted consistently in children. Studies from North America, New Zealand and Britain have demonstrated this relation, which is present at ages 4, 5 to 7, and 10 years (Simpson et al., 1981; Cater

& Gill, 1984; Whincup, Cook & Shaper, 1989). Childhood blood pressure is higher by 1.5 to 2 mm Hg for each kg that birthweight is lower (Whincup et al., 1989).

Blood pressure is also related to a child's size throughout childhood. In adults, blood pressure is positively related to fatness (Chiang, Perlman & Epstein, 1969) but not height (Dyer, Elliott & Shipley, 1990). In children, blood pressure is positively related to height as well as ponderosity (Voors et al., 1977; de Swiet, Fayers & Shinebourne, 1984). Whereas in adults weight is a function of height and fatness, in children it is a measure of biological maturity, in addition to height and fatness. At any given chronological age, a heavier, taller child is likely to be more biologically mature than a lighter, shorter child, and this has led to recommendations that, in clinical practice, a child's blood pressure should be considered in relation to his or her size rather than age (Dillon, 1988). Thus, developmental differences may dominate blood pressure variation in children, but may have no prognostic significance for adult life. As weight during childhood is positively correlated with both birthweight and biological age, it is important to allow for current size in any analysis of children's blood pressure. This enables assessment of the independent associations with birthweight. Table 11.3 shows systolic blood pressure by birthweight and current weight in 3591 boys and girls aged 5 to 7 years (Whincup et al., 1989).

The relations between children's blood pressure, and both birthweight and size during childhood lead to the prediction that children's blood pressure would vary internationally, as birthweight and childhood growth are known to differ from place to place (Eveleth, 1986). Unfortunately, international comparisons of absolute blood pressure levels are difficult, because of the variety of equipment and techniques used for measurement, and the likelihood of systematic differences arising between methods and observers (Grimley Evans & Rose, 1971). However, within the UK, reliable methodology has shown that there is variation in children's blood pressure from place to place. This parallels differences in adult blood pressure and cardiovascular mortality (Whincup et al., 1988).

Birthweight is a summary measure of fetal growth, which includes head size, length and fatness. In order to understand the mechanisms operating in fetal life and leading to raised blood pressure subsequently, it is necessary to refine the relation between blood pressure and fetal growth.

Table 11.3. *Mean systolic blood pressure (mm Hg) by birthweight and current weight as fifths of their distributions in boys and girls, aged 5 to 7 years*

Birthweight (g)	Current weight (kg)					Mean (SD)
Boys (n = 1789)						
	13.1–18.8	18.9–20.4	20.5–21.7	21.8–23.7	23.8–47.8	
1190–2999	96.5	100.6	100.8	103.1	108.6	100.2 (9.0)
3000–3289	97.3	99.9	100.4	103.6	106.5	101.0 (8.6)
3290–3529	94.8	98.9	100.5	102.6	106.8	101.1 (9.2)
3530–3799	96.0	99.7	100.3	102.3	104.3	101.1 (8.5)
3800–5469	96.4	98.0	99.7	100.8	104.4	101.0 (8.0)
Mean (SD)	96.4 (8.3)	99.6 (7.6)	100.2 (7.7)	102.5 (8.2)	105.4 (8.7)	
Girls (n = 1802)						
	13.3–18.1	18.2–20.0	20.1–21.4	21.5–23.6	23.7–47.0	
1040–2819	97.7	99.7	102.6	105.3	105.5	101.1 (9.4)
2820–3169	97.7	100.1	100.8	102.0	107.8	101.0 (9.2)
3170–3389	94.5	97.7	100.6	103.2	103.7	100.0 (8.8)
3390–3659	96.6	99.0	99.7	102.4	105.8	101.0 (8.0)
3660–5299	95.6	97.9	98.9	99.5	104.5	100.4 (8.9)
Mean (SD)	96.8 (9.0)	98.9 (8.2)	100.4 (7.6)	102.1 (8.4)	105.2 (8.8)	

Placental weight and blood pressure

In Sharoe Green Hospital in Preston, England, detailed measurements of mother and baby have been made at birth and recorded from 1932 onwards. 449 men and women, who were still living in the Preston area, were visited at home when they were around 50 years of age (Barker et al., 1990). Table 11.4 shows mean blood pressure, measured at the home visit according to birthweight and placental weight. Although birthweight and placental weight were strongly positively related to each other, their individual relations with blood pressure were in opposite directions. Thus blood pressure fell with increasing birthweight and rose with increasing placental weight. The highest pressures were found in the group with the smallest birthweight and the largest placental weight, and the lowest pressures were found in the group who had the largest birthweight and the smallest placental weight. These relations were not dependent on gestation: adjustment for gestational age, and consideration of term

Table 11.4. *Mean systolic and diastolic pressures (mm Hg) of men and women aged 46 to 54 years according to placental weight and birthweight*

Birthweight (pounds)	Placental weight (pounds)				
	−1.0	−1.25	−1.5	>1.5	All
Systolic pressure					
−5.5	152	154	153	206	154
	(26)	(13)	(5)	(1)	(45)
−6.5	147	151	150	166	151
	(16)	(54)	(28)	(8)	(106)
−7.5	144	148	145	160	149
	(20)	(77)	(45)	(27)	(169)
>7.5	133	148	147	154	149
	(6)	(27)	(42)	(54)	(129)
All	147	149	147	157	150
	(68)	(171)	(120)	(90)	(449)
Diastolic pressure					
−5.5	84	87	87	97	86
−6.5	84	88	85	93	87
−7.5	84	84	84	90	85
>7.5	78	85	85	88	86
All	84	86	85	89	86

Note: Numbers of people in parentheses.
(1 pound = 0.45 kg).

babies only, gave similar results. The risk of hypertension (defined as systolic pressure >160 mm Hg) was similarly negatively related to birthweight and positively related to placental weight.

Most of those who were hypertensive had not been babies considered to be growth-retarded in utero on conventional clinical grounds because their birthweight was above the 10th centile. Their distinguishing feature was the large placental size compared to that expected for their birthweight. Thus they might be considered to be growth retarded in relative terms, in that fetal growth had not matched that of the placenta.

The relation between blood pressure and placental and birthweights were stronger than those with current body mass index or alcohol consumption. Blood pressure was, on average, 5 mm Hg higher in moderate and heavy consumers of alcohol compared with mild consumers, whereas the difference in blood pressure between the lightest and heaviest groups was 12 mm Hg for placental weight and 10 mm Hg for birthweight.

The relation between birthweight and blood pressure has also been studied in 405 four year old children born and still resident in Salisbury,

Table 11.5. *Mean change (95% confidence interval) in systolic pressure associated with weight at four, birthweight* and placental weight**

	n	Systolic pressure (mm Hg)
Weight at four (kg)		
≤16.5	108	0.0 (baseline)
−17.5	92	0.1 (−2.6 to 2.9)
−18.5	66	0.3 (−2.7 to 3.4)
>18.5	98	3.7 (0.8 to 6.5)
Birthweight (g)		
≤3000	75	0.0 (baseline)
−3300	102	−0.8 (−3.7 to 2.2)
−3600	82	−0.9 (−4.1 to 2.4)
>3600	105	−2.6 (−6.0 to 0.8)
Placental weight (g)		
≤550	96	0.0 (baseline)
−650	102	−0.1 (−3.0 to 2.7)
−750	83	0.6 (−2.5 to 3.7)
>750	83	2.6 (−0.8 to 6.0)

* Birthweight and placental weight are adjusted for gestational age.

England (Law et al., 1991*a*). Table 11.5 shows the simultaneous effects of weight at four and birthweight and placental weight (adjusted for gestational age) on child's systolic pressure at four years of age. Variables were grouped into approximate fourths, with the lowest fourth as the baseline: the systolic pressure in each group is given as its difference from the baseline. Systolic blood pressure rose with increasing weight, with a pronounced rise in the heaviest group. Blood pressure fell as birthweight increased and rose as placental weight increased. It can be seen that the relationships between blood pressure and placental and birthweights, although in the same direction as those in adults, were of much smaller magnitude, even allowing for the smaller variation in children's blood pressure.

Head size and length at birth, and blood pressure

The association between systolic blood pressure and size at birth was also examined in the Salisbury study by analysing birthweight in relation to length and head circumference at birth, after adjustment for gestational age. Systolic pressure was inversely related to ponderal index (weight/length^3) (Table 11.6). Babies with a low ponderal index tended to have below average measurements of head circumference but normal length. The same association between low ponderal index and high blood pressure was found in adults in Preston, but only amongst those who had placentas of below average weight (Barker et al., 1991). Thus, patterns of fetal growth may allow identification of babies at risk of higher blood pressure in childhood and hypertension in adulthood. Research can now focus on the intrauterine processes which lead to particular birth measurements, and hence on the maternal influences which may determine hypertension in the next generation.

Table 11.6. *Mean systolic blood pressure (mm Hg) in children aged 4 years*

Ponderal index at birth (adjusted for gestation)	Mean systolic blood pressure	SD	Number of subjects
≤23	106.9	10.9	81
−25	106.1	10.2	90
−27.5	104.6	8.8	99
>27.5	103.2	9.2	89
All	105.2	9.8	359

Tracking

It has been argued that the relative weakness of tracking of blood pressure suggests that early influences are not important for adult blood pressure. Tracking is the persistence of rank order of an individual, relative to others, in the population. For blood pressure, it is evident from 6 months of age but becomes more marked as age increases (Labarthe, Eissa & Varas, 1991). The correlation coefficients are relatively low: for example, the correlation coefficient of systolic pressure at three years with that at four years is of the order of 0.5 (de Swiet, Fayers & Shinebourne, 1980). However, it has been shown that placental weight and birthweight have similar relationships to blood pressure in children and adults whereas the relationships between blood pressure and current body size very markedly according to biological maturity. Blood pressure is strongly related to weight and height in childhood, but only to measures of fatness in adult life, and not even to these measures in the elderly (Chiang et al., 1969). Given the potential of biological maturation to perturb blood pressure relationships during childhood, low correlation coefficients for tracking would be expected.

Programming

The long-term relation between impaired fetal growth and subsequent blood pressure, and the importance to this relation of qualitative differences in growth, suggest that the pathophysiology of hypertension may be based on restraint of tissue growth by an adverse environment during a critical, possibly brief, period of fetal development (Barker, 1991). The tissues affected, and the extent of the effect, depend upon the nature of the adverse influence and its timing. The phenomenon of programming has been demonstrated on a range of structures and functions in experimental animals (Dubos, Savage & Schaedler, 1966; Kahn, 1968; Mott, Lewis & McGill, 1991). It may also occur widely in human development and have important effects on the development of degenerative disease. Long-term studies are needed to extend the knowledge of the occurrence of programming, and give insight into the timing of the critical periods, before precise primary prevention can take place.

Maternal nutrition and blood pressure

The balance of evidence from studies of many types suggests that fetal growth, rather than growth in childhood or adult lifestyle, is important in determining adult blood pressure. The mother exerts a profound effect upon fetal growth. Studies of the birthweights of first born children of mothers and daughters suggest that genetic factors play only a small part in determining birthweight (Carr-Hill et al., 1987). Maternal nutrition may be one of the factors which, if adverse, is reflected in impaired fetal growth, and ultimately results in hypertension in the offspring. The evidence to support this hypothesis is fourfold.

First, the geographical differences in death rates from stroke in England and Wales can be related to past differences in maternal nutrition and health. In the early part of the century, rates of maternal mortality differed markedly from one place to another. A series of reports from 1911 onwards showed that these rates were highest in areas where maternal health and physique were poor (Campbell, Cameron & Jones, 1932). Recent mortality from stroke is positively correlated with maternal mortality earlier in the century (Barker & Osmond, 1987). Interestingly, mortality from stroke has no relation with differences in postneonatal mortality, which is further evidence that the critical period in blood pressure development occurs before birth.

Secondly, in the 50-year-old adults in Preston, hypertension was associated with high placental weight and low birthweight (Barker et al., 1990). The causes of large placental size are mostly unknown; fewer mothers (7%) in social classes I and II had placentas weighing more than one and a half pounds compared with mothers in social classes III, IV and V (24%). A study of 8684 recent births in Oxford showed that large placental weight was associated with low maternal haemoglobin recorded during pregnancy, and with a fall in maternal mean cell volume (Godfrey et al., 1991). The highest ratio of placental weight to birthweight was found in the most anaemic women with the largest falls in mean cell volume. Anaemia and iron deficiency are commoner in the lower social classes and reflect maternal nutritional deficiency.

Thirdly, recent work on the four-year-old children in Salisbury has shown that the children of mothers who were anaemic in pregnancy had higher blood pressure at four years of age than did the children of mothers who had not been anaemic (Law et al., 1991a). Table 11.7 shows mean systolic pressure in these children grouped by haemoglobin concentration during pregnancy: systolic pressure is presented as its unadjusted value, as well as after adjustment for current weight and maternal blood pressure, which are the two strongest correlates of children's blood pressure at four. Maternal anaemia in pregnancy was associated with higher childhood blood pressure subsequently. This relation was also

Table 11.7. *Mean child's systolic pressure (mm Hg), unadjusted and adjusted both for weight at four and for mother's systolic pressure*

Lowest haemoglobin during pregnancy g/dl	Unadjusted			Adjusted	
	n	Mean	SD	Mean	SD
<10	36	108.1	10.9	108.1	10.7
−10.9	88	105.8	10.0	105.9	9.3
−11.9	164	104.8	9.7	104.7	9.3
≥12	106	105.2	9.6	104.6	9.4
Total	394	105.4	9.9	105.3	9.5

found to be independent of size at birth and placental weight. It did not reach statistical significance, and further work is in progress to confirm it.

Fourthly, a survey of blood pressure in children living in a rural community in the Gambia, West Africa, also showed a relation between a measure of maternal nutrition (weight gain in the third trimester of pregnancy) and subsequent blood pressure in the offspring (Margetts et al., 1991). In children aged 8 to 9 years, failure of mothers to gain weight during the last trimester was associated with increased systolic pressure. Childhood systolic blood pressure was an average of 5.6 mm Hg higher if the mother's weight gain had been in the lowest third (weight loss, or gain of less than 0.8 kg) compared to children whose mother's weight gain had been in the highest third (1.65 to 5.3 kg). Interestingly, these relations were not seen in younger children, and follow-up work is in progress to see if they will become manifest with age, or are specific to the birth cohort in which they were first found.

Further work is required to confirm these findings, many of which have been demonstrated recently for the first time. If confirmed, they will have major implications for the antenatal care of women, for they suggest that improvement of maternal nutrition before and during pregnancy may lower the distribution of blood pressure in the next generation.

Maternal smoking and blood pressure

Maternal smoking during pregnancy is associated with reduced placental weight and, thus, cannot explain the strong association between large placental size and blood pressure (Barker et al., 1990). There were no data on maternal smoking in Preston, although it is likely to have been relatively rare in young women in the 1930s. However, in Salisbury, smoking habit was recorded in the obstetric notes and by recall at interview of the mothers. There was no relation between maternal smoking during pregnancy and systolic pressure in the offspring at the age of four (Law et al., 1991*a*).

Child health surveillance and adult disease

There is now considerable evidence that factors operating in utero and early life are important in establishing risk of adult disease. In the Salisbury study, maternal anaemia was associated with a 2 to 3 mm Hg increase in systolic pressure, about a quarter of a standard deviation at four years of age (Law et al., 1991). Since differences in blood pressure between individuals increase with age, small differences in childhood may be magnified in adult life. Thus, factors acting in fetal life, but manifest in adulthood, might have far larger effects on adult blood pressure than those which exert their influence mostly in adult life, such as salt intake. This raises the question as to whether the monitoring and surveillance of children is given sufficient importance and is done with sufficient regard to future health.

Conclusion

First, it has been shown that birthweights at the lower end of the normal distribution are associated with an increased risk of adult hypertension. The acceptance of any birthweight which is usual as biologically satisfactory is outmoded. Achievement of average growth, in utero and in childhood, may be insufficient when the end point is risk of adult disease. Secondly, measures at birth, in addition to weight, allow stronger prediction of subsequent blood pressure and the risk of hypertension. It is necessary to know how these patterns of fetal growth, such as low ponderal index, are linked to the development of blood vessels. An understanding of the nature and timing of the possible maternal influences which give rise to differences in fetal growth may enable primary prevention of hypertension in future generations.

References

Barker, D. (1991). The intrauterine origins of cardiovascular and obstructive lung disease in adult life. *Journal of the Royal College of Physicians*, **25** (2), 129–33.

Barker, D., Bull, A., Osmond, C. & Simmonds, S. (1990). Fetal and placental size and risk of hypertension in adult life. *British Medical Journal*, **301**, 259–62.

Barker, D., Godfrey, K., Osmond, C. & Bull, A. (1991). The relation of fetal length, ponderal index and head circumference to blood pressure and the risk of hypertension in adult life. *Paediatric and Perinatal Epidemiology*, **6**, 35–44.

Barker, D. & Osmond, C. (1987). Death rates from stroke in England and Wales predicted from past maternal mortality. *British Medical Journal*, **295**, 83–6.

Barker, D., Osmond, C., Golding, J., Kuh, D. & Wadsworth, M. (1989). Growth in utero, blood pressure in childhood and adult life, and mortality from cardiovascular disease. *British Medical Journal*, **298**, 564–7.

Campbell, J., Cameron, D. & Jones, D. (1932). Ministry of Health reports on public health and medical subjects, No. 68. High maternal mortality in certain areas. HMSO, London.

Carr-Hill, R., Campbell, D., Hall, M. & Meredith, A. (1987). Is birthweight determined genetically? *British Medical Journal*, **295**, 687–9.

Cater, J. & Gill, M. (1984). The follow-up study: medical aspects. In *Low Birthweight, a Medical Psychological and Social Study*, ed. R. Illsley & R. Mitchell. pp. 191–205. John Wiley, Chichester.

Chiang, B., Perlman, L. & Epstein, F. (1969). Overweight and hypertension: a review. *Circulation*, **39**, 403–21.

de Swiet, M., Fayers, P. & Shinebourne, E. (1980). Value of repeated blood pressure measurement in children – the Brompton study. *British Medical Journal*, **280**, 1567–9.

de Swiet, M., Fayers, P. & Shinebourne, E. (1984). Blood pressure in four and five year old children. The effects of environment and other factors in its measurement. *Journal of Hypertension*, **2**, 501–5.

Dillon, M. (1988). Blood pressure. *Archives of Disease in Childhood* **63**, 347–9.

Dubos, R., Savage, D. & Schaedler, R. (1966). Biological Freudianism: lasting effects of early environmental influences. *Pediatrics*, **38**, 789–800.

Dyer, A., Elliott, P. & Shipley, M. (1990). For the Intersalt Cooperative Research Group. Body Mass Index versus height and weight in relation to blood pressure. *American Journal of Epidemiology*, **131**, 589–96.

Eveleth, P. (1986). Population differences in growth: environmental and genetic factors. In *Human Growth, Volume 3*. ed. F. Falkner & J. Tanner. pp. 221–239. Plenum Press, New York.

Godfrey, K., Redman, C., Barker, D. & Osmond, C. (1991). The effect of maternal anaemia and iron deficiency on the ratio of fetal weight to placental weight. *British Journal of Obstetrics and Gynaecology*, **98**, 886–91.

Grimley Evans, J. & Rose, G. (1971). Hypertension. *British Medical Bulletin*, **27**, 37–41.

HMSO Office of Population Censuses and Surveys (1991). Mortality statistics 1989: cause. Series DH2 no. 16. London.

Kahn, A. (1968). Embryogenic effect on post-natal changes in haemoglobin with time. *Growth*, **32**, 13–22.

Labarthe, D., Eissa, M. & Varas, C. (1991). Childhood precursors of high blood pressure and elevated cholesterol. *Annual Review of Public Health*, **12**, 519–41.

Law, C., Barker, D., Bull, A. & Osmond, C. (1991a). Maternal and fetal influences on blood pressure. *Archives of Disease in Childhood*, **66**, 1291–5.

Law, M., Frost, C. & Wald, N. (1991b). By how much does dietary salt reduction lower blood pressure: analysis of data from trials of salt reduction. *British Medical Journal*, **302**, 819–24.

MacMahon, S., Peto, R., Cutler, J., Collins, R., Sorlie, P., Neaton, J., Abbott, R., Godwin, J., Dyer, A. & Stamler, J. (1990). Blood pressure, stroke and coronary heart disease. Part I, prolonged differences in blood pressure: prospective observational studies corrected for regression dilution bias. *Lancet*, **335**, 765–74.

Margetts, B., Rowland, M., Foord, F., Cruddas, A., Cole, T. & Barker, D. (1991). The relation of maternal weight to the blood pressure of Gambian children. *International Journal of Epidemiology*, **20**, 938–43.

Mott, G., Lewis, D. & McGill, H. (1991). Programming of cholesterol metabolism by breast or formula feeding. In *The Childhood Environment and Adult Disease. Ciba Symposium* 156. John Wiley, Chichester.

Simpson, A., Mortimer, J., Silva, P., Spears, G. & Williams, S. (1981). In *Hypertension in the young and old*, ed. G. Onesti & K. Kim. pp. 153–166. Grune and Stratton, New York.

Voors, A., Webber, L., Frerichs, R. & Berenson, G. (1977). Body height and body mass as determinants of basal blood pressure in children – The Bogalusa heart study. *American Journal of Epidemiology*, **106**, 101–8.

Whincup, P., Cook, D., Shaper, A., MacFarlane, D. & Walker, M. (1988). Blood pressure in British children: associations with adult blood pressure and cardiovascular mortality. *Lancet*, **i**, 890–3.

Whincup, P., Cook, D. & Shaper A. (1989). Early influences on blood pressure: a study of children aged 5–7 years. *British Medical Journal*, **299**, 587–91.

Clinical applications

12

Recording and analysis of fetal heart rate variation

TIMOTHY WHEELER

The development of FHR monitoring techniques

'Monitoring' implies that the fetal heart rate (FHR) is recorded continuously from one beat to the next. For this purpose one brief event unique to each heart cycle has to be identified so that the duration of successive heart intervals can be measured. The first recordings of this nature were published by Hon in 1958 and were obtained from an electrode attached directly to the fetus using the R wave of the fetal electrocardiogram (ECG) to trigger a cardiotachometer (Fig. 12.1). The fetal R wave recorded in this way has an amplitude of between 100 and 400 μV (Figueroa-Longo et al., 1966; Hon, 1967) with a good signal to noise ratio so that its detection is relatively simple. As no detail in the ECG complex is required other than the R wave, baseline wander can be eliminated with appropriate filtering and the R wave detected, for example, by threshold crossing.

The first non-invasive recordings of the FHR were also made in 1958 by Hellman et al., who used a phonocardiographic technique to detect the heart sounds across the maternal abdomen. In comparison to the R wave of the fetal ECG, heart sounds are complex signals (Fig. 12.1) requiring sophisticated processing before the FHR can be recorded.

When FHR monitors were first marketed in the late 1960s, most was known about their potential use during labour. The pioneering research of Hon (1959) and Caldeyro-Barcia et al. (1967) had clearly demonstrated that changes in the FHR during contractions, which could not be detected by auscultation, were associated with fetal distress; thus monitoring offered the prospect of earlier diagnosis of this problem and improvements in its management. Bipolar electrodes, making contact with the fetus and with the mother (across the vagina), produced ECGs of satisfactory quality for recording the FHR (Hon, 1963). The first elec-

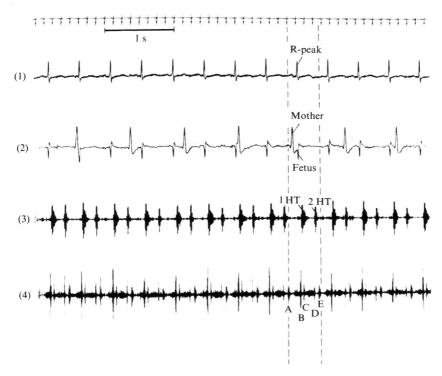

Fig. 12.1. Signals from the fetal heart. (1) Fetal ECG from electrode attached directly to fetus. (2) Fetal and maternal ECGs from electrodes on the maternal abdomen. (3) Fetal phonocardiogram. (4) Doppler ultrasound signal. (From 'Kardiotokographie', ed W.M. Fisher, 1973, reproduced with permission from Georg Thieme Verlag, Stuttgart.)

trodes were similar to surgical skin clips and attached to the fetus in the same way; these have since been replaced by needle electrodes, which are easier to apply.

The possible benefits of antenatal monitoring of the FHR were first described by Hammacher et al., in 1968. For this purpose the fetal heart beat must be detected on the surface of the mother. The R wave of the fetal ECG is not suitable as it is attenuated at the maternal skin surface, with an amplitude of only 5–25 μV, smaller than the maternal QRS complex which is also present (Fig. 12.1). The size of the fetal ECG is also related to gestation with a decrease between 28 and 34 weeks (Fig. 12.2); this may be related to the formation of vernix caseosa. In the earlier days of FHR monitoring considerable efforts were made to remove the

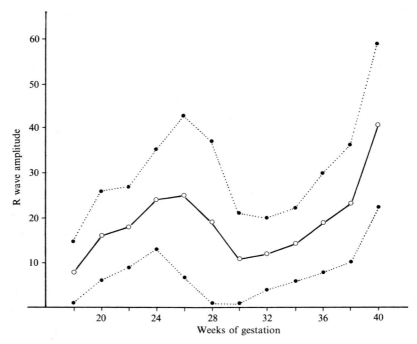

Fig. 12.2. Fetal R wave amplitude related to gestation. (Data from Bolte, 1969, reproduced with permission.)

maternal ECG from the recordings so that the fetal ECG alone would be available for analysis. Details of a subtraction technique for this purpose were published by Sureau and Trocellier in 1961 and with modifications the technique was used by Wheeler, Murrills & Shelley (1978) to study the FHR during pregnancy. The authors admit however that the technique has a high failure rate due to the low signal to noise ratio and that it is really only suitable for research. Whereas the aim of the subtraction technique is to reveal all the fetal R waves including those occurring by coincidence in the maternal QRS complexes, 'blanking' techniques remove all the maternal signals and interpolate fetal information when necessary. Certain FHR monitors have been supplied with this facility including the Hewlett Packard 8020A and the Brattle monitor (Van Horn, Epstein & Phillips, 1974). The high recording success rates found by Ruttgers et al. (1974) for the Hewlett Packard (80%) and by Leventhal et al. (1975) for the Brattle monitor (87%) did not take into account fetal maturity and are unlikely to be representative of the problem as a whole.

Phonocardiography, another method of recording the FHR externally, is based upon the detection of the heart sounds on the maternal abdomen. One difficulty in analysing such signals was to determine whether one or two heart sounds had been detected during each cardiac cycle. In 1962 Hammacher described a suitable technique for this purpose, which was later to be used in the first FHR monitors manufactured by Hewlett Packard in 1968. Recordings for at least some min can be made from most patients in this manner but outside noise or fetal movements readily disturb the system. Ruttgers et al. (1970) claimed a 70–80% yield of successful data.

The major breakthrough for external monitoring of the FHR was made possible with the use of Doppler ultrasound (Callagan, Rowland & Goldman, 1964). Initially narrow beamed continuous ultrasound was passed across the fetal chest where complex signals (Fig. 12.1) derived from the movements of the heart wall, and sometimes heart valves, could be detected (Abelson & Balin, 1972). Higher frequency components of the signal were due to the movement of blood cells, whose flow could be additionally modulated by fetal breathing (Boyce et al., 1976). As with phonocardiography, fetal movement could easily disturb the recordings and the complicated nature of the Doppler signals made signal processing difficult. One visual appraisal of the Hewlett Packard narrow beam ultrasound system (Wheeler & Guerard, 1974) showed that 60% of the FHR data was satisfactory while the remainder was disturbed by artefact (30%) or was missing (10%). Though never formally compared with phonocardiography, Doppler ultrasound was recognized as a superior system and introduced widely as the system of choice for external monitoring. Wide angle ultrasound transducers were designed (around 1973) which enabled the heart to be detected more successfully during fetal movement. The complexity of the signals remained a problem and led to mistriggering of the ratemeter, giving a characteristic artefact described as 'jitter'. For a limited period Roche Medical Electronics marketed a pulsed Doppler system, able to select both the recording depth and the direction of the movement chosen to record the heart (Lauersen et al., 1978). It was claimed that good quality recordings were obtained but extra supervision during the recordings was required. However two separate developments, introduced around 1982, have substantially improved the quality of ultrasound recordings. These are firstly the insonation of a wider area of the uterus achieved by using an array of crystals within the ultrasound transducer, pulsed to transmit and receive alternately; and secondly on-line autocorrelation of the signals.

Autocorrelation compares the signal with itself and has the effect of reducing errors due to random noise (e.g. that due to fetal movement) whilst enhancing the repetitive components of the signal (e.g. those due to fetal heart activity). The resultant autocorrelation function, which oscillates between a maximum value when consecutive portions of the signal most closely match, and a minimum value when the signal is least closely matched, has a time period identical to the repetitive components of the signal. Furthermore signal quality can be indicated so that the ultrasound transducer can be positioned to obtain the best signals from the fetal heart. Unlike phonocardiography, ultrasound passes a small amount of energy across the fetus. This is not believed to be harmful but there were, and anecdotally still are, reports that ultrasound causes an increase in fetal activity (David, Weaver & Pearson, 1975). However, a randomized and double blind study has shown that such an effect is most unlikely (Murrills et al., 1983). The actual levels of ultrasound intensity (typically <1 mW/cm^2, SPTA) are substantially below the limit of 100 mW/cm^2 recommended by the American Institute of Ultrasound in Medicine.

Efficient though FHR monitoring now appears, an important misre-presentation of the data is possible. When the fetus is dead, both direct electrocardiography and ultrasound can detect the maternal heart and process the signals so that a recording is produced. Clearly, if this is not appreciated, it is possible for the situation to be seriously mismanaged.

The accuracy of FHR measurements

Today the processing of the signals from the fetal heart is computerized and each heart cycle is available as a digital measurement. This means that assessments of data quality can be made objectively by computer rather than by 'eyeballing' recordings. Data obtained from the fetal ECG remains the 'gold standard' to which the external systems of FHR monitoring are compared. The precision with which each R-R interval can be measured depends upon the signal to noise ratio of the fetal ECG; from good quality abdominal recordings the accuracy is in the order of 1 to 2 milliseconds (Fig. 12.3). Signal loss is potentially an important problem especially with external systems of recording the FHR; for example an average of 40% of the data is lost using continuous wave ultrasound (Dawes et al., 1981) but this has improved tenfold with the use of pulsed ultrasound and autocorrelation (Dawes, Redman & Smith, 1985). A number of studies have investigated the accuracy of FHR data,

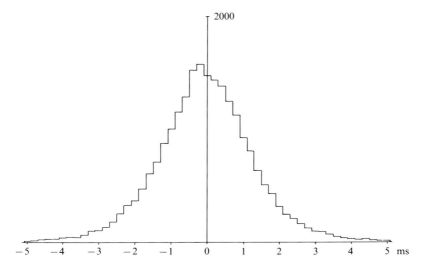

Fig. 12.3. Distribution of interval differences due to noise. Distribution of the time differences (in milliseconds) from interval to interval due to noise on the abdominal fetal ECG. The 20,000 differences were obtained from 5 different fetuses, each monitored for approximately 30 minutes. (From Murrills & Wheeler, 1980, reproduced with permission from Pitman Medical Limited, London.)

obtained by ultrasound and processed by autocorrelation, in comparison to simultaneous recordings of the FHR made from the fetal ECG. There is a close correlation of the average FHR and long term variation (Lawson et al., 1985) but not with beat to beat variation (Fig. 12.4). An increase in signal loss reduces the correlation between ultrasound and ECG measurements of FHR variation (Spencer, Belcher & Dawes, 1987).

Analysis of the fetal heart rate

The first major study of the FHR during pregnancy was instigated by the Fels Institute and performed by Sontag and Richards in 1938. The results were published in a monograph entitled *Fetal Heart Rate as a Behavioural Indicator*. The observations were based upon estimates of the FHR made every ten heart beats; the heartbeats were counted using a stethoscope. The decrease in heart rate as gestation advanced was established and it was also found that within any minute the heart rate showed an 8–9% variation around its mean. During fetal activity both the average heart

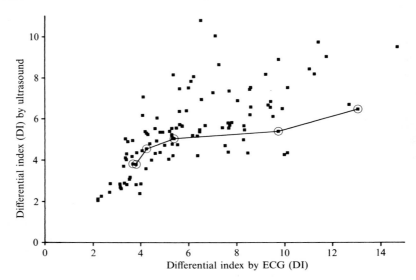

Fig. 12.4. Beat to beat variation. Measurements of the differential index (Yeh et al., 1973) over periods of 5 minutes obtained from 25 subjects between 34 and 42 weeks of gestation. A poor correlation was found between the ultrasound data (obtained by autocorrelation using a Hewlett Packard 8040A) and the abdominal fetal ECG data. 6 values from one fetus over a 30 minute period are linked and show a range from 4.1 ms to 13.2 ms (discussed in text). (From Murrills et al., 1986, reproduced with permission from Butterworths.)

rate and its variation were observed to increase. Phonocardiographic recordings which plotted the heart rate from beat to beat (Hellman et al., 1958) showed that a pattern of oscillations (about six per min) modulated the FHR; these were described in more detail by Hammacher et al. (1968) according to their amplitude. Visual appraisal of the cardiotoco-gram remains the most common method of assessing the FHR but of concern is the evidence of interobserver variation when this is done (Trimbos & Keirse, 1978; Borgotta, Shrout & Divon, 1988).

In recent years, computer systems have been developed enabling sophisticated analyses of FHR data during pregnancy (Dawes et al., 1985). Fundamental to such analyses is the identification of the baseline FHR (Dawes et al., 1982); this normally represents the modal value of the FHR and specifically excludes accelerations or decelerations. The variation of the heart rate is measured as long-term or short-term variation. Many expressions for long-term variation have been published

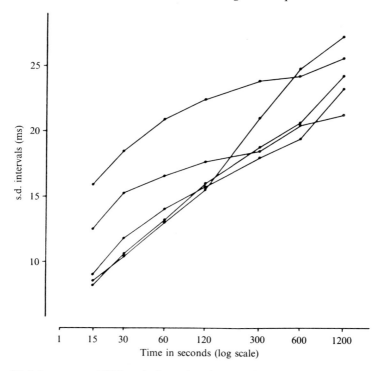

Fig. 12.5. Long term FHR variation related to epoch. The relationship between the standard deviation of the heart intervals (a measure of long term variation) and observational epoch. Data from 5 abdominal recordings of the fetal ECG, each over a period of one hour. The values obtained over each epoch were averaged and plotted on a logarithmic time scale. (From Wheeler et al., 1979, reproduced with permission from Blackwell Scientific Publications.)

and several have been compared and reviewed by Laros et al. (1977). Long term FHR variation is positively correlated with the period of time over which it is measured (Fig. 12.5). A recent computer analysis of long-term FHR variation during pregnancy has shown an important correlation between this and the fetal PO_2 (Fig. 12.6).

The term 'short-term' heart rate variation has been interpreted loosely in the literature; it may certainly include the change in heart rate from one beat to the next ('beat to beat variation'). Measurements of beat to beat variation are only possible when the trigger pulses for each heart cycle are derived from the R wave of the fetal ECG. Typical differences in heart

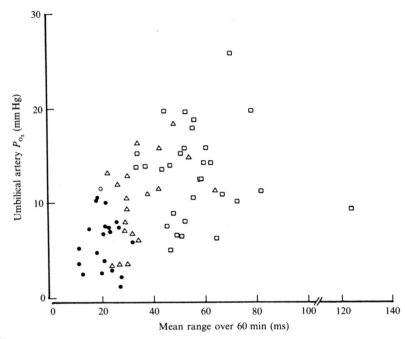

Fig. 12.6. Relationship between umbilical artery oxygen tension at delivery and the mean range of the fetal heart rate before delivery. Solid circles denote fetuses delivered because of suspected fetal compromise, triangles denote delivery undertaken for urgent maternal reasons, open circles denote a healthy fetus in whom delivery was undertaken to by-pass possible mechanical problems in labour. The FHR was recorded by Doppler ultrasound and autocorrelation; each recording lasted for 60 minutes. The range of the baseline FHR, including any accelerations, was calculated (in ms) for each minute and expressed as a mean for the whole recording. (From Smith et al., 1988, reproduced with permission from Blackwell Scientific Publications.)

intervals from beat to beat are shown in Fig. 12.7 and it can be seen that 10–20% of such differences are at a level that is indistinguishable from that caused by noise. Beat to beat variation is related to the average heart rate, more variation occurring at the lower rates in any given recording (Fig. 12.8). The value of measuring beat to beat variation is uncertain; Kariniemi and Ammala (1981) measured the differential index (Yeh, Forsythe & Hon, 1973) over epochs of 5 min and reported that this provided a reliable prediction of fetal welfare. However other studies of the same index (Murrills, Wilmshurst & Wheeler, 1986) have shown that large changes in its value may occur from one epoch to the next (Fig.

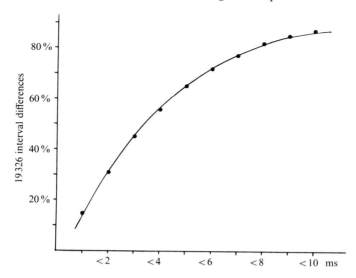

Fig. 12.7. Interval differences. Cumulative distribution of 19,326 interval differences obtained from 5 abdominal recordings of the fetal ECG made after 36 weeks of gestation. Each recording lasted approximately 30 minutes. (From Wheeler et al., 1979, reproduced with permission from Blackwell Scientific Publications.)

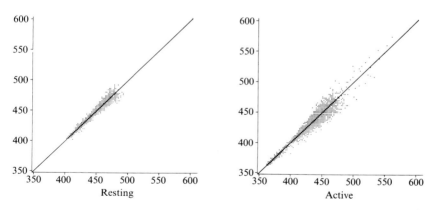

Fig. 12.8. 2-Dimensional plot of fetal heart intervals. Heart interval data plotted according to the 2-dimensional system of de Haan et al. (1971). Each point represents the relationship between pairs of successive heart intervals (T1 & T2, T2 & T3, etc). If 2 successive intervals are of the same value the point will be plotted on the line of equality; large differences between pairs are reflected in points further away from that line. The plots were obtained from the same fetus, recorded at term during periods of rest and activity.

12.4). More recently Street et al. (1991) have examined FHR variation
between short epochs of 3.75 s. Although not a measure of beat-to-beat
variation, this description of short-term variation adds helpful information to that provided by variation over epochs of one min (Dawes et
al., 1985).

Studies have been made of the rhythms within the FHR, which are not
revealed by summary (overall) descriptions of heart rate variation and
ideally require spectral analysis. By term, a diurnal variation in heart rate
is apparent with the greatest variation occurring during the night (Visser
et al., 1982*a*). There are also 'quasi-periodic' (Campbell, MacNeill &
Patrick, 1981) cycles of fetal rest and activity, which cause a detectable
effect on the FHR by 27 weeks of gestation (Visser, Dawes & Redman,
1981). By the end of gestation, the cycle length (measured from FHR
variation) is similar in duration to the cycle of REM and non-REM sleep
found in the newborn, which suggests that these effects are mediated
through the CNS (Visser et al., 1982*b*). Two other rhythms of shorter
duration are present in the human FHR. 'Oscillations' with a range of 3 to
10 cycles per min were noted by Hammacher et al. (1968). The origin and
control of these is uncertain but may be related to sympathetic activity
since in the newborn respiration and heart rate are modulated at similar
frequencies, which in turn are related to sleep state (deHaan et al., 1977).
In the lamb fetus there is more direct evidence which links sympathetic
tone to sleep state (Zhu & Szeto, 1987). Fetal breathing increases beat to
beat variation (Wheeler et al., 1980) and is represented by a pattern of
respiratory sinus arrhythmia (frequency 40–70 cycles per min). The
mechanism behind this is uncertain but it could be accounted for by a
local response to stretching of the heart wall caused by the increased
venous return during inspiration.

Conclusions

Technically the problems of fetal heart rate (FHR) monitoring are
determined by the nature of the signals, which originate from the heart
and which are used to derive its rate. When FHR monitors became
available in the late 1960s, interest was principally in their role in the
detection of intrapartum fetal distress. Once the membranes had rup-
tured in labour, an electrode could be attached to the fetus to record the
fetal ECG which provided a well-defined timing point (the R wave) from
which the duration of each heart cycle could be measured. Since then the
developing role of antenatal cardiotocography has led to the need for

high quality FHR recordings during pregnancy. Doppler ultrasound has replaced phonocardiography as the more reliable method of detecting the fetal heart across the maternal abdomen but, only recently, with the processing of the complex Doppler signals by autocorrelation have good quality recordings been possible.

Further technical problems are now the focus of research. These include automated methods of FHR analysis and presentation. And a practical problem for which solutions exist but have yet to be implemented, is that of data storage. It is a legal requirement (in the UK) that FHR records are stored for 25 years after delivery; paper recordings may get lost, destroyed or fade with time.

References

Abelson, D. & Balin, H. (1972). Analysis of the Doppler signals from the fetal heart. *American Journal of Obstetrics and Gynecology,* **112**, 796.

Bolte, A. (1969). Die pranatale fetale elektrokardiographie. *Gynakologe,* **2**, 63.

Borgotta, L., Shrout, P. E. & Divon, M. Y. (1988). Reliability and reproducibility of nonstress test readings. *American Journal of Obstetrics and Gynecology,* **159**, 554–8.

Boyce, E. S., Dawes, G. S., Gough, J. D. & Poore, E. R. (1976). Doppler ultrasound method for detecting human fetal breathing in utero. *British Medical Journal,* **2**, 17–18.

Caldeyro-Barcia, R., Casacuberta, C., Bustos, R. et al. (1967). Correlation of intrapartum changes in fetal heart rate with fetal blood oxygen and acid-base state. In *Diagnosis and Treatment of Fetal Disorders,* ed. K. Adamsons. pp. 212–222. Springer-Verlag.

Callagan, D. A., Rowland, T. C. & Goldman, D. E. (1964). Ultrasonic Doppler observation of the fetal heart. *Obstetrics and Gynecology,* **23**, 637.

Campbell, K., MacNeill, I. & Patrick, J. (1981). Time series analysis of ultrasonic observations of gross fetal body movements during the last 10 weeks of pregnancy. *Ultrasonic Imaging,* **3**, 330–41.

David, H., Weaver, J. B. & Pearson, J. F. (1975). Doppler ultrasound and fetal activity. *British Medical Journal,* **ii**, 62–4.

Dawes, G. S., Visser, G. H. A., Goodman, J. D. S. & Redman, C. W. G. (1981). Numerical analysis of the human fetal heart rate: the quality of ultrasound records. *American Journal of Obstetrics and Gynecology,* **141**, 43–52.

Dawes, G. S., Houghton, C. R. S. & Redman, C. W. G. (1982). Baseline in human fetal heart rate recordings. *British Journal of Obstetrics and Gynaecology,* **89**, 270–5.

Dawes, G. S., Redman, C. W. G. & Smith, J. H. (1985). Improvements in the registration and analysis of fetal heart rate records at the bedside. *British Journal of Obstetrics and Gynaecology,* **92**, 317–25.

deHaan, R., Patrick, J., Chess, G. F. & Jaco, N. J. (1977). Definition of sleep state in the newborn by heart rate analysis. *American Journal of Obstetrics and Gynecology,* **127**, 753–8.

de Haan, J., van Bemmel, J. H., Versteeg, B., Veth, A. F. L., Stolte, L. A. M., Janssens, J. & Eskes, T. K. A. B. (1971). Quantitative evaluation of the fetal heart rate patterns. 1. Processing methods. *European Journal of Obstetrics and Gynecology,* **1**, 95.

Figueroa-Longo, J. G., Poseiro, J. J., Alvarez, L. O. & Caldeyro-Barcia, R. (1966). Fetal electrocardiogram at term obtained with subcutaneous fetal electrodes. *American Journal of Obstetrics and Gynecology,* **96**, 556.

Hammacher, K. (1962). Neue methode zur selektiven registrierung der herzschlagfrequenz. *Geburtshilfe Frauenheilkd,* **22**, 1542.

Hammacher, K., Huter, K. A., Bokelmann, J. & Werners, P. H. (1968). Fetal heart frequency and perinatal condition of the fetus and newborn. *Gynaecologia,* **166**, 349.

Hellman, L. M., Schiffer, M. A., Kohl, S. G. & Tolles, L. G. (1958). Studies in fetal well-being: variations in fetal heart rate. *American Journal of Obstetrics and Gynecology,* **76**, 998.

Hon, E. H. (1958). The electronic evaluation of the fetal heart; preliminary report. *American Journal of Obstetrics and Gynecology,* **75**, 1215.

Hon, E. H. (1959). Observations on 'pathologic' fetal bradycardia. *American Journal of Obstetrics and Gynecology,* **77**, 1084–99.

Hon, E. H. (1963). Instrumentation of fetal heart rate and fetal electrocardiography. II A vaginal electrode. *American Journal of Obstetetrics and Gynecology,* **86**, 772–84.

Hon, E. H. (1967). Fetal ECG electrodes: further observations. *Obstetrics and Gynecology,* **30**, 281.

Kariniemi, V. & Ammala, P. (1981). Short-term variability of fetal heart rate during pregnancy with normal and insufficient placental function. *American Journal of Obstetrics and Gynecology,* **139**, 33–7.

Laros, R. K., Wong, W. S., Heilbron, D. C., Parer, J. T., Schnider, S. M., Naylor, H. & Butler, J. (1977). A comparison of methods for quantitating fetal heart rate variability. *American Journal of Obstetrics and Gynecology,* **128**, 381–92.

Lauersen, N. H., Hochberg, H. M., George, M. E. D., Tegge, C. S. & Meighan, J. J. (1978). Technical aspects of ranged directional Doppler: a new Doppler method of fetal heart rate monitoring. *Journal of Reproductive Medicine,* **20**, 77–83.

Lawson, G. W., Belcher, R., Dawes, G. S. & Redman, C. W. G. (1985). A comparison of ultrasound (with autocorrelation) and direct electrocardiogram fetal heart rate detector systems. *American Journal of Obstetrics and Gynecology,* **147**, 721–2.

Leventhal, J. M., Brown, W. U., Weiss, J. B. & Alper, M. H. (1975). A new method of fetal heart rate monitoring. *Obstetrics and Gynecology,* **45**, 494.

Murrills, A. J., Barrington, P., Harris, P. D. & Wheeler, T. (1983). Influence of Doppler ultrasound on fetal activity. *British Medical Journal,* **286**, 1009–12.

Murrills, A. J. & Wheeler, T. (1980). Measurement of heart rate variation from abdominal fetal ECG signals. In *Fetal and Neonatal Physiological Measurements*, ed. P. Rolfe. pp. 1–8. Pitman Medical Books, London.

Murrills, A. J., Wilmshurst, T. H. & Wheeler, T. (1986). Antenatal measurement of beat to beat variation: accuracy of the Hewlett Packard ultrasound auto-correlation technique. In *Fetal Physiological Measurements*, ed. P. Rolfe. pp. 36–44. Butterworths, London.

Ruttgers, H., Kubli, F., Hinselmann, M. & Grund, K. (1970). Continuous monitoring of the instantaneous fetal heart rate by Doppler-ultrasound. Conference on Ultrasonics in Biology and Medicine, Warsaw, pp. 195.

Ruttgers, H., Meyer-Menk, W., Stagel, A., Spangler, W. & Kubli, F. (1974). Instantaneous fetal heart rate measurement using the abdominal ECG. *Gynakologische Rundschau,* **14**, 79.

Smith, J. H., Anand, K. J. S., Cotes, P. M., Dawes, G. S., Harkness, R. A., Howlett, T. A., Rees, L. H. & Redman, C. W. G. (1988). Antenatal fetal heart rate variation in relation to the respiratory and metabolic status of the compromised human fetus. *British Journal of Obstetrics and Gynaecology,* **95**, 980–9.

Sontag, L. W. & Richards, T. W. (1938). Fetal heart rate as a behavioural indicator. *Monographs of the Society for the Research in Child Development,* **3**, No. 4 (Serial No 17).

Spencer, J. A. D., Belcher, R. & Dawes, G. S. (1987). The influence of signal loss on the comparison between computer analyses of the fetal heart rate in labour using pulsed Doppler ultrasound (with autocorrelation) and simultaneous scalp electrocardiogram. *European Journal of Obstetrics, Gynecology and Reproductive Biology,* **25**, 29–34.

Street, P., Dawes, G. S., Moulden, M. & Redman, C. W. G. (1991). Short term variation in abnormal fetal heart rate records. *American Journal of Obstetrics and Gynecology* (in press).

Sureau, C. & Trocellier, R. (1961). Un probleme technique d'electrocardiographie foetale. Note sur l'elimination de l'electrocardiogramme maternel. *Gynecologie et Obstetrique,* **60**, 43.

Trimbos, J. B. & Keirse, M. J. N. C. (1978). Observer variability in assessment of antepartum cardiotocograms. *British Journal of Obstetrics and Gynaecology,* **85**, 900–6.

Van Horn, J. M., Epstein, P. & Phillips, P. G. (1974). Biological signals monitor. *United States Patent* 3, 811, 428.

Visser, G. H. A., Dawes, G. S. & Redman, C. W. G. (1981). Numerical analysis of the normal human antenatal fetal heart rate. *British Journal of Obstetrics and Gynaecology,* **88**, 792–802.

Visser, G. H. A., Goodman, J. D. S., Levine, D. & Dawes, G. S. (1982*a*). Diurnal and other cyclic variations in human fetal heart rate near term. *American Journal of Obstetrics and Gynecology,* **142**, 535–44.

Visser, G. H. A., Carse, E. A., Goodman, J. D. S. & Johnson, P. (1982*b*). A comparison of episodic heart-rate patterns in the fetus and newborn. *British Journal of Obstetrics and Gynaecology,* **89**, 50–5.

Wheeler, T. & Guerard, P. (1974). Fetal heart rate during late pregnancy. *Journal of Obstetrics and Gynaecology of the British Commonwealth,* **81**, 348–56.

Wheeler, T., Murrills, A. & Shelley T (1978). Measurement of the fetal heart rate during pregnancy by a new electrocardiographic technique. *British Journal of Obstetrics and Gynaecology,* **85**, 12–17.

Wheeler, T., Cooke, E. & Murrills, A. (1979). Computer analysis of fetal heart rate variation during normal pregnancy. *British Journal of Obstetrics and Gynaecology,* **86**, 186–97.

Wheeler, T., Gennser, G., Lindvall, R. & Murrills, A.J. (1980). Changes in the fetal heart rate associated with fetal breathing and fetal movement. *British Journal of Obstetrics and Gynaecology,* **87**, 1068–79.

Yeh, S-Y., Forsythe, A. & Hon, E. H. (1973). Quantification of fetal heart beat-to beat interval differences. *Obstetrics and Gynecology,* **41**, 355–63.

Zhu, Y. & Szeto, H. H. (1987). Cyclic variation in fetal heart rate and sympathetic activity. *American Journal of Obstetrics and Gynecology,* **156**, 1001–5.

13

Fetal heart rate monitoring: application in clinical practice

JOHN A. D. SPENCER

Antepartum fetal monitoring

Definitions and classification

The parameters of the fetal heart rate (FHR) seen on the cardiotocograph (CTG) include baseline rate, baseline variability, accelerations and decelerations. Variability and accelerations cannot be recorded easily by intermittent auscultation unless repeated at frequent short intervals (Steer & Beard, 1970). The accuracy and reproducibility of auscultation, even in experienced hands, have been questioned (Day, Maddern & Wood, 1968).

Classification of CTG traces has been the subject of discussion in the literature for two decades (Spencer, 1990). One of the most common methods used during pregnancy, introduced in the mid-1970s, relies on the presence of accelerations associated with fetal movements – a so-called reactive trace (Lee, DiLoreto & O'Lane, 1975; Flynn & Kelly, 1977) – to identify normality. Others at this time were introducing scoring systems (Fischer, Stude & Brandt, 1976; Pearson & Weaver, 1978) or alternative descriptive classifications (Visser & Huisjes, 1977). Recently, FIGO (1987) has published guidelines for the use of FHR monitoring (Table 13.1).

Changes in normal pregnancy

As pregnancy progresses the FHR gradually falls such that, after 28 weeks, the normal range is 110 – 150 beats per min (Wheeler & Murrills, 1978; FIGO, 1987). After 30 weeks the continuing fall in FHR is confined to episodes of low variability (Dawes et al., 1982), associated with fetal quiescence.

281

Table 13.1. *Guidelines for FHR monitoring*

Interpretation	Baseline (bpm)	Variability (bpm)	Accelerations (per 10 min)	Decelerations
Normal	110–150	5–25	2 or more	Absent
Suspicious	100–110 or 150–170	5–10 >40 min or >25	Absent >40 min	Sporadic, small
Pathological	<100 or >170	<5 >40 min or sinusoidal >20 min	Absent	Repeated (any) or sporadic, large prolonged or late

Source: Int. J. Gynaecol. Obstet. (1987), **25**, 159.

After 28 weeks there are predominantly two patterns of FHR variability: saltatory, produced by frequent accelerations above the baseline during periods of fetal activity (Wheeler & Guerard, 1974), and undulatory episodes, usually with variability between 5 and 15 beats per min and lasting between 10 and 40 min, associated with a stable baseline during periods of fetal quiescence (Wheeler & Murrills, 1978; Dawes et al., 1982).

The cardinal feature of normality on a record of the FHR in late pregnancy is the presence of accelerations associated with fetal movements. Such a FHR pattern is termed reactive and is generally associated with normal baseline variability. There is, however, considerable variation in the definition of a normal FHR record in terms of the number, amplitude and duration of accelerations and the duration of the recording (Spencer, 1990) and, similarly, the application of the method and management of non-reactive traces is far from uniform (Thacker & Berkelman, 1986). False-positive rates exceed 50% for morbidity and 80% for mortality. False-negative rates are less than 10% for morbidity and less than 2% for mortality. Sensitivity is around 50% and specificity exceeds 80% (Thacker & Berkelman, 1986).

Influence of fetal activity

The number of accelerations and degree of FHR variability are significantly influenced by the presence or absence of fetal activity (Dawes et al., 1982) and periods of fetal quiescence, with few accelerations and reduced variability, are a major cause of false positive FHR records during pregnancy. Such records cannot be called either normal or abnormal and have been labelled doubtful (Fischer et al., 1976), non-reactive (Rochard et al., 1976; Flynn & Kelly, 1977), suboptimal (Visser & Huisjes, 1977), suspicious (Trimbos & Keirse, 1978), suspect or flat (Flynn, Kelly & O'Conor, 1979) and prepathologic (Lyons et al., 1979). The combination of reduced baseline variability and absence of accelerations alone accounts for more than 80% of these patterns. Such records were found on at least one occasion in 37% and twice or more in 9% of normal pregnancies (Trimbos & Keirse, 1978). The incidence of a suspicious record in normal pregnancies is about 7% whereas in high-risk pregnancies it is 17% with a much higher recurrence rate (Keirse & Trimbos, 1981). It was found that adequate follow-up of such records allowed the majority of cases which did not need intervention to be distinguished from those which did. In a similar way, extending the recording time to 120 min was shown to improve the positive predictive value of a non-reactive FHR record for fetal morbidity or mortality to 86% and the negative predictive value of a reactive record to 98.5% (Brown & Patrick, 1981). Recently, vibro-acoustic stimulation applied to the maternal abdomen has also been shown to significantly improve the predictive value by reducing both the incidence of non-reactive tests and the overall testing time (Ohel et al., 1986).

Antepartum fetal stimulation

In the presence of a non-reactive FHR, manual manipulation of the fetus through the maternal abdomen was used in an attempt to alter the fetal state from quiescence to activity. However, prospective studies showed that this was not of significant value and appeared to work only by chance (Richardson et al., 1981). Sound (Read & Miller, 1977) was found to be more effective and, more recently, vibro-acoustic stimulation has become the method of choice, particularly in the USA. Irrespective of fetal state, vibro-acoustic stimulation produces a transient episode of fetal wakefulness after which the fetus remains in the active state. Thus, the disturbance to fetal behaviour is greater when the stimulation is performed during quiescence but subsequent rest–activity cycles are not influenced (Spencer et al., 1991a).

Oxytocin stress test

The provocation of uterine activity by oxytocin became popular in the USA during the 1970s as a method for assessing fetal well-being in high risk pregnancy (Freeman, 1975). FHR decelerations occurring after contractions were considered to be an indication of poor fetal reserve for labour. However, extensive study of the FHR record prior to oxytocin-induced uterine contractions showed that the combination of minimal baseline variability and lack of accelerations with fetal movement increased the likelihood of the occurrence of late decelerations with oxytocin-induced uterine contractions. Conversely, the presence of FHR accelerations associated with fetal movements was not associated with late decelerations during the subsequent oxytocin stress test (Trierweiler, Freeman & James, 1976). Others also showed the reliability of non-stressed records of the FHR if accelerations in response to movements were present and recommended that the oxytocin-induced contraction stress test be reserved to evaluate further a non-reactive record (Evertson et al., 1979). The stress-test has never been popular in the UK.

FHR changes associated with IUGR

The characteristic changes in the FHR associated with the progressive effects of chronic placental failure and fetal growth retardation include loss of accelerations associated with a reduction in fetal movements, a baseline variability below 5 beats per min and the onset of recurrent decelerations (Rochard et al., 1976; Visser & Huisjes, 1977; Flynn et al., 1979). Such a pathological FHR record has been considered as evidence of critical fetal reserve (Beischer et al., 1983) and delivery by Caesarean section, if the fetus is viable, is indicated. The quality of survival of these infants was found to be satisfactory. At delivery a significantly higher incidence of metabolic acidosis was found to be associated with such FHR patterns (Visser et al., 1980) but when delivery was expedited prior to a pathological FHR pattern then fetal decompensation into metabolic acidaemia had not occurred (Henson, Dawes & Redman, 1983). One of the major indications for an antenatal CTG is the identification of chronic placental failure in pregnancies complicated by hypertension and fetal growth retardation (FIGO, 1987).

Predictive value in pregnancy

Approximately 85–90% of CTG traces performed in high-risk pregnancies are normal (Oats, Chew & Rarren, 1987). The false negative rate of a reactive CTG is low (e.g. 3 per 1000 excluding lethal fetal malformations, Oats et al., 1987) and the negative predictive value has been reported as greater than 96% in most studies (Devoe et al., 1985). Reports of the positive predictive value of a non-reactive CTG have varied between 11 and 53% (Devoe et al., 1985) which indicates a large number of false positive traces.

Approximately 32% of one antenatal population were considered sufficiently 'at risk' to merit an antenatal CTG at some stage: 8% indicated reduced fetal reserve and 1% indicated critical reserve (Oats et al., 1987). The incidence of small babies was 8% if the CTG was normal, 11% if suspicious and 30% if pathological. The rates of Caesarean section were 16, 27 and 62% respectively, and the perinatal mortality rates were 0.8, 4 and 20% respectively.

Use in pregnancy

Pooled analysis of data from four small randomized trials of routine weekly screening of high-risk obstetric outpatients (Flynn et al., 1982; Brown et al., 1982; Lumley et al., 1983; Kidd, Patel & Smith, 1985) showed that more women were allowed to continue their pregnancy as an outpatient but there was a slightly ($P < 0.05$) greater risk of perinatal death if the CTG report was available (Grant & Mohide, 1982). It would appear that false reassurance from the CTG may have kept some high risk pregnancies out of hospital, to their detriment.

Antepartum FHR monitoring should be used for diagnostic purposes only and the result needs to be interpreted in the light of the clinical indication for performing the test (FIGO, 1987). The main objective is to detect placental dysfunction. Thus, evaluation of fetal well-being in acute circumstances such as antepartum haemorrhage (Fig. 13.1) and chronic situations such as pre-eclampsia, suspected fetal growth retardation, and postdates pregnancy, are common indications (Oats et al., 1987).

A recent survey of UK consultant units revealed that 92% considered the CTG, alone or in combination with other tests, to be the most reliable method of detecting fetal distress before labour (Wheble et al., 1989).

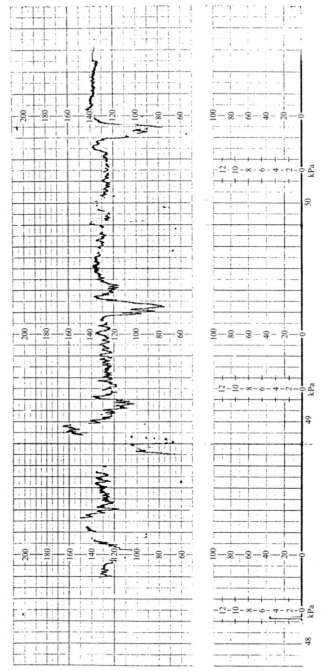

Fig. 13.1. CTG record illustrating the fetal response to a moderate abruption at 36 weeks gestation. The woman presented with antepartum haemorrhage and the fetal response prompted an emergency Caesarean section. An appropriately grown baby was delivered, acidaemic but in good clinical condition.

Fetal monitoring in labour

Classifications

Intrapartum classifications of the association between uterine contractions and decelerations began with Caldeyro-Barcia et al. (1966) and Hon (1968). Type 1 (early) and type 2 (late) decelerations were soon ascribed diagnostic and prognostic significance despite the poor correlation between such changes and fetal acidaemia (Beard et al., 1971). Many FHR decelerations are a feature of fetal adaptation to uterine contractions, such changes being part of the fetal cardiovascular response to hypoxaemia which help to maintain oxygen supply to the fetal brain. Many of these changes occur without fetal acidaemia (Fig. 13.2). The FIGO guidelines (1987) recommend the use of fetal blood sampling when suspicious or pathological fetal heart rate patterns are noted in labour.

Normal labour

The FHR in normal labour continues to show alternating episodes of high and low variability, the latter often being less than 5 beat per min amplitude for up to 40 min duration (Spencer & Johnson, 1986). Accelerations often continue during labour and have always been associated with a fetal pH above 7.20 (Kubli et al., 1969; Beard et al., 1971) as well as higher mean Apgar scores at one min after birth (Mendez-Bauer et al., 1967; Tejani, Mann & Bhakthavathsalan, 1976).

Intrapartum fetal stimulation

A FHR acceleration in response to scalp stimulation at the time of fetal scalp blood sampling during labour is rarely associated with fetal acidaemia (pH less than 7.20) (Clark, Grimovsky & Miller, 1984; Rice & Benedetti, 1986). However, absence of an acceleration also occurs in many non-acidaemic fetuses and this may relate to analgesia usage (Spencer, 1991). Fetal stimulation could be used to reduce fetal blood sampling in cases which respond with a FHR acceleration but further investigation of non-responders would still be necessary. Similar results have been obtained using vibro-acoustic stimulation prior to fetal blood sampling (Edersheim et al., 1987; Ingemarsson & Arulkumaran, 1989).

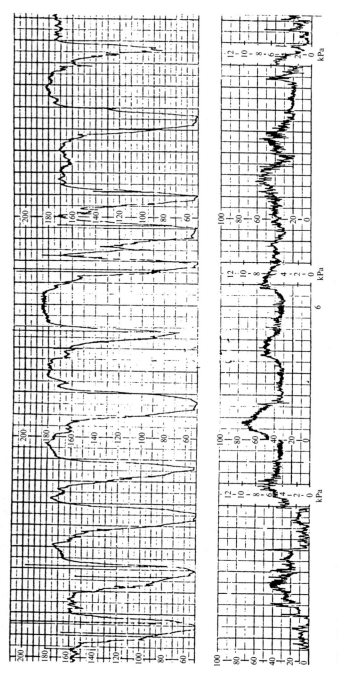

Fig. 13.2. A complicated baseline tachycardia with large, late, variable decelerations from a spontaneous preterm labour at 32 weeks. Repeated fetal scalp blood samples confirmed that the pH remained normal and resulted in a normal vaginal delivery of an appropriately grown, healthy, preterm baby.

Predictive value in labour

Although the association between FHR abnormalities during labour and fetal acidaemia is not good, the chance of the fetus being acidaemic is higher when there are more 'abnormalities' of the FHR pattern in high risk labours (Beard et al., 1971). The positive predictive value of late decelerations for fetal acidaemia is only between 30 and 40% (Beard et al., 1971; Young et al., 1980). Low variability alone is very poorly predictive of fetal acidaemia (Low et al., 1981), with a positive predictive value of around 5%.

The reported association between late decelerations and a 1 min Apgar score of less than 7 at delivery fell from greater than 70% (Beard et al., 1971), in high risk cases, to less than 20% (Curzen et al., 1984) as the use of continuous FHR monitoring was increasingly used in all labours. Positive predictive value has fallen with the decrease in prevalence due to lower overall risk in the population of labours monitored. Predictive value was only reasonable in the studies of high-risk patients which suggests that the occurrence of decelerations is not related to fetal risk. Late decelerations commonly occur after epidural analgesia (Fig. 13.3) and relate poorly to neonatal condition (Spencer, Koutsoukis & Lee, 1991*b*). It is clear that differentiation between significant (followed by birth asphyxia) and non-significant CTG changes in labour continues to pose great difficulties (Murphy et al., 1990).

Use in labour

Continuous FHR monitoring was originally applied to high-risk labours. Data from published studies do not justify the use of routine FHR monitoring in all labours (Shy et al., 1990). When the results of nine controlled trials of the use of continuous FHR monitoring during labour were pooled for analysis it was found that the perinatal mortality was not decreased. However, although the neonatal seizure rate was decreased, even with the use of fetal blood sampling, the Caesarean section and forceps delivery rates were increased (Thacker, 1991).

Fetal blood sampling is necessary for optimal management of labour, particularly in view of the large number of false positive changes seen on the CTG (Beard et al., 1971; Thacker, 1991). However, in practice, less than half the units in the UK which perform continuous FHR monitoring during labour also measure the fetal scalp pH during labour (Wheble et al., 1989).

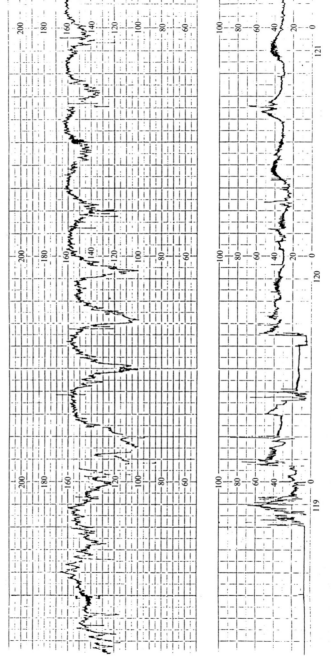

Fig. 13.3. A transient episode of late decelerations following an epidural in labour. A fetal scalp blood sample revealed a normal pH and the labour was allowed to continue.

Outcome

The biggest problem in evaluating the use of continuous FHR monitoring has been deciding upon the outcome criteria by which to judge its potential value. FHR changes do not correlate well with either fetal pH during labour or Apgar scores at delivery, which is not surprising since low fetal pH (umbilical artery at delivery) itself does not correlate well with low Apgar scores (Sykes et al., 1982; Dijxhoorn et al., 1986). Neither of these parameters perform well at predicting neonatal neurological morbidity (Dijxhoorn et al., 1986) or perinatal brain damage (Ruth & Raivio, 1988) and so it is not surprising that intrapartum events, suggestive of transient hypoxia, bear no significant relationship to subsequent neurodevelopmental outcome (Low et al., 1981; Painter et al., 1988). In fact, a recent follow-up study suggested that fetal acidaemia at birth indicated an ability to respond appropriately to intrapartum hypoxia as judged by the long term outcome (Dennis et al., 1989). Continuous FHR monitoring has been shown to significantly reduce the incidence of neonatal seizures but not the incidence of subsequent cerebral palsy (Grant et al., 1989).

Although evidence for improved quality of survivors seems lacking, the introduction of continuous FHR monitoring during high risk labour was associated with a reduction in the incidence of fetal and neonatal deaths related to labour (Paul & Hon, 1974; Johnstone, Campbell & Hughes, 1978). Continuous FHR monitoring in labour would appear to be beneficial for one baby per 1000 monitored labours (Johnstone et al., 1978; Neutra et al., 1978). However, there is overwhelming evidence that the incidence of Caesarean section and forceps deliveries has increased as a result of such practice (Thacker, 1991).

References

Beard, R. W., Filshie, G. M., Knight, C. A. & Roberts, G. M. (1971). The significance of the changes in the continuous fetal heart rate in the first stage of labour. *Journal of Obstetrics and Gynaecology of the British Commonwealth*, **78**, 865–81.

Beischer, N. A., Drew, H. J., Ashton, P. W., Oats, J. N., Gaudry, E., Chew, F. T. K. & Parkinson, P. (1983). Quality of survival of infants with critical fetal reserve detected by antenatal cardiotocography. *American Journal of Obstetrics and Gynecology*, **146**, 662–70.

Brown, R. & Patrick, J. (1981). The nonstress test: how long is enough? *American Journal of Obstetrics and Gynecology*, **141**, 646–51.

Brown, V. A., Sawers, R. S., Parsons, R. J., Duncan, S. L. B. & Cooke, I. D.

(1982). The value of antenatal cardiotocography in the management of high-risk pregnancy: a randomised controlled trial. *British Journal of Obstetrics and Gynaecology,* **89**, 716–22.

Caldeyro-Barcia, R., Mendez-Bauer, C., Poseiro, J.J., Escarcena, L. A., Pose, S. V., Bieniarz, J., Arnt, I., Gulin, L. & Althabe, O. (1966). Control of human fetal heart rate during labour. In *The Heart and Circulation in the Newborn and Infant*, ed. D.E. Cassels. pp. 7–36. Grune and Stratton, New York.

Clark, S. L., Grimovsky, M. L. & Miller, F. C. (1984) The scalp stimulation test: a clinical alternative to fetal scalp blood sampling. *American Journal of Obstetrics and Gynecology,* **148**, 274–7.

Curzen, P., Bekir, J. S., McLintock, D. G. & Patel, M. (1984). Reliability of cardiotocography in predicting baby's condition at birth. *British Medical Journal,* **289**, 1345–7.

Dawes, G. S., Houghton, C. R. S., Redman, C. W. G. & Visser, G. H. A. (1982). Pattern of the normal human fetal heart rate. *British Journal of Obstetrics and Gynaecology,* **89**, 276–84.

Day, E., Maddern, L. & Wood, C. (1968). Auscultation of foetal heart rate: an assessment of its error and significance. *British Medical Journal,* **4**, 422–4.

Dennis, J., Johnson, A., Mutch, L., Yudkin, P. & Johnson, P. (1989). Acid-base status at birth and neurodevelopmental outcome at four and one-half years. *American Journal of Obstetrics and Gynecology,* **66**, 213–20.

Devoe, L. D., McKenzie, J., Searle, N. & Sherline, D. M. (1985). Nonstress test: dimensions of normal reactivity. *Obstetrics and Gynecology,* **66**, 617–20.

Dijxhoorn, M. J., Visser, G. H. A., Fidler, V. J., Touwen, B. C. L. & Huisjes, H. J. (1986). Apgar score, meconium and acidaemia at birth in relation to neonatal neurological morbidity in term infants. *British Journal of Obstetrics and Gynaecology,* **93**, 217–22.

Edersheim, T. G, Hutson, J. M., Druzin, M. L. & Kogut, E. A. (1987). Fetal heart rate response to vibratory acoustic stimulation predicts fetal pH in labour. *American Journal of Obstetrics and Gynecology,* **157**, 1557–60.

Evertson, L. R., Gauthier, R. J., Schifrin, B. S. & Paul, R. H. (1979). Antepartum fetal heart rate testing 1. Evolution of the nonstress test. *American Journal of Obstetrics and Gynecology,* **133**, 29–33.

FIGO News (1987). Guidelines for the use of fetal monitoring. *International Journal of Gynaecology and Obstetrics,* **25**, 159–67.

Fischer, W. M., Stude, I. & Brandt, H. (1976). A suggestion for the evaluation of the antepartum cardiotocogram. *Zeitschrift fur Geburtshilfe und Perinatologie,* **180**, 117–23.

Flynn, A. M. & Kelly, J. (1977). Evaluation of fetal wellbeing by antepartum fetal heart monitoring. *British Medical Journal,* **1**, 936–9.

Flynn, A. M., Kelly, J. & O'Conor, M. (1979). Unstressed antepartum cardiotocography in the management of the fetus suspected of growth retardation. *British Journal of Obstetrics and Gynaecology,* **86**, 106–10.

Flynn, A. M., Kelly, J., Mansfield, H., Needham, P., O'Conor, M. & Viegas, O. (1982). A randomized controlled trial of non-stress antepartum cardiotocography. *British Journal of Obstetrics and Gynaecology,* **89**, 427–33.

Freeman, R. K. (1975). The use of the oxytocin challenge test for antepartum clinical evaluation of uteroplacental respiratory function. *American Journal of Obstetrics & Gynecology,* **121**, 481–9.

Grant, A. & Mohide, P. (1982). Screening and diagnostic tests in antenatal care. In *Effectiveness and Satisfaction in Antenatal Care*, ed. M. Enkin & I. Chalmers. pp. 22–59. William Heinemann, London.

Grant, A., O'Brien, N., Joy, M. T., Hennessy, E. & MacDonald, D. (1989). Cerebral palsy among children born during the Dublin randomised trial of fetal monitoring. *Lancet*, **ii**, 1233–5.

Henson, G. L., Dawes, G. S. & Redman, C. W. G. (1983). Antenatal fetal heart-rate variability in relation to fetal acid-base status at Caesarean section. *British Journal of Obstetrics and Gynaecology*, **90**, 516–21.

Hon, E. H. (1968). *An Atlas of Fetal Heart Rate Patterns*. Harty Press, New Haven.

Ingemarsson, I. & Arulkumaran, S. (1989). Reactive fetal heart rate response to vibroacoustic stimulation in fetuses with low scalp blood pH. *British Journal of Obstetrics and Gynaecology*, **96**, 562–5.

Johnstone, F. D., Campbell, D. M. & Hughes, G. J. (1978). Has continuous intrapartum monitoring made any impact on fetal outcome? *Lancet*, **i**, 1298–300.

Keirse, M. J. N. C. & Trimbos, J. B. (1981). Clinical significance of suspicious antepartum cardiotocograms: a study of normal and high-risk pregnancies. *British Journal of Obstetrics and Gynaecology*, **88**, 739–46.

Kidd, L. C., Patel, N. B. & Smith, R. (1985). Non-stress antenatal cardiotocography – a prospective randomized clinical trial. *British Journal of Obstetrics and Gynaecology*, **92**, 1156–9.

Kubli, F. W., Hon, E. H., Khazin, A. F. & Takemura, H. (1969). Observations on heart rate and pH in the human fetus during labour. *American Journal of Obstetrics and Gynecology*, **104**, 1190–206.

Lee, C. Y., DiLoreto, P. C. & O'Lane, J. M. (1975). A study of fetal heart rate acceleration patterns. *Obstetrics and Gynecology*, **45**, 142–6.

Low, J. A., Cox, M. J., Karchmar, E. J., McGrath, M. S., Pancham, S. R. & Piercy, W. N. (1981). The prediction of intrapartum fetal metabolic acidosis by fetal heart rate monitoring. *American Journal of Obstetrics and Gynecology*, **139**, 299–305.

Lumley, J., Lester, A., Anderson, I., Renou, P. & Wood, C. (1983). A randomized trial of weekly cardiotocography in high-risk obstetric patients. *British Journal of Obstetrics and Gynaecology*, **90**, 1018–26.

Lyons, E. R., Bylsma-Howell, M., Shamsi, S. & Towell, M. E. (1979). A scoring system for nonstressed antepartum fetal heart rate monitoring. *American Journal of Obstetrics and Gynecology*, **133**, 242–6.

Mendez-Bauer, C., Arnt, I. C., Gulin, L., Escarcena, L. & Caldeyro-Barcia, R. (1967). Relationship between blood pH and heart rate in the human fetus during labour. *American Journal of Obstetrics and Gynecology*, **97**, 530–45.

Murphy, K. W., Johnson, P., Moorcraft, J., Pattinson, R., Russell, V. & Turnbull, A. (1990). Birth asphyxia and the intrapartum cardiotocograph. *British Journal of Obstetrics and Gynaecology*, **97**, 470–9.

Neutra, R. R., Fienberg, S. E., Greenland, S. & Friedman, E. A. (1978). Effect of fetal monitoring on neonatal death rates. *New England Journal of Medicine*, **299**, 324–6.

Oats, J. N., Chew, F. T. K. & Rarren, V. J. (1987). Antepartum cardiotography – an audit. *Australian and New Zealand Journal of Obstetrics and Gynaecology*, **154**, 619–21.

Ohel, G., Birkenfeld, A., Rabinowitz, R. & Sadovsky, E. (1986). Fetal

294   *John A. D. Spencer*

response to vibratory acoustic stimulation in periods of low heart rate reactivity and low activity. *American Journal of Obstetrics and Gynecology*, **154**, 619–21.

Painter, M. J., Scott, M., Hirsch, R. P., O'Donoghue, P. & Depp, R. (1988). Fetal heart rate patterns during labour: neurologic and cognitive development at six to nine years of age. *American Journal of Obstetrics and Gynecology*, **159**, 854–5.

Paul, R. H. & Hon, E. H. (1974). Clinical fetal monitoring V. Effect on perinatal outcome. *American Journal of Obstetrics and Gynecology*, **118**, 529–33.

Pearson, J. F. & Weaver, J. B. (1978). A six-point scoring system for antenatal cardiotocograms. *British Journal of Obstetrics and Gynaecology*, **85**, 321–7.

Read, J. A. & Miller, F. C. (1977). Fetal heart rate acceleration in response to acoustic stimulation as a measure of fetal well-being. *American Journal of Obstetrics and Gynecology*, **129**, 512–17.

Rice, P. E. & Benedetti, T. J. (1986). Fetal heart rate acceleration with fetal blood sampling. *Obstetrics and Gynecology*, **68**, 469–72.

Richardson, B., Campbell, K., Carmichael, L. & Patrick, J. (1981). Effects of external physical stimulation on fetuses near term. *American Journal of Obstetrics and Gynecology*, **139**, 344–52.

Rochard, F., Schifrin, B. S., Goupil, F., Legrand, H., Blottiere, J. & Sureau, C. (1976). Nonstressed fetal heart rate monitoring in the antepartum period. *American Journal of Obstetrics and Gynecology*, **126**, 699–706.

Ruth, V. J. & Raivio, K. O. (1988). Perinatal brain damage: predictive value of metabolic acidosis and Apgar score. *British Medical Journal*, **297**, 24–7.

Shy, K. K., Luthy, D. A., Bennett, F. C., Whitfield, M., Larson, E. B., van Belle, G., Hughes, J. P., Wilson, J. A. & Stenchever, M. A. (1990). Effects of electronic fetal-heart-rate monitoring, as compared with periodic auscultation, on the neurologic development of premature infants. *New England Journal of Medicine*, **322**, 588–93.

Spencer, J. A. D. & Johnson, P. (1986). Fetal heart rate variability changes and fetal behavioural cycles during labour. *British Journal of Obstetrics and Gynaecology*, **93**, 314–21.

Spencer, J. A. D. (1990). Antepartum cardiotocography. In *Modern Antenatal Care of the Fetus*, ed. G. Chamberlain. pp. 163–188. Blackwell Scientific Publications, Oxford.

Spencer, J. A. D. (1991). Predictive value of a fetal heart rate acceleration at the time of fetal blood sampling in labour. *Journal of Perinatal Medicine*, **19**, 207–15.

Spencer, J. A. D., Deans, A., Nicolaides, P. & Arulkumaran, S. (1991*a*). Fetal heart rate response to vibro-acoustic stimulation during low and high heart rate variability episodes in late pregnancy. *American Journal of Obstetrics and Gynecology*, **165**, 86–90.

Spencer, J. A. D., Koutsoukis, M. & Lee, A. (1991*b*). Fetal heart rate and neonatal condition related to epidural analgesia in women reaching the second stage of labour. *European Journal of Obstetrics, Gynecology and Reproductive Biology*, **41**, 173–8.

Steer, P. J. & Beard, R. W. (1970). A continuous record of fetal heart rate obtained by serial counts. *Journal of Obstetrics and Gynaecology of the British Commonwealth*, **77**, 908–14.

Sykes, G. S., Molloy, P. M., Johnson, P., Gu, W., Ashworth, F., Stirvat, G.

M., & Turnbull, A. C. (1982). Do Apgar Scores indicate asphyxia? *Lancet*, **i**, 494–6.

Tejani, N., Mann, L. I. & Bhakthavathsalan, A. (1976). Correlation of fetal heart rate patterns and fetal pH with neonatal outcome. *Obstetrics and Gynecology*, **48**, 460–3.

Thacker, S. B. (1991). Effectiveness and safety of intrapartum fetal monitoring. In *Fetal Monitoring*, ed. J. A. D. Spencer. pp. 211–217. Oxford University Press, Oxford.

Thacker, S. B. & Berkelman (1986). Assessing the diagnostic accuracy and efficacy of selected antepartum fetal surveillance techniques. *Obstetric and Gynecological Survey*, **41**, 121–41.

Trierweiler, M. W., Freeman, R. K. & James, J. (1976). Baseline fetal heart rate characteristics as an indicator of fetal status during the antepartum period. *American Journal of Obstetrics and Gynecology*, **125**, 618–23.

Trimbos, J. B. & Keirse, M. J. N. C. (1978). Significance of antepartum cardiotocography in normal pregnancy. *British Journal of Obstetrics and Gynaecology*, **85**, 907–13.

Visser, G. H. A. & Huisjes, H. J. (1977). Diagnostic value of the unstressed antepartum cardiotocogram. *British Journal of Obstetrics and Gynaecology*, **84**, 321–6.

Visser, G. H. A., Redman, C. W. G., Huisjes, H. J. & Turnbull, A. C. (1980). Nonstressed antepartum heart rate monitoring: Implications of decelerations after spontaneous contractions. *American Journal of Obstetrics and Gynecology*, **138**, 429–35.

Wheble, A. M., Gillmer, M. D. G., Spencer, J. A. D. & Sykes, G. S. (1989). Changes in fetal monitoring practice in the UK: 1977–1984. *British Journal of Obstetrics and Gynaecology*, **96**, 1140–7.

Wheeler, T. & Guerard, P. (1974). Fetal heart rate during late pregnancy. *Journal of Obstetrics and Gynaecology of the British Commonwealth*, **84**, 348–56.

Wheeler, T. & Murrills, A. (1978). Patterns of fetal heart rate during normal pregnancy. *British Journal of Obstetrics and Gynaecology*, **85**, 18–27.

Young, D. C., Gray, J. H., Luther, E. R. & Reddle, L. J. (1980). Fetal scalp blood pH sampling: Its value in an active obstetric unit. *American Journal of Obstetrics and Gynecology*, **136**, 276–81.

14

Doppler ultrasonography: techniques

KAREL MARŠÁL

Historical considerations

The Austrian scientist, Christian Doppler (1803–53), when professor of physics at the Technical Institute of Prague, published a paper in 1842 describing a principle that has since been named after him – the Doppler effect (Doppler, 1842). The Doppler principle involves the change in frequency of wave energy when reflected by a moving object, the frequency shift being proportional to the velocity of the reflector. The Doppler principle is valid for all types of wave propagation, light, sound, microwaves and ultrasonic waves, and is utilized by such animals as bats for localization purposes.

In obstetrics, since Satomura (1956) showed it to be possible to detect blood flow by means of ultrasound Doppler frequency shifts, the ultrasonic Doppler effect has been used to monitor fetal heart activity in utero (Callagan, Rowland & Goldman, 1964). The first reports on recording blood flow signals from the umbilical artery in utero, published in the late 1970s (Fitzgerald & Drumm, 1977; McCallum et al., 1978), were soon followed by others describing the estimation of blood flow both in the umbilical vein (Gill, 1978) and in the fetal descending aorta (Eik-Nes, Brubakk & Ulstein, 1980). Subsequent empirical evidence of the existence of relationships between velocity waveform changes and pregnancy outcome aroused the interest of perinatologists in the recording of velocity waveforms from the fetal and uteroplacental arteries (Jouppila & Kirkinen, 1984; Trudinger, Giles & Cook, 1985). The recent advent of the colour Doppler mode has enabled blood flow signals to be recorded even from such very small vessels as fetal renal arteries (Vyas, Nicolaides & Campbell, 1989).

A growing amount of published data suggests that, when properly applied in monitoring fetal health, ultrasound Doppler velocimetry might be a useful aid in managing high-risk pregnancies (Laurin et al., 1987; Trudinger et al., 1987). Naturally, this is contingent upon the primary velocity signals being of good quality, and caution with interpretation of results which, in turn, presupposes the availability of high quality equipment in the hands of skilful and experienced operators well aware of the various potential sources of error inherent in the method.

Physics of Doppler ultrasound

The Doppler principle concerns the relationship between the velocity of a moving reflector and the change in frequency of the transmitted wave, e.g. a sound wave. When the reflector is moving toward the source of sound, the reflected sound will be received at a frequency higher than that transmitted. Conversely, if the reflector is moving away from the source, the frequency of the received sound will be lower than that transmitted. A similar effect also occurs when the source is moving in relation to a stationary reflector. The change in the frequency is called the Doppler shift (f_d) and is described by the equation:

$$f_d = 2 \cdot f_o \cdot V \cdot \cos \theta / c \qquad (1)$$

where f_o = the frequency of the transmitted sound, V = the velocity of the moving reflector, θ = the angle between the sound beam and the velocity vector of the moving reflector, and c = the velocity of sound in the medium. For blood flow velocity measurement, ultrasound is transmitted by a piezo-electric crystal into the tissue at a frequency f_o, is reflected by the moving red cells within the vessel and is received at a different frequency (Fig. 14.1). The velocity of the blood flow (V) can be calculated from the equation:

$$V = f_d \cdot c / 2 \cdot f_o \cdot \cos \theta \qquad (2)$$

Thus, at a given frequency f_o and a constant sound velocity c, the measured velocity is directly proportional to the Doppler frequency shift (f_d) and inversely proportional to the cosine of the insonation angle (cos θ). The ultrasound frequency used in clinical practice is typically 1 to 10 MHz which results in a Doppler shift, caused by blood flow within the audible frequency range. The detected Doppler shift is a spectrum of frequencies rather than a single frequency, as it originates from red cells moving at various velocities within the lumen of the vessel.

As passage of the ultrasound wave through the tissue causes a partial loss of ultrasound energy, penetration of the ultrasound is limited. The

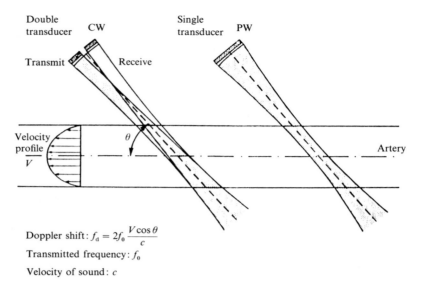

Doppler shift: $f_d = 2f_0 \dfrac{V \cos \theta}{c}$

Transmitted frequency: f_0

Velocity of sound: c

Fig. 14.1. Principle of the ultrasonic Doppler blood velocity measurement with continuous (CW) and pulsed (PW) wave technique. (From Hatle, L. & Angelsen, B. (1985). Reprinted with permission.)

depth of penetration of ultrasound is inversely related to the ultrasound frequency. Accordingly, for measurements of blood flow in deep-lying vessels, low frequency ultrasound is be used. For use on fetal and uteroplacental vessels, an ultrasound frequency of 2 to 4 MHz is usually suitable.

Doppler ultrasound instruments

The continuous wave (CW) Doppler technique

A CW Doppler flowmeter contains two piezo-electric crystals, one continuously transmitting ultrasound signals, the other functioning as a receiver (Fig. 14.1). The recorded spectrum of Doppler frequencies contains information on the movements of all interfaces traversed by the ultrasound beam and the sampling is thus non-discriminative. As the construction of the CW Doppler instrument is technically quite simple, it is cheaper than the more complicated pulsed wave Doppler instrument. However, owing to the lack of range resolution, the application of CW Doppler is limited; in obstetrics, its use is virtually confined to vessels where interference by signals from nearby vessels is not imminent, e.g.

the umbilical artery and the uterine artery. An advantage of the CW Doppler technique is that there is no limitation of the highest blood velocity which can be measured.

The pulsed wave (PW) Doppler technique

PW Doppler instruments permit the option of sampling from a given depth range within the tissue. In other words, using this technique, blood velocity signals from a specific vessel can be assured. The signal-to-noise ratio is usually better in the PW than in the CW Doppler mode.

In the PW technique, a single piezo-electric crystal is used alternately as a transmitter and receiver (Fig. 14.1). The ultrasound is transmitted in a short pulse. The transducer gate is then closed for a period corresponding to the time required for the ultrasound pulse to travel to the vessel of interest and back. Then the gate opens again to receive the ultrasound echoes returning from a defined region within the tissue, the so-called sample volume. The size of the sample volume is determined by the size of the emitting crystal, the shape of the ultrasound beam and the duration of the pulse. The positioning of the sample volume is governed by setting the interval between transmitting and receiving the ultrasound signals, i.e. between opening and closing of the transducer gate.

The PW Doppler technique is limited with regard to the maximum detectable velocity, owing to the fact that the maximum Doppler shift frequency to be unambiguously detected is one half of the pulse repetition frequency (the Nyquist limit). At high Doppler frequencies, the aliasing phenomenon arises, i.e. the misinterpretation of high velocities as being of opposite polarity. However, aliasing is seldom a problem in obstetrics, as the peak velocities in the fetoplacental and uteroplacental vessels do not usually exceed 1.5–2.0 m/s. It is important that the instrument allows optimization of the depth–velocity product, by adjustment of the pulse repetition frequency. Aliasing, when it occurs, can be avoided by changing the insonation angle or the instrument settings (scale, baseline position).

Processing of Doppler signals

A relatively simple way of processing the Doppler signals is the determination of zero-crossing frequency, i.e. the number of zero crossings per unit time. However, this method is quite inaccurate, and is dependent on

Karel Maršál

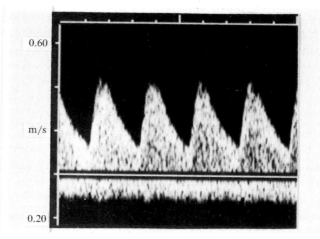

Fig. 14.2. Doppler shift frequency spectrum recorded from the umbilical cord of a 35-week old fetus. Pulsatile signals of the flow velocity in the umbilical artery in the upper part, continuous non-pulsatile signals of the flow in the umbilical vein in the lower part of the picture.

the blood velocity profile. Modern instruments are designed to be capable of more sophisticated analysis of the Doppler spectrum by digitising the signals for spectral analysis by Fast Fourier Transform. In this way, all information contained in the complex Doppler signal is retrieved. The frequency distribution of the Doppler signal is presented graphically, the average power of each frequency being indicated on a grey scale (Fig. 14.2).

The appearance of the Doppler spectrum is related to the blood velocity profile over the cross-section of the vessel. A plug or flat velocity profile (e.g. signals recorded from the fetal aorta during systole) gives a narrow spectrum with no low frequencies; a flow with a parabolic profile (e.g. fetal aortic flow during diastole or flow in the umbilical vein) produces a broadening of the spectrum.

Good quality of the primary Doppler signals recorded from the vessel under examination is crucial for obtaining correct results. The choice of a proper insonation angle, and in the PW mode, the size and positioning of the sample volume, must be carefully controlled. Real-time control during recording is mandatory, with the operator listening to the audible Doppler signals and observing the Doppler spectrum analysed on-line and displayed on a monitor.

From the Doppler spectrum both the maximum velocity (i.e. the envelope of the spectrum) and the mean velocity (i.e. the weighted average Doppler shift frequency) can be estimated. The waveform of the maximum velocity recorded from arteries can be further characterised by various indices (see below). A time-averaged mean velocity is used for estimation of volume flow.

The received Doppler signals are usually passed through a high-pass filter to eliminate signals from any slow-moving interfaces in the path of the ultrasound beam. When a high-pass filter with a high cut-off level is used, most of the low velocity flow signals will be eliminated. This results in overestimation of the mean velocity, and may lead to an erroneous diagnosis of absent end-diastolic flow. Therefore, it has been recommended that the use of high-pass filters, with cut-off levels exceeding 100 Hz, should be avoided (*Eur. Assn. Perinat. Med.,* 1989). When examining fetal vessels, very little disturbance is produced by the elastic vessel walls and so no high-pass filtering is necessary.

Duplex systems

The Doppler instruments, both CW and PW, can be used without imaging, the Doppler signals being monitored by ear. This approach is limited in application and, in obstetrics, is virtually confined to recordings from the umbilical artery and uterine/uteroplacental vessels. In duplex ultrasound systems, an imaging ultrasound scanner is combined either with a PW or a CW Doppler instrument. The vessel of interest is visualized and the Doppler ultrasound beam easily directed. In the PW mode the sample volume can be properly localised with help of a cursor displayed on the image. The two ultrasound systems are mutually exclusive and cannot be used simultaneously. During the Doppler recording, the two-dimensional image is frozen; during updating of the image, the recording of Doppler signals is interrupted. The use of electronic real-time scanners enables rapid switches to be made from one system to the other.

Doppler instruments can be combined either with linear array transducers or with sector transducers (phased array or mechanical). The combination of an off-set PW Doppler transducer and a linear array transducer not only enables a longer section of the vessel to be visualized, but also allows a suitable angle of insonation to be selected. Both of these features are advantageous when, for example, examining the fetal descending aorta. One of the image lines of a sector real-time scanner is usually used for Doppler recording in a duplex system which is superior when examining small vessels such as fetal cerebral arteries.

Colour flow imaging

The advent of the colour Doppler technique has extended the scope of ultrasound examination of the fetal and uteroplacental circulation. Colour flow imaging is based on PW Doppler ultrasound for detection of flow signals from a sectional area within the tissue. The flow signals are colour coded according to the direction of flow (usually red for flow toward the transducer, and blue for flow away from the transducer), velocity (low velocity, dark colour; high velocity, bright colour) and variance. Flow in the vessels is visualized in colour in the two-dimensional sectional real-time image, enabling swift localization of even very small vessels and a rapid estimation of the flow direction. For quantification purposes, the spectral PW Doppler mode is used. With the colour Doppler mode, there is a risk of aliasing when the blood velocities exceed certain depth-dependent limits. The flow is then depicted in the wrong colour, thus giving a false indication of opposite direction of flow. Like the spectral PW Doppler technique, the colour flow imaging is vulnerable to the effects of the filters incorporated, and the possibility of errors due to filtering needs to be borne in mind.

Blood flow estimation

Blood volume flow in a vessel (Q), i.e. the amount of blood passing through the cross-section of the vessel per unit of time, can be estimated from the ultrasonically measured diameter of the vessel (d) and the time-averaged mean Doppler velocity (V) recorded with Doppler ultrasound. The shift can be converted to the mean blood velocity using the equation.

$$Q = \frac{V}{\cos \theta} \cdot \pi \cdot \left(\frac{d}{2}\right)^2 \qquad (3)$$

Vessel diameter is measured in the frozen images of the vessel section. Usually, an average value of several measurements is utilized to minimize the effect of diameter changes in vessels with pulsatile flow. To enable comparison between intra-individual measurements at different stages of gestation and between fetuses, the flow is related to the ultrasonically estimated fetal weight and expressed in ml/min per kg.

The measurement of vessel diameter has been found to be the major source of error in estimating flow (Eik-Nes et al., 1982), the risk of error being especially pronounced in vessels of small calibre (less than 6 mm). Therefore, the application of the method during pregnancy is limited to large fetal vessels (the descending aorta [Eik-Nes et al., 1980], and the intra-abdominal part of the umbilical vein [Gill, 1978]). Precision in measuring the diameter of pulsating vessels might be improved by using automatic phase-locked echo-tracking systems (Stale, Maršál & Gennser, 1990).

Recording and estimation of the mean velocity is also susceptible to several sources of possible error. Uniform insonation of the whole cross-section of the vessel is a prerequisite, as is accurate positioning of the sample volume which needs to be of suitable size (Gill, 1982). The recorded Doppler shift is corrected for the insonation angle. At large angles of insonation, error in the estimation of true velocity might be considerable (Fig. 14.3), and thus Doppler examinations should not be performed at insonation angles greater than 55° (*Eur. Assn. Perinat. Med.*, 1989).

The inherent sources of error, outlined above, have led to the abandonment of volume flow estimation in obstetrics. During recent years the interest of researchers and clinicians has concentrated on velocity waveform analysis. However, as waveform analysis is not directly related to

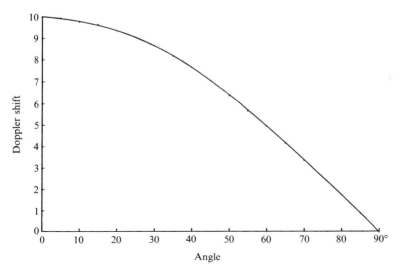

Fig. 14.3. Doppler shift as a function of angle as determined by the Doppler equation. (From Kremkau, F.W. (1985). Reprinted with permission.)

the blood flow, a renewal of interest in measuring flow in obstetrics is to be expected when the accuracy of estimating volume blood flow is improved in the future.

Velocity waveform analysis

The early reports on Doppler studies in fetuses showed relationships between unfavourable fetal outcome and some typical changes of the velocity waveforms recorded from fetal aorta (Jouppila & Kirkinen, 1984; Lingman, Laurin & Maršál, 1986) or umbilical artery (Trudinger et al., 1985). Experience of the diagnostic use of Doppler ultrasound in peripheral vessels indicated that important information on circulation might be gained by analysing the maximum velocity waveforms (Gosling & King, 1975). In fetal arterial waveform analysis, many of the possible errors involved in volume flow estimation are avoided; there is no need to control the insonation angle, to measure vessel diameter, or to estimate fetal weight. A number of formulae and indices have been evolved to characterize the waveform mathematically. However, despite the wide use of waveform analysis, there would seem to be little agreement as to the interpretation and definitions of waveform indices.

Most of the waveform indices express the degree of pulsatility of the velocity waveform. Some of them make use of only two points on the curve, e.g. the systolic-to-diastolic ratio (A/B ratio) (Stuart et al., 1980) or the resistance index (RI) according to Pourcelot (1974); some include the average velocity over the heart cycle in the calculation, e.g. the pulsatility index (PI) (Gosling & King, 1975) (Fig. 14.4). The object of such indices is to eliminate the effect of the insonation angle by calculating a ratio.

The shape of the velocity waveform recorded from the fetal arteries is dependent on several factors: heart action, blood velocity, vessel wall compliance, and both proximal and distal resistance to flow. The vascular resistance peripheral to the site of measurement mainly affects the diastolic part of the velocity waveform – an increase in resistance causing a decrease in diastolic flow.

Owing to the presence of the placental vascular bed, the fetal circulation as a whole is a low resistance system (Dawes, 1968). When resistance in the placental vasculature increases (e.g. in pregnancies with hypertension or intra-uterine growth retardation), diastolic flow in the umbilical artery and the fetal descending aorta decreases and may even be absent (Jouppila & Kirkinen, 1984; Lingman, Laurin & Maršál, 1986;

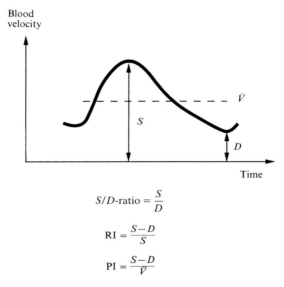

$$S/D\text{-ratio} = \frac{S}{D}$$

$$RI = \frac{S-D}{S}$$

$$PI = \frac{S-D}{\bar{V}}$$

Fig. 14.4. Waveform analysis of the maximum blood velocity. *S*: peak systolic velocity; *D*: the least diastolic velocity; *V*: mean velocity over the heart cycle; RI: resistance index according to Pourcelot; PI: pulsatility index according to Gosling.

Rochelson et al., 1987). With increasing peripheral resistance, the values of the waveform indices increase. When the end-diastolic flow is absent, the *A/B* ratio becomes infinite and thus not discriminative, and the RI is then equal to 1.0. The PI reflects also the area under the curve and is superior to the other two indices for practical purposes (*Eur. Assn. Perinat. Med.*, 1989). The disadvantage of the PI is that it entails more complex computation than does the *A/B* ratio or the RI.

In healthy fetuses during the second half of gestation, diastolic flow is always present in the descending aorta and umbilical artery during fetal apnoea (Lingman & Maršál, 1986*b*; Gudmundsson & Maršál, 1988*a*). Conversely, absence of diastolic flow is often associated with adverse outcome of pregnancy, e.g. intrauterine growth retardation and fetal hypoxia (Laurin et al., 1987; Rochelson et al., 1987; Gudmundsson & Maršál, 1988*b*). In extreme cases, a diastolic flow can even be reversed (Lingman et al., 1986), the extremely altered velocity waveform sometimes being referred to as ARED flow (i.e. absent or reverse end-diastolic flow).

The appearance of the diastolic part of the velocity waveform is thus a

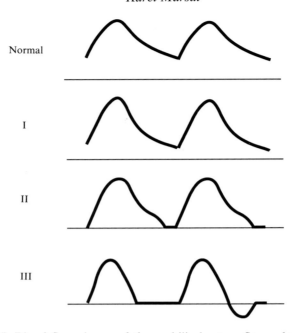

Fig. 14.5. Blood flow classes of the umbilical artery flow velocity waveforms (BFC). BFC normal: positive flow throughout the heart cycle and a normal pulsatility index; BFC I: positive flow throughout the cycle and a pulsatility index ⩾ mean + 2 SD of the normal population; BFC II: non-detectable end-diastolic velocity; BFC III: absence of positive flow throughout the diastole and/or reverse flow in diastole.

clinically important prognostic feature. On the basis of earlier findings that the degree of intrauterine and neonatal morbidity is reflected in the degree of pathological changes of the fetal aortic velocity waveform, a semi-quantitative method of assessing the waveform was designed (Laurin et al., 1987) (Fig. 14.5). Four blood flow classes (BFC) were defined as follows: BFC normal, positive flow throughout the heart cycle, and a normal PI; BFC I, positive flow throughout the cycle, and a PI ⩾ mean + 2 SD of the normals; BFC II, non-detectable end-diastolic velocity; and BFC III, absence of positive flow throughout diastole and/or reverse flow in diastole. This simple system of pattern recognition has been further refined and computerized, using a classification based on ten curve types (Malcus et al., 1991).

Validation of the Doppler ultrasound method

Measurement of flow

The estimation of flow in fetal vessels from the mean velocity measured by Doppler ultrasound and vessel diameter measured in the real-time image is open to many possible sources of error: change in the insonation angle causes error in the estimated velocity; too small or too large a sample volume can give erroneous Doppler signals, as can a wrongly positioned sample volume; non-uniform insonation of the vessel does not yield representative Doppler signals; and too high a cut-off level of the high-pass filter causes overestimation of the mean velocity. The principal source of error, however, is the measurement of the vessel diameter by ultrasound, as the radius is squared when calculating the cross-sectional area of the vessel. An additional possible source of error in Doppler measurement of fetal blood flow is the fetal weight estimation by ultrasound fetometry.

Each of the factors listed above has been evaluated separately. It was found that the insonation angle can be kept within ±5°. The accuracy of vessel diameter measurement has been tested in both in vitro and in vivo studies, and the maximum error found to be 0.4 mm (Eik-Nes et al., 1982).

The reproducibility of each of the measurement procedures and of the total flow estimation was found acceptable in vitro (Eik-Nes et al., 1982). It is difficult to evaluate intra- and interindividual reproducibility in vivo, however, as the biological variability of fetal flow with time cannot be controlled. It is also very difficult in the clinical situation to assess overall error in volume flow estimation. As compared with electromagnetic flow measurement, the Doppler method shows a good agreement – in an in vivo animal model the correlation coefficient was 0.91 (Eik-Nes et al., 1981).

Blood velocity waveform analysis

Waveform analysis has been evaluated from several points of view: the various waveform indices have been compared, and the reproducibility of estimating maximum velocity from the Doppler spectrum and of calculating the indices has been studied, as has the dependence of the waveform shape and waveform indices on various flow factors (e.g. preload, heart rate, downstream impedance, blood viscosity). Recordings performed using CW versus PW Doppler ultrasound have been found to be fully comparable (Mehalek et al., 1988; Gudmundsson et al., 1990).

Several reproducibility studies of various waveform indices and various vessels have been published. Very good reproducibility of the indices in the umbilical artery, both regarding the intra- and interobserver variability was found (Pearce et al., 1988; Maulik et al., 1989a; Davies, Lee & Spencer, 1990; Gudmundsson et al., 1990), the coefficients of variation being reported to be below 10%.

The number of waveforms calculated and averaged to obtain the index value differs from one research group to another, often depending on the equipment used. Without any doubt, a large number of cycles improves the accuracy, the use of ten consecutive cycles being probably the best, although laborious, approach. Provided that the Doppler velocity recording is stable and the waveforms uniform, five cycles have been found to be as representative as ten or more (Spencer & Price, 1989). In one study, a sequence of six heart cycles was found to be acceptably reproducible, even during periods of fetal breathing and fetal movements (Spencer et al., 1991b). It is important, however, to bear in mind that a Doppler recording made during a period of fetal breathing is not representative, as the breathing movements have a marked effect on blood flow (Maršál et al., 1984).

Fetal breathing movements modulate very profoundly the blood velocities, not only in the venous circulation – in the umbilical vein and inferior vena cava – but also in the descending aorta, umbilical artery and other fetal arteries (Maršál et al., 1984). The increase in time-averaged mean blood velocity in the fetal aorta during breathing is dependent on the amplitude of breathing. As the vessel diameter cannot be measured simultaneously with the blood velocity, it is not possible to draw any conclusions as to the effect of breathing on the venous return to the fetal heart or on fetal cardiac output. As the velocity waveforms in the fetal vessels are modulated during breathing, measurements taken during breathing are unacceptable for the purpose of waveform analysis. While recording signals from the umbilical artery, the possible presence of fetal breathing can easily be recognized in the tracing of the umbilical venous blood velocity (Fig. 14.6).

Fetal blood velocity waveforms have been examined during different fetal behavioural states (van Eyck et al., 1985, 1987), identified from the recordings of FHR variability, fetal breathing, fetal movements and fetal eye movements, as defined by Nijhuis et al. (1982). In the internal carotid artery and descending aorta of the fetuses, the PI levels changed with

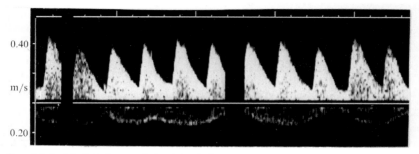

Fig. 14.6. Modulations of the blood flow velocity signals recorded from the umbilical artery (upper tracing) and umbilical vein (lower tracing) caused by fetal breathing movements.

fetal behavioural state, being higher during quiet sleep (state F1) than during active sleep (state F2). In the umbilical artery, no such difference was found. For strictly controlled physiological studies, it might be of interest to record the behavioural states. However, in a clinical context, the changes in the waveform indices due to pathological processes will exceed the changes due to fetal behaviour. It might therefore be sufficient to ensure that recordings are made during fetal quiescence, i.e. during periods of fetal apnoea and without the occurrence of general movements.

In both maternal and fetal vessels, waveform indices (A/B ratio, RI & PI) have been found to be inversely correlated to the heart rate. With increasing heart rate, the beat-to-beat interval shortens and the diastolic flow velocity increases relative to the peak velocity. An opposite effect is seen in bradycardia. For both the fetal descending aorta and the umbilical artery this effect has been found to be not too pronounced provided the fetal heart rate (FHR) is within normal limits (120–160 beats/min) (Lingman & Maršál, 1986*b*; Thompson, Trudinger & Cook, 1986; Gudmundsson & Maršál, 1988*a*). Although some other investigators have reported finding a strong negative correlation (Mulders et al., 1986; Mires et al., 1987), their data also included cases of FHR outside the normal limits. The relationship between FHR and PI would not appear to be linear, as profound changes in fetal PI have been found both in extreme bradycardia and in tachycardia (Lingman & Maršál, 1986*c*).

Many reference values of waveform indices have been published for various fetal vessels, and all three indices (A/B ratio, RI & PI) have been found to be profoundly dependent on gestational age. Indeed, gestational age and FHR appear to be the predominant determinants of the variance of umbilical artery waveform indices (Maulik et al., 1989*a*). In the umbilical artery (Schulman et al., 1984; Pearce et al., 1988; Thompson et al., 1988; Gudmundsson & Maršál, 1988*a*), fetal renal artery (Vyas et al., 1989), common and internal carotid arteries (Maršál, Lingman & Giles, 1984*b*; Wladimiroff, Tonge & Stewart, 1986) and cerebral arteries (Woo et al., 1987; Kirkinen et al., 1987; Årström et al., 1989), the indices have been found to decrease steadily with gestational age throughout the last trimester of pregnancy. Thus, when relating results of Doppler waveform analysis to reference values, curves corrected for gestational age should always be used.

Although, as already discussed, waveform analysis is much less prone to error than is the estimation of fetal blood flow, nonetheless there are some pitfalls to be borne in mind. The importance of fetal apnoea and quiescence for recording reproducible Doppler signals has already been stressed. The small sample volume of some duplex scanners needs careful positioning in the axis of the vessel for proper detection of the maximum velocity; for this purpose on-line control of the Doppler spectrum is invaluable.

Clinically, the most important possible error is obtaining false positive findings of missing end-diastolic velocities. When the diastolic velocity is low, it may fall below the cut-off level of the high-pass filter, and a waveform with erroneously missing end-diastolic flow will appear. The risk of this error increases with increasing insonation angle, as the shifted frequency of the recorded velocities decreases as the angle increases (Fig. 14.3): the cut-off level of the filter then corresponds to much higher velocities than at low insonation angles. The risk of falsely missing diastolic velocities is most pronounced in situations where the insonation angle is unknown, e.g. in recordings of signals from the umbilical artery. Therefore, a finding of missing diastolic flow should be verified from at least two different insonation angles.

The efficacy of the velocity waveform indices as indicators of peripheral vascular resistance – in the case of the umbilical artery of the resistance in the placental circulation – has been tested in a number of studies. Both with in vitro (Legarth & Thorup, 1989; Spencer, Price & Lee, 1991*b*) and computer models (Adamson et al., 1989; Thompson & Stevens, 1989), an increase in the resistance peripheral to the site of measurement has been shown to result in an increase in the value of waveform indices (PI, RI, S/D ratio), when other features (e.g. the pulse rate or pressure) remained constant. Similar findings have also been reported from animal models, where placental resistance was increased either by embolising the fetal side of the placenta using microspheres (Trudinger et al., 1987*b*; Morrow et al., 1989) or by constricting the umbilical vein (Maulik et al., 1989*b*; Fouron et al., 1991). It may thus be concluded that the waveform indices are mainly, though not solely, determined by the peripheral vascular resistance.

Doppler velocimetry applied to various fetal vessels

Umbilical vein

During the last trimester of gestation, the mean blood velocity in the intra-abdominal part of the umbilical vein remains fairly stable at about 12 cm/s (Lingman & Maršál, 1986*a*). Volume blood flow increases with gestational age up to 36 weeks, after which it decreases towards term. When related to the fetal weight, a continuous and linear decrease with gestational age is seen. Flow has been reported to be better correlated with placental weight (r = 0.83) than with fetal weight (r = 0.45) (Lingman & Maršál, 1986*a*), a finding which agrees with experimental data from fetal sheep (Clapp, 1989). Flow related to placental weight was 51 ml/min per 100g (Lingman & Maršál, 1986*a*).

Reported data on umbilical venous flow have been quite similar, within the relatively narrow range of 106 to 139 ml/min/kg (Table 14.1), which is in accord with the minimum need of the human fetus as calculated by Dawes (1968).

In healthy fetuses during fetal apnoea, flow in the umbilical vein is of low velocity, and continuous without pulsations. If pressure in the inferior vena cava increases umbilical venous blood velocity may become pulsatile (Hasaart & de Haan, 1986). These pulsations are synchronous with the heart and are transmitted in a retrograde manner. In human fetuses the finding of pulsatile flow in the umbilical vein usually signals fetal asphyxia (Lingman et al., 1986).

Inferior vena cava

The velocity trace recorded from the inferior vena cava of a fetus shows typical biphasic pulsations, reflecting the function of the right atrium (Griffin, Cohen-Overbeek & Campbell, 1983). Recently, attempts have been made to quantify changes in the velocity waveform of the inferior vena cava, especially in fetuses developing heart insufficiency.

Table 14.1. *Volume flow values in the umbilical vein and fetal descending aorta according to literature*

Author	Year	Gestational age (weeks)	Blood flow (ml/min/kg)	
			Umbilical vein	Descending aorta
Gill	1979	25–40	104	
Eik-Nes et al.	1980	32–41	110	191
Gill et al.	1981	26–35	120	
		36–40	106	
Jouppila et al.	1981	30–36	108	
Kurjak & Rajhvajn	1982	30–41	107	
Griffin et al.	1983	24–42	122	
Maršál et al.	1984a	27–40		246
van Lierde, Oberweis & Thomas	1984	37–40		240
Erskine & Ritchie	1985a	28–40	117	216
Lingman & Maršál	1986a	27–36	125	206
		37–38	115	238
		39–40	76	221
Gerson et al.	1987	20	65	213
		30	153	
		40	131	
			108	

Table 14.2. *Waveform indices of blood velocity recorded from fetal arteries according to literature*

Author	Year	Index	Gestational age (weeks)	Index value
Descending aorta				
Lingman & Maršál	1986*a*	PI	28–40	1.96
Wladimiroff et al.	1986	PI	24–40	1.8
Bilardo et al.	1988	PI	24–40	2.1
Årström et al.	1989	PI	24–40	1.9
Common carotid artery				
Lingman & Maršál	1989	PI	34–41	1.89
Internal carotid artery				
Wladimiroff et al.	1986	PI	28–40	1.6
Simonazzi, Wladimiroff & van Eyck	1989	PI	39–40	1.3
Middle cerebral artery				
Kirkinen et al.	1987	RI	28–40	0.80
Woo et al.	1987	S/D	24	6.9
			40	4.2
Årström et al.	1989	PI	28	2.98
			40	1.52
Renal artery				
Veille & Kanaan	1989	PI	31	2.34
Vyas, Nicolaides & Campbell	1989	PI	28	2.65
			40	2.17
Arduini & Rizzo	1990	PI	28	2.35
			40	2.11
Umbilical artery				
Fitzgerald et al.	1984	RI	28	0.71
			40	0.57
Thompson et al.	1988	RI	28	1.0
			40	0.52
Reuwer et al.	1986	PI	28	1.00
			40	0.80
Erskine & Ritchie	1985*b*	PI	28	1.0
			40	0.65
Wladimiroff et al.	1986	PI	28	1.3
			40	0.7
Gudmundsson & Maršál	1988*b*	PI	28	1.15
			40	0.80
Pearce et al.	1988	PI	28	1.0
			40	0.8
Schulman et al.	1984	S/D	28	2.8
			40	2.3
Gerson et al.	1987	S/D	28	3.1
			40	1.7
Al-Ghazal, Chapman & Allan	1988	S/D	28	3.5
			40	2.2
Gudmundsson & Maršál	1988*b*	S/D	28	3.9
			40	2.4

Note: PI: pulsatility index; RI: resistance index; S/D = systolic to diastolic ratio.

Fetal descending aorta

The diameter of the aorta increases with advancing gestational age, but the cross-sectional area of the vessel related to fetal weight remains constant (Lingman & Maršál, 1986*b*). The mean velocity is constant during the third trimester (34 cm/s). Weight-related flow also remains constant during the last four weeks of gestation (Table 14.1). The pulsatility index in the thoracic descending aorta does not change significantly with gestational age between 28 weeks and term (Lingman & Maršál, 1986*b*; Årström et al., 1989) (Table 14.2). The waveform of the blood velocity recorded from the thoracic descending aorta is highly pulsatile with low diastolic flow. In the abdominal descending aorta of the fetus, the proportion of diastolic flow is higher and the PI value generally lower than in the thoracic aorta – possibly due to the low vascular resistance in the placenta.

From flow values recorded in the same fetus at different sites (umbilical vein, thoracic and abdominal descending aorta) it is possible to calculate the percentage distribution of aortic flow to different vascular beds. The proportion of aortic flow to the placenta diminishes from 59% at 28 weeks to 33% at term (Lingman & Maršál, 1986*a*).

Cerebral arteries

Reports have been published on velocity recordings from the common carotid artery (Maršál, Lingman & Giles, 1984; Arabin, Bergmann & Saling, 1987), internal carotid artery (Wladimiroff et al., 1986), and the middle cerebral artery (Woo et al., 1987; Kirkinen et al., 1987; Årström et al., 1989) (Fig. 14.7). The colour Doppler technique has also enabled velocity signals to be detected from the anterior and posterior cerebral arteries. In all cerebral vessels, diastolic velocities are low before 28 weeks of gestation and PI values are relatively high. During the third trimester a continuous decrease in PI has been observed (Table 14.2). Some investigators have speculated that this decrease is due to changing levels of fetal oxygenation (Bilardo, Campbell & Nicolaides, 1988).

Renal arteries

Colour Doppler ultrasound enables renal arteries of the fetus to be examined (Vyas et al., 1989). The waveform of the renal blood velocity changes with increasing gestational age, the diastolic flow increasing and the PI decreasing.

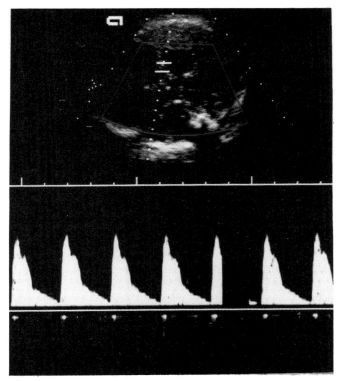

Fig. 14.7. Doppler recording of the blood velocity in the middle cerebral artery of a fetus at 28 weeks of gestation. *Upper part:* Two-dimensional image of the transverse section through the fetal head. Two parallel lines indicate the position of Doppler sample volume. *Lower-part:* Doppler shift spectrum.

Umbilical artery

Doppler velocity signals from umbilical arteries are readily obtainable even with simple Doppler instruments. In uncompromised fetuses they can be recognized by their typical 'soft-blowing' sound. When recording Doppler signals from an umbilical artery, without the support of imaging, the presence in the Doppler spectrum of continuous venous flow in the opposite direction confirms that the signals emanate from the umbilical cord (Fig. 14.2). The proportion of diastolic flow increases with increasing gestational age and values of the waveform indices (PI, RI, S/D ratio) decrease progressively (Schulman et al., 1984; Pearce et al., 1988; Thompson et al., 1988; Gudmundsson & Maršál, 1988a). Reported reference ranges for the umbilical artery are in a very good agreement

Karel Maršál

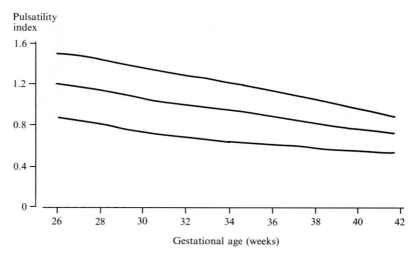

Fig. 14.8. Reference curve of the pulsatility index recorded by Doppler ultrasound from the umbilical artery of normal Swedish population (mean ±2 SD). Based on the values published by Årström et al., 1989.

(Table 14.2) (Fig. 14.8). The decrease in the waveform indices is interpreted as a reflection of decreasing vascular resistance in the placental bed towards term.

Usually, Doppler signals of the umbilical arteries are recorded from the middle portion of the cord which is freely floating in the amniotic fluid. It has been shown that higher values of waveform indices (PI, RI, S/D ratio) are obtained close to the fetal abdomen, whereas lower values are obtained close to the placental insertion of the cord (Mehalek et al., 1989).

Safety aspects

As high intensity levels of ultrasound have known biological effects, e.g. thermal effects and cavitation (Miller, Church & Barnett, 1987), researchers, ultrasound societies and health authorities are constantly alert to the possibility of adverse effects of diagnostic ultrasound. Hitherto, no harmful effects of ultrasound on mammalian tissues have been found at the intensities used for diagnostic purposes (Br. Inst. Radiol., 1987). Epidemiological follow-up studies have failed to elicit any evidence of adverse effects of exposure to diagnostic ultrasound in utero. Nevertheless, it is recommended that intensities of the spatial-peak temporal-average (SPTA) exceeding 94 mW/cm^2 in situ should be avoided (FDA, 1987; AIUM, 1988) and patients should be exposed to ultrasound only for valid clinical reasons (WHO, 1982).

It is important that users of Doppler ultrasound during pregnancy are aware of the output ultrasound energy of the Doppler equipment they are using and that they use the mode with the lowest energy when applied to a fetus. Output energy data should be provided by the manufacturers. Owing to the specific physical conditions of a fetus in utero, Doppler signals of high quality can usually be obtained even when using low intensity output energy.

References

Adamson, S. L., Morrow, R. J., Bascom, P. A., Mo, L. Y. & Ritchie, J. W. (1989). Effect of placental resistance, arterial diameter, and blood pressure on the uterine arterial velocity waveform: a computer modeling approach. *Ultrasound in Medicine and Biology,* **15**, 437–42

AIUM, American Institute of Ultrasound in Medicine, Bioeffects Committee (1988). Bioeffects considerations for the safety of diagnostic ultrasound. *Journal of Ultrasound in Medicine,* **7** (supplement).

Al-Ghazali, W., Chapman, M. G. & Allan, L. D. (1988). Doppler assessment of the cardiac and uteroplacental circulations in normal and complicated pregnancies. *British Journal of Obstetrics and Gynaecology,* **95**, 575–80.

Arabin, B., Bergmann, P. L. & Saling, E. (1987). Qualitative Analyse von Blutflußspektren uteroplazentarer Gefäße, der Nabelarterie, der fetalen Aorta und der fetalen Arteria carotis communis in normaler Schwangerschaft. *Ultraschall Klin Prax,* **2**, 114–19

Arduini, D. & Rizzo, G. (1990). Normal values of pulsatility index from fetal vessels: A cross-sectional study on 1566 healthy fetuses. *Journal of Perinatal Medicine,* **18**, 165–72.

Årström, K., Eliasson, A., Hareide, J. H. & Maršál, K. (1989). Fetal blood velocity waveforms in normal pregnancies. A longitudinal study. *Acta Obstetricia et Gynecologica Scandinavica,* **68**, 171–8.

Bilardo, C. M., Campbell, S. & Nicolaides, K. H. (1988). Mean blood velocities and flow impedance in the fetal descending thoracic aorta and common carotid artery in normal pregnancy. *Early Human Development,* **18**, 213–21.

British Institute of Radiology (1987). The Safety of Diagnostic Ultrasound, *British Journal of Radiology,* Suppl. No. 20, ed. P.N.T. Wells. pp. 1–43.

Callagan, D. A., Rowland, T. C. Jr. & Goldman, D. E. (1964). Ultrasonic Doppler observation of the fetal heart. *Obstetrics and Gynecology,* **23**, 637.

Clapp III, J. P. (1989). Utero-placental blood flow and fetal growth. In *Fetal Growth,* ed. F. Sharp, R. B. Fraser & R. D. G. Milner. pp. 235–244. Royal College of Obstetricians and Gynaecologists, London.

Davies, J. A., Lee, A. & Spencer, J. A. D. (1990). Variability of continuous-wave Doppler flow velocity waveform indices from the umbilical artery. *Obstetrics and Gynecology,* **76**, 366–9.

Dawes, G. S. (1968). *Foetal and Neonatal Physiology*. YearBook Publishers Inc., Chicago.

Doppler, C. (1842). Ueber das farbige Licht der Doppelsterne und einiger anderer Gestirne des Himmels. *Abhandlungen königlich böhmischen Gesellschaft der Wissenschaften*, **2**, 465–82

Eik-Nes, S. H., Brubakk, A. O. & Ulstein, M. (1980). Measurement of human fetal blood flow. *British Medical Journal*, **1**, 283–4.

Eik-Nes, S. H., Maršál, K., Kristoffersen K. & Vernersson, E. (1981). Noninvasive Messung des fetalen Blutstromes mittels Ultraschall. *Ultraschall in der Medizin*, **2**, 226–31.

Eik-Nes, S. H., Maršál, K., Brubakk, A. O., Kristofferson, K. & Ulstein, M. (1982). Ultrasonic measurement of human fetal blood flow. *Journal of Biomedical Engineering*, **4**, 28–36.

Erskine, R. L. A. & Ritchie, J. W. K. (1985*a*). Quantitative measurement of fetal blood flow using Doppler ultrasound. *British Journal of Obstetrics and Gynaecology*, **92**, 600–4.

Erskine, R. L. A. & Ritchie, J. W. K. (1985*b*). Umbilical artery blood flow characteristics in normal and growth-retarded fetuse. *British Journal of Obstetrics and Gynaecology*, **92**, 605–10.

European Association of Perinatal Medicine (1989). Regulation for the use of Doppler technology in perinatal medicine. Consensus of Barcelona. Instituto Dexeus, Barcelona, 1989.

FDA/CDRH 510 K (1987). Guidelines for measuring and reporting acoustic output of diagnostic ultrasound medical devices.

Fitzgerald, D. E. & Drumm, J. E. (1977). Non-invasive measurement of human fetal circulation using ultrasound: a new method. *British Medical Journal*, **ii**, 1450–1.

Fitzgerald, D. E., Stuart, B., Drumm, J. E. & Duignan, N. H. (1984). The assessment of fetal–placental circulation with continuous wave Doppler ultrasound. *Ultrasound in Medicine and Biology*, **10**, 371–6.

Fouron, J. C., Teyssiger, G., Maroto, E., Lessard, M. & Marquette, G. (1991). Diastolic circulatory dynamics in the presence of elevated placental resistance and retrograde diastolic flow in the umbilical artery: a Doppler echographic study in lambs. *American Journal of Obstetrics and Gynecology*, **164**, 195–203.

Gerson, A. G., Wallace, D. M., Stiller, R. J., Paul, D., Weiner, S. & Bolognese, R. J. (1987). Doppler evaluation of umbilical venous and arterial blood flow in the second and third trimesters of normal pregnancy. *Obstetrics and Gynecology*, **70**, 622–6.

Gill, R. W. (1978). Quantitative blood flow measurement in deep-lying vessels using pulsed Doppler with the Octoson. *Ultrasound in Medicine and Biology*, **4**, 341–5.

Gill, R. W. (1979). Pulsed Doppler with B-mode imaging for quantitative blood flow measurement. *Ultrasound in Medicine and Biology*, **5**, 223–35.

Gill, R. W. (1982). Accuracy calculations for ultrasonic pulsed Doppler blood flow measurements. *Australasian Physical and Engineering Sciences in Medicine*, **5**, 51–7.

Gill, R. W., Trudinger, B. J., Garrett, W. J., Kossoff, G. & Warren, P. S. (1981). Fetal umbilical venous flow measured in utero by pulsed Doppler and B-mode ultrasound. *American Journal of Obstetrics and Gynecology*, **139**, 720–5.

Gosling, R. G. & King, D. H. (1975). Ultrasonic angiology. In *Arteries and Veins*, ed. A. W. Harcus & L. Adamson. pp. 61–98. Churchill-Livingstone, Edinburgh.

Griffin, D., Cohen-Overbeek, T. & Campbell, S. (1983). Fetal and utero-placental blood flow. *Clinical Obstetrics and Gynecology*, **10**, 565–602.

Gudmundsson, S., Fairlie, F., Lingman, G. & Maršál, K. (1990). Recording of blood flow velocity waveforms in the uteroplacental and umbilical circulation – reproducibility study and comparison of pulsed and continuous wave Doppler ultrasound. *Journal of Clinical Ultrasound*, **18**, 97–101.

Gudmundsson, S. & Maršál, K. (1988*a*) Umbilical artery and uteroplacental circulation in normal pregnancy – a cross-sectional study. *Acta Obstetricia et Gynecologica Scandinavica*, **67**, 347–54.

Gudmundsson, S. & Maršál, K. (1988*b*) Umbilical and uteroplacental blood flow velocity waveforms in pregnancies with fetal growth retardation. *European Journal of Obstetrics, Gynecology and Reproductive Biology*, **27**, 187–96.

Hasaart, T. H. & de Haan, J. (1986). Phasic blood flow patterns in the common umbilical vein of fetal sheep during umbilical cord occlusion and the influence of autonomic nervous system blockade. *Journal of Perinatal Medicine*, **14**, 19–26.

Hatle, L. & Angelsen, B. (1985). *Doppler Ultrasound in Cardiology. Physical Principles and Clinical Applications*. 2nd edn. p. 35. Lea & Febiger, Philadelphia.

Jouppila, P. & Kirkinen, P. (1984). Increased vascular resistance in the descending aorta of the human fetus in hypoxia. *British Journal of Obstetrics and Gynaecology*, **91**, 853–6.

Jouppila, P., Kirkinen, P., Eik-Nes, S. & Koivula, A. (1981). Fetal and intervillous blood flow measurements in late pregnancy. In *Recent Advances in Ultrasound Diagnosis*, ed. A. Kurjak & A. Kratochwil. *Excerpta Medica*, pp. 226–233, Amsterdam.

Kirkinen, P., Müller, R., Huch, R. & Huch, A. (1987). Blood flow velocity waveforms in human fetal intracranial arteries. *Obstetrics and Gynecology*, **70**, 617–21.

Kremkau, F. W. (1985). Seeing and hearing blood flow noninvasively using the doppler shift. *Diagnostic Imaging*, **7**, 131.

Kurjak, A. & Rajhvajn, B. (1982). Ultrasonic measurements of umbilical blood flow in normal and complicated pregnancies. *Journal of Perinatal Medicine*, **10**, 3–16.

Laurin, J., Lingman, G., Maršál, K. & Persson, P.-H. (1987). Fetal blood flow in pregnancies complicated by intrauterine growth retardation. *Obstetrics and Gynecology*, **69**, 895–902.

Legarth J. & Thorup, E. (1989). Characteristics of Doppler blood-velocity waveforms in a cardiovascular in vitro model. II. The influence of peripheral resistance, perfusion pressure and blood flow. *Scandinavian Journal of Clinical Laboratory Investigation*, **49**, 459–64.

Lingman, G., Laurin, J. & Maršál, K. (1986). Circulatory changes in fetuses with imminent asphyxia. *Biology of the Neonate*, **49**, 66–73.

Lingman, G. & Maršál, K. (1986*a*). Fetal central blood circulation in the third trimester of normal pregnancy. I. Aortic and umbilical blood flow. *Early Human Development*, **13**, 137–50.

Lingman, G. & Maršál, K. (1986*b*). Fetal central blood circulation in the third trimester of normal pregnancy. Longitudinal study. II. Aortic blood velocity waveform. *Early Human Development,* **13**, 151–9.

Lingman, G. & Maršál, K. (1986*c*). Circulatory effects of fetal heart arrhythmia. *Journal of Pediatric Cardiology,* **7**, 67–74.

Lingman, G. & Maršál, K. (1989). Non-invasive assessment of the cranial blood circulation in the fetus. *Biology of the Neonate,* **56**, 129–35.

Malcus, P., Andersson, J., Maršál, K. & Olofsson, P-Å. (1991). Waveform pattern recognition – A new semiquantitative method for analysis of fetal aortic and umbilical artery blood flow velocity recorded by Doppler ultrasound. *Ultrasound in Medicine and Biology,* **17**, 453–60.

Maršál, K., Lindblad, A., Lingman, G. & Eik-Nes, S. H. (1984*a*). Blood flow in the fetal descending aorta; intrinsic factors affecting fetal blood flow, i.e., fetal breathing movements and cardiac arrhythmia. *Ultrasound in Medicine and Biology,* **10**, 339–48.

Maršál, K., Lingman, G. & Giles, W. B. (1984*b*). Evaluation of the carotid, aortic and umbilical blood velocity waveforms in the human fetus. In *Proceedings, XI Annual Conference, Society for the Study of Fetal Physiology,* Oxford, C33.

Maulik, D. Yarlagadda, A. P., Youngblood, J. P. & Willoughby, L. (1989*a*). Components of variability of umbilical arterial Doppler velocimetry – A prospective analysis. *American Journal of Obstetrics and Gynecology,* **160**, 1406–12.

Maulik, D., Yarlagadda, P., Nathanielsz, P. W. & Figueroa, J. P. (1989*b*). Hemodynamic validation of Doppler assessment of fetoplacental circulation in a sheep model system. *Journal of Ultrasound in Medicine,* **8**, 177–81.

McCallum, W. D., Williams, C. S., Napel, S. & Daigle, R. E. (1978). Fetal blood velocity waveforms. *American Journal of Obstetrics and Gynecology,* **132**, 425–9.

Mehalek, K. E., Berkowitz, G. S., Chitkara, U., Rosenberg, J. & Berkowitz, R. L. (1988). Comparison of continuous-wave and pulsed Doppler S/D ratios of umbilical and uterine arteries. *Obstetrics and Gynecology,* **72**, 603–6.

Mehalek, K. E., Rosenberg, J., Berkowitz, G. S., Chitkara, U. & Berkowitz, R. L. (1989). Umbilical and uterine artery flow velocity waveforms. Effect of the sampling site on Doppler ratios. *Journal of Ultrasound in Medicine,* **8**, 171–6.

Miller, M. W., Church, C. C. & Barnett, S. B. (1987). Bioeffects of Doppler ultrasound in the maternal-fetal context. In *Doppler Ultrasound Measurement of Maternal-Fetal Hemodynamics,* ed. D. Maulik & D. McNellis. pp. 105–114. Perinatology Press, Ithaca, N.Y.

Mires, G., Dempster, J., Patel, N. B. & Crawford, J. W. (1987). The effect of fetal heart rate on umbilical artery flow velocity waveforms. *British Journal of Obstetrics and Gynaecology,* **94**, 665–9.

Morrow, R. J., Adamson, S. L., Bull, S. B. & Ritchie, J. W. K. (1989). Effect of placental embolization on the umbilical arterial velocity waveform in fetal sheep. *American Journal of Obstetrics and Gynecology,* **161**, 1055–60.

Mulders, L. G. M., Muijers, G. J. J. M., Jongsma, H. W., Nijhuis, J. G. & Hein, P. R. (1986). The umbilical artery blood flow velocity waveform in relation to fetal breathing movements, fetal heart rate and fetal behavioral states in normal pregnancy at 37–39 weeks. *Early Human Development,* **14**, 283–93.

Nijhuis, J. G., Prechtl, H. F., Martin, C. B. Jr & Bots, R. S. (1982). Are there behavioural states in the human fetus? *Early Human Development,* **6**, 177–95.

Pearce, J. M., Campbell, S., Cohen-Overbeek, T., Hackett, G., Hernandez, J. & Royston, J. P. (1988). References ranges and sources of variation for indices of pulsed Doppler flow velocity waveforms from the uteroplacental and fetal circulation. *British Journal of Obstetrics and Gynaecology,* **95**, 248–56.

Pourcelot, L. (1974). Aplications clinique de l'examen Doppler transcutane. In *Velocimetric ultrasonore Doppler,* ed. P. Peronneau. pp. 213–240. INSERM, Paris.

Reuwer, P. J., Nuyen, W. C., Beijer, H. J., Heethaar, R. M., Haspels, A. A. & Bruinse, H. W. (1986). Feto-placental circulatory competence. *European Journal of Obstetric and Gynecological Reproductive Biology,* **21**, 15–26.

Rochelson, B., Schulman, H., Farmakides, G., Bracero, L., Ducey, J., Fleischer, A., Penny, B. & Winter, D. (1987). The significance of absent end-diastolic velocity in umbilical artery velocity waveforms. *American Journal of Obstetrics and Gynecology,* **156**, 1213–18.

Satomura, S. (1956). A study on examining the heart with ultrasonics. I. Principles. II. Instruments. *Japanese Circulation Journal,* **20**, 227–39.

Schulman, H., Fleischer, A., Stern, W., Farmakides, G., Jagani, N. & Blattner, P. (1984). Umbilical velocity wave ratios in human pregnancy. *American Journal of Obstetrics and Gynecology,* **148**, 985–90.

Simonazzi, E., Wladimiroff, J. W. & van Eyck, J. (1989). Flow velocity waveforms in the fetal internal carotid artery relative to fetal blood gas and acid–base measurements in normal pregnancy. *Early Human Development,* **19**, 111–15.

Spencer, J. A. D. & Price, J. (1989). Intraobserver variation in Doppler ultrasound indices of placental perfusion derived from different numbers of waveforms. *Journal of Ultrasound in Medicine,* **8**, 197–9.

Spencer, J. A. D., Giussani, D. A., Moore, P. J. & Hanson, M. A. (1991a). In vitro validation of Doppler indices using blood and water. *Journal of Ultrasound in Medicine,* **10**, 305–8.

Spencer, J. A. D., Price, J. & Lee, A. (1991b). Influence of fetal breathing and movements on variability of umbilical Doppler indices using different numbers of waveforms. *Journal of Ultrasound in Medicine,* **10**, 37–41.

Stale, H., Maršál, K. & Gennser, G. (1990). Blood flow velocity and diameter changes in the fetal descending aorta: A longitudinal study. *American Journal of Obstetrics and Gynecology,* **163**, 26–9.

Stuart, B., Drumm, J., Fitzgerald, D. E. & Diugnan, N.M. (1980). Fetal blood velocity waveforms in normal pregnancy. *British Journal of Obstetrics and Gynaecology,* **87**, 780–5.

Thompson, R. S. & Stevens, R. J. (1989). Mathematical model for interpretation of Doppler velocity waveform indices. *Medical and Biological Engineering and Computing,* **27**, 269–76.

Thompson, R. S., Trudinger, B. J. & Cook, C. M. (1986). A comparison of Doppler ultrasound waveform indices in the umbilical artery. I. Indices derived from the maximum velocity waveform. *Ultrasound in Medicine and Biology,* **12**, 835–44.

322 *Karel Maršál*

Thompson, R. S., Trudinger, B. J., Cook, C. M. & Giles, W. B. (1988). Umbilical artery velocity waveforms: normal reference values for A/B ratio and Pourcelot ratio. *British Journal of Obstetrics and Gynaecology,* **95**, 589–91.

Trudinger, B. J., Giles, W. B. & Cook, C. M. (1985). Flow velocity waveforms in the maternal uteroplacental and fetal umbilical placental circulations. *American Journal of Obstetrics and Gynecology,* **152**, 155–63.

Trudinger, B. J., Giles, W. B., Cook, C. M., Connely, A. & Thompson, R. S. (1987a). Umbilical artery flow velocity waveforms in high-risk pregnancy. *Lancet,* **i**, 188–90.

Trudinger, B. J., Stevens, D., Connelly, A., Hales, J. R., Alexander, G., Bradley, L., Fawcett, A. & Thompson, R. S. (1987b). Umbilical artery flow velocity waveforms and placental resistance: the effects of embolization of the umbilical circulation. *American Journal of Obstetrics and Gynecology,* **157**, 1443–8.

van Eyck, J., Wladimiroff, J. W., Noordam, M. J., Tonge, H. M. & Prechtl, H. F. (1985). The blood flow velocity waveform in the fetal descending aorta: its relationship to fetal behavioural states in normal pregnancy at 37–38 weeks. *Early Human Development,* **12**, 137–43.

van Eyck, J., Wladimiroff, J. W., van den Wijngaard, J. A., Noordam, M. J. & Prechtl, H. F. (1987). The blood flow velocity waveform in the fetal internal carotid and umbilical artery; its relation to fetal behavioural states in normal pregnancy at 37–38 weeks. *British Journal of Obstetrics and Gynaecology,* **94**, 736–41.

van Lierde, M., Oberweis, D. & Thomas, K. (1984). Ultrasonic measurement of aortic and umbilical blood flow in the human fetus. *Obstetrics and Gynecology,* **63**, 801–5.

Veille, J. C. & Kanaan, K. (1989). Duplex Doppler ultrasonographic evaluation of the fetal renal artery in normal and abnormal fetuses. *American Journal of Obstetrics and Gynecology,* **161**, 1502–7.

Vyas, S., Nicolaides, K. H. & Campbell, S. (1989). Renal artery flow-velocity waveforms in normal and hypoxemic fetuses. *American Journal of Obstetrics and Gynecology,* **161**, 168–72.

WHO, World Health Organization (1982). *Environmental Health Criteria 22 – Ultrasound.* WHO, Geneva.

Wladimiroff, J. W., Tonge, H. M. & Stewart, P. A. (1986). Doppler ultrasound assessment of cerebral blood flow in the human fetus. *British Journal of Obstetrics and Gynaecology,* **93**, 471–5.

Woo, J. S. K., Liang, S. T., Roxy, L. S. & Chan, F. Y. (1987). Middle cerebral artery Doppler flow velocity waveforms. *Obstetrics and Gynecology,* **70**, 613–16.

15

Doppler ultrasonography: applications in clinical practice

BRIAN J. TRUDINGER

Introduction

Doppler ultrasound has provided the ability to study fetal and placental circulations in a non-invasive manner. It has been adopted by obstetricians, who for so long had postulated inadequate circulation as the underlying disturbance of placental insufficiency and had wondered about fetal responses.

Two avenues have been explored. Assessment of volume flow in large fetal vessels, the umbilical vein and aorta (Gill, 1979; Eik-Nes, Brubakk & Ulstein, 1980), soon indicated that this technique had problems of accuracy when applied to the clinical domain and early results did not substantiate the expected clinical discrimination. Analysis of the flow velocity waveform (FVW) was a far simpler technique which was improved by the development of real time spectrum analysers.

After descriptive studies of the possibility of recording from the umbilical circulation (Fitzgerald & Drumm, 1977; McCallum et al., 1978), the first systematic studies in complicated pregnancy (Giles, Trudinger & Cook, 1982; Trudinger & Cook, 1982; Trudinger et al., 1985a) provided very encouraging results. Indices of resistance which had already been described for the study of peripheral vascular disease were used. This remains the major application for Doppler ultrasound in obstetric practice, although the study of FVWs in the fetal arteries and the uterine circulation has also developed. Doppler is also an integral part of the detailed examination of the fetal heart.

The umbilical circulation

Studies of the umbilical artery FVW are increasingly being incorporated into the clinical management of high fetal risk pregnancies. There has

323

been considerable progress towards understanding the basis of the change seen in complicated pregnancy. Clinical correlation studies with adverse fetal outcome have been reported and several randomised clinical trials have supported the use in high risk pregnancy.

The meaning of umbilical artery FVW patterns

The indices of resistance described in the previous chapter have been widely applied to studies of the umbilical circulation. These indices should not be equated with volume flow. Rather they relate to downstream resistance. Strictly, the term resistance should only be used for steady flow in rigid pipes. Impedance is the more appropriate term since blood flow is pulsatile. The blood flow velocity waveform depends not only on the downstream vascular bed, but also the upstream pressure pump, the elasticity or distensibility of vessel walls and the viscous properties of blood. In the umbilical circulation in disease (rather than physiological experiments), the extent, and so the influence, of changes in the downstream vascular bed is so large in comparison to these other considerations that it is the major determinant of changes in the waveform pattern.

Throughout pregnancy the placenta grows with an increase in size and number of villi. The resistance vessels of the placenta are the small arterial and arteriolar channels in the tertiary villi. It is across this generation of vessels that the greatest drop in pressure occurs. The decreasing vascular resistance in the umbilical placental circulation seen through pregnancy (Dawes, 1968) is attributable to the increase in the number of these channels occurring with growth. In addition, there is a small increase in the number of arterial channels in the tertiary stem villi (Giles, Trudinger & Cook, 1985b). A study to correlate the umbilical artery FVW pattern with these 'resistance' vessels in the placenta has been carried out. The modal tertiary villus small arterial vessel count was significantly less in a group of patients with abnormal (high resistance index) umbilical artery Doppler FVW patterns in contrast to normal (1–2 to 7–8 arteries/high power field). This placental lesion of vascular sclerosis with obliteration of the small muscular arteries of the tertiary villi could be expected to increase flow resistance. It is the Doppler-defined lesion of umbilical placental insufficiency.

There is also support for the concept of a reduction in small arterial channels in the placenta from physical modelling studies. Using a lumped electrical circuit equivalent, Thompson and Stevens (1989) developed a computer-based model of the placental vasculature. This has proved to

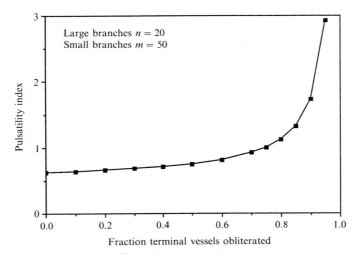

Fig. 15.1. The change in umbilical artery pulsatility index resulting from progressive obliteration of an increasing fraction of the umbilical vascular bed.

be a very valuable approach and has produced realistic data in a variety of tests. Using this model it can be shown that the pulsatility index of the FVW is related to the size of the downstream vascular bed. This index will increase as the fraction of terminal vessels obliterated is increased, but this is not a linear relationship (Thompson & Trudinger, 1990). Initially there was little change and indeed it was not until the extent of reduction exceeded 50% that the pulsatility index increased beyond the normal range (Fig. 15.1). It is widely believed that umbilical artery Doppler studies provide an early sign of fetal adaptation and potential fetal compromise, and data from the results of mathematical models of the placenta indicate the extent to which the pathology may be established before clinical detection occurs.

The concept that the various indices of resistance derived from the umbilical Doppler FVW relate to the size (number of vascular channels) of the downstream bed is also supported by experimental studies in fetal lambs. Microsphere embolization of the umbilical cotyledonary circulation produced an increase in these indices (Trudinger et al., 1987a).

Clinical correlations of abnormal umbilical Doppler studies

The use of umbilical Doppler FVW studies in clinical practice can be simply summarized by:

Placental lesion → Fetal effect

Brian J. Trudinger

As described above, umbilical Doppler studies detect a reduction in the placental vasculature. It is this lesion that is believed to deprive or constrain the fetus. On this basis it can be appreciated that umbilical Doppler studies are not a 'fetal test'. The pregnancies identified as abnormal will include those in which the fetus has been affected and those in which a process is occurring, but the fetus is not yet affected. However, not unexpectedly the most abnormal Doppler results will correlate with the greatest fetal effect (Fig. 15.2).

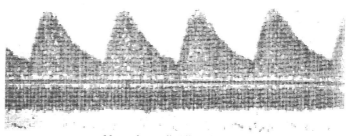

Normal systolic/diastolic ratio

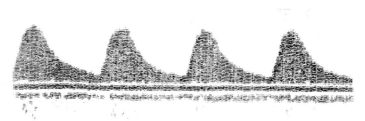

High systolic/diastolic ratio

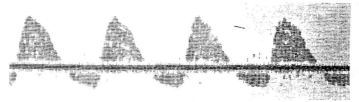

Extreme systolic/diastolic ratio

Fig. 15.2. An example of a normal, high, and extreme resistance flow velocity waveform recorded from the umbilical artery at 32 weeks. The lowermost panel illustrates reversal of flow velocities in diastole.

Many early studies correlated abnormal umbilical artery Doppler results with fetal growth retardation and the birth of an infant small for gestational age (Reuwer et al., 1984; Schulman et al., 1984; Erskine & Ritchie, 1985; Trudinger et al., 1985*a*; Gudmundsson & Maršál, 1988). However, what matters most to the obstetrician is not the recognition of the small fetus, but rather of the fetus at risk of death in utero, distress in labour, and neonatal morbidity. The author has reviewed the clinical outcome of all studies in high risk pregnancy in his laboratory (2178 patients) over a five-year period (Trudinger et al., 1991)(Table 15.1).

The significant differences in size at birth and duration of neonatal intensive care remained when analysis of covariance was carried out to eliminate the effects of gestational age.

The author has also analysed the value of using serial studies of the umbilical Doppler FVW to determine a trend (Trudinger et al., 1991). The rationale for this is that an increasing index of resistance suggests vessel obliteration whereas a decrease is indicative of placental growth with vascular expansion. In comparison to the single (abnormal) last study result, the use of an upward trend of serial studies showed stronger correlations for adverse outcome in terms of perinatal mortality or duration of neonatal intensive care nursery stay. In contrast, a downward trend, even if the values were outside the normal range, was associated with an outcome little different from normal.

Umbilical Doppler studies and other fetal assessments

The relationship of change in umbilical Doppler studies to tests of fetal welfare has been reported in a number of studies. In comparison to non-stressed fetal heart rate monitoring the umbilical Doppler waveform is a more sensitive indicator of size at birth (Trudinger et al., 1986; Farmakides et al., 1988). Although it is important to identify the small fetus it is more important to identify those at risk of morbidity. Size may not be the most important fetal end-point. Higher sensitivity extends to such measures of 'asphyxia' as operative delivery for fetal distress, low 5 min Apgar score and admission to neonatal intensive care. Non-stressed FHR monitoring and umbilical Doppler had similar predictive values. In current obstetric practice monitoring is widely used to confirm well-being or otherwise in a fetus considered to be at risk. For that reason the published results revealing a higher sensitivity (without additional false positive cases) of umbilical Doppler studies are noteworthy.

Table 15.1. *Outcome in 2178 pregnancies by result of last umbilical artery flow velocity waveform (FVW) study*

	Whole group	Systolic:diastolic ratio centile			
		<95th (normal)	95–99th (elevated)	>99th (high)	ADF (extreme)
Number of pregnancies	2178	1650 (76%)	193 (9%)	239 (11%)	96 (4%)
Gestational age at delivery (weeks)	37.7	38.3	37.6[c]	35.8[d]	31.1[d]
Onset of labour					
Spontaneous	790	691 (42%)	56 (29%)	35 (15%)	8 (8%)[a]
Induced	818	642 (39%)	86 (45%)	85 (36%)	5 (5%)[a]
Mode of delivery					
Elective CS	570	317 (19%)	51 (26%)	119 (50%)	83 (86%)[a]
Vaginal	1371	1145	122	95	9
Emergency CS	237	188	20	25	4
Newborn					
Birthweight (g)	2875	3097	2713[d]	2148[d]	1198[d]
Length (cm)	47.8	48.8	47[d]	44.2[d]	37.6[d]
Ponderal index	26.0	26.4	25.9	24.6[d]	21.8[d]
Birthweight centile	36.2	41.9	27.0[d]	15.1[d]	9.0[d]
Number of SGA infants					
<10th centile	588 (27%)	293 (18%)	73 (38%)	144 (60%)	78 (81%)[e]
<5th centile	389 (18%)	165 (10%)	44 (23%)	111 (46%)	69 (72%)[e]

Apgar score ≤6					
At 1 min	531 (24%)	335 (20%)	53 (27%)	78 (33%)	65 (68%)[e]
At 5 min	131 (6%)	62 (4%)	16 (8%)	27 (11%)	26 (27%)[e]
Admission to NICU					
Number admitted	548	303	45	113	87[a]
Mean stay (days)	18.5	10.0	18.9[a]	25.0[d]	43.7[d]
Perinatal deaths					
Stillbirths	21	8	4	3	6
Neonatal deaths					
Day 0–7	38	16	4	9	9
Day 8–28	10	2	0	0	8
PNM rate/1000	31.7	15.8	41.5	50.2	239.6[a]
Corrected PNM	18.2	7.9	21.2	13.0	206.5[a]

Note: Results shown are mean values or number (% of group) as appropriate. Significance of difference compared with the normal group.
[a] $P < 0.05$.   [b] $P < 0.01$.   [c] $P < 0.001$.   [d] $P < 0.0001$ (ANOVA with Bonferroni correction).   [e] $P < 0.0001$ (χ^2 for categorical data).
ADF = absent diastolic flow; CS = Caesarean section; corrected PNM = perinatal mortality rate/1000 total births corrected for fetal anomaly.

Ultrasound biometry is widely used in the third trimester to identify the SGA fetus. The abdominal circumference is the most widely measured fetal dimension for this purpose. Not unexpectedly this measurement was shown to be more sensitive than umbilical Doppler in identifying the SGA fetus (Berkowitz et al., 1988; Chambers et al., 1989). However, Doppler studies were shown to identify small fetuses at risk of subsequent perinatal asphyxia and morbidity (Maršál & Persson, 1988). When a screening of an unselected population was conducted in the third trimester of pregnancy, umbilical Doppler ultrasound and ultrasonic measurement of fetal abdominal circumference were shown to be identical in terms of their sensitivity, specificity and predictive value when birthweight less than the tenth centile was combined with evidence of fetal hypoxia as end-point (Newnham et al., 1990).

Blood gas tensions have been measured in relation to umbilical Doppler studies. Such studies are observational and depend upon the existence of a reason for percutaneous umbilical blood sampling. Hypoxaemia is a feature of small fetuses with absent end diastolic flow velocities in the umbilical FVW, although not all fetuses were hypoxaemic (Soothill et al., 1986; Nicolaides et al., 1988; Bilardo, Nicolaides & Campbell, 1990). Blood gas analysis of cord blood taken at delivery (Tyrrell, Obaid & Lilford, 1989) revealed similar findings. Again this data involves a bias in that the fetuses had been selected for elective Caesarean section.

Umbilical Doppler studies in specific pregnancy complications

Information has been collected on umbilical Doppler studies in pregnancies with a particular problem. All published series of high risk pregnancies include cases with maternal hypertension. In these cases it has been demonstrated that an abnormal Doppler result is associated with the expected fetal morbidity and mortality. Interestingly, there was no relationship between the duration of hypertension and the umbilical FVW result (Trudinger & Cook, 1990). The author has also noted that in many cases the abnormal fetal Doppler result precedes maternal disease. In diabetes, fetal size does not correlate well with the Doppler result. Abnormal results predict failure of ultrasonically measured growth or finding a non-reactive, non-stressed FHR tracing. In multiple pregnancy umbilical Doppler studies are very useful in predicting fetal growth restriction (Giles et al., 1985*b*, 1988, 1990; Farmakides et al., 1985). Umbilical Doppler measurements are simpler to make than ultrasound measurements of size in this situation. In the antiphospholipid antibody syndrome, fetal deterioration may also be predicted by umbilical Doppler FVW (Trudinger et al., 1988*a*). It appears that umbilical Doppler findings are normal in association with fetal anaemia, whether as a result of autoimmunization or a feto-maternal haemorrhage. There are also reports of normal findings in association with placental abruption.

Randomized trials of umbilical Doppler studies

To date, there have been four reports evaluating umbilical Doppler studies through the conduct of a randomized trial. It is important to understand that any such trial is specific in design and clinical setting and the findings cannot be extrapolated without further test. The author conducted a study (Trudinger et al., 1987*b*) in which clinicians had access to all fetal welfare assessments, but access to umbilical Doppler findings was randomised. Availability of a Doppler result was not associated with earlier delivery. Intervention rate was similar in the groups which had access to Doppler results to that in the group which did not. However, there was a significantly lower incidence of fetal distress during labour and in emergency Caesarean section in the group to which Doppler findings were available, and neonates spent less time in the Level three nursery. A Dutch study (Omtzigt, 1990) was performed in which patients were randomized at the outset of pregnancy as to whether Doppler studies would be performed should an indication occur during the pregnancy. All other fetal welfare assessments were available. There was a significant reduction in fetal deaths in the group with access to umbilical Doppler findings. In a study (Newnham et al., 1991) of high risk patients referred to an ultrasound department for biometry, umbilical Doppler studies were not shown to be associated with differences in outcome. These are interesting results and suggest that umbilical Doppler adds little to clinical management if detailed fetal biometry is also available. Umbilical Doppler was compared to non-stressed FHR monitoring in a Swedish study (Almstrom et al., 1991) as a method of surveillance of fetuses identified as small by third trimester biometry. The Doppler group had a smaller incidence of emergency Caesarean section for fetal distress and neonates required less Level three care. Similarly, a reduction in the number of babies admitted for neonatal care was found in a large (2600 patients) randomised trial of routine pregnancy screening by Doppler ultrasound in a total obstetric population (Spencer, Davies & Gallivan, 1991) although there were no differences in modes of delivery between the two groups.

Clinical strategies incorporating umbilical Doppler information

The approach of the obstetrician to fetal compromise progresses through a sequence of steps which can be summarized as follows:

1. Recognition of high risk pregnancy through history and/or clinical examination.
2. Determination of whether the fetus is affected in the high risk situation.
3. Quantification of the degree of fetal compromise.
4. Minimising fetal compromise by therapies aimed at improving the intrauterine environment.
5. Delivery if the intrauterine risk to the fetus is greater than the risk of delivery.

Doppler umbilical studies provide important information which fits well into this scheme in two ways:

(a) Clinical recognition of a potential at risk pregnancy. Umbilical Doppler studies allow confirmation that placental pathology is present and that the fetus is truly at risk. It thus identifies fetuses for intensive surveillance.
(b) The umbilical placental vascular lesion identified by Doppler studies is associated with reduced fetal platelet count (Wilcox et al., 1989; Wilcox & Trudinger, 1990) and vessel obliteration (Giles, Trudinger & Baird, 1985a). Low dose aspirin may be used to treat this. Such therapy is associated with a 25% increase in fetal weight and a 30% increase in placental size (Trudinger et al., 1988b).

Fetal arterial blood flow

Studies of major arteries within the fetus have been carried out by several workers. Most attention has been directed to studies of the fetal aorta and cerebral circulation, although other vessels such as the renal and femoral arteries have also been examined. All these studies require the use of a pulsed Doppler system (see Chapter 14).

The fetal aorta

The pulsatility index of the descending thoracic aorta changes little during the second half of pregnancy (Maršál et al., 1984). In fetal growth retardation the pulsatility index is increased (Griffin et al., 1984; Jouppila & Kirkinen, 1984). This probably reflects an increase in placental vascular resistance since the greatest part of flow is directed to that bed. There is no evidence that analysis of aortic FVW in this way provides superior or more discriminatory information compared to analysis of umbilical flow. One group (Soothill et al., 1986; Bilardo et al., 1990) has assessed peak mean aortic velocity and demonstrated a correlation between this index and fetal hypoxia and hypercapnia. Such studies have not been evaluated in terms of clinical decision-making. Possibly changes in this index reflect late changes in association with developing fetal hypoxaemia.

Fetal cerebral blood flow

The internal carotid arteries and all the arteries of the circle of Willis can be imaged and so yield Doppler FVW. In normal pregnancy these vessels show a low resistance FVW waveform pattern. There is a small change with advancing gestation (van den Winjngaard et al., 1989). In fetal growth retardation it has been shown that this index is decreased (Arbeille et al., 1987). The separation is not as complete as one would like for a diagnostic test and this has limited its clinical application. It has been clearly shown that the more hypoxaemic the fetus the greater is the decrease in indices of resistance (Vyas et al., 1990). The decrease in pulsatility index is assumed to be the result of cerebral vasodilatation. It is popular to associate this with an increase in blood flow. The term 'centralization of fetal flow' has been coined to describe the presumed redistribution of cardiac output to maintain oxygen delivery to the fetal brain (see Chapters 2, 8 and 9).

Other fetal vessels

Studies of the fetal femoral artery FVW have been carried out (Mari, 1991). A high resistance waveform was seen and the pattern changed during gestation, reflecting increasing resistance. In fetal growth failure, little change was seen.

Reports of recordings from fetal renal arteries have not yet provided a clear picture of any changes in fetal growth retardation (Vyas, Nicolaides & Campbell, 1989).

The maternal uteroplacental circulation

Both pulsed (Campbell et al., 1983) and continuous wave (Trudinger et al., 1985*b*; Schulman et al., 1986) Doppler have been used to study the uterine circulation. A low resistance FVW is recorded, although in the first trimester high resistance patterns are seen. The waveforms recorded from the main uterine arterial trunk and its branches in the placental bed differ (Chambers et al., 1988) so that the index of resistance used is lower in recordings from the placental bed. Recordings with continuous wave ultrasound lack certainty about the site from which readings are made. Published studies associate adverse pregnancy (outcome in terms of maternal hypertension or fetal growth retardation) with a high resistance waveform pattern. Others, however, have disputed this (Hanretty, Whittle & Rubin, 1988; Jacobson et al., 1990; Newnham et al., 1990). There has been recent interest in the presence of a dicrotic notch in the waveform as a further marker of high resistance in the downstream bed.

It is assumed that the change in the uterine artery FVW in normal pregnancy is due to a fall in resistance associated with trophoblastic invasion of the spiral arteries. This has not been established. Based on this assumption, it was postulated that an increase in indices of the resistance of the uterine waveform might predict mothers who will develop hypertension (Campbell et al., 1986). This study has been confirmed (Steel et al., 1990). Uterine artery FVW patterns at 18 and 24 weeks have been reported to identify 63% of mothers who will develop proteinuric hypertension and 33% of fetuses born SGA but there is not universal agreement on this question (Newnham et al., 1990). It has been suggested that such a method could be used to provide an indicator for low dose aspirin therapy and such therapy has been show to reduce the incidence of hypertension in this group (McParland, Pearce & Chamberlain, 1990).

References

Almstrom, H., Axelsson, O., Cnattingius, S., Ekman, G., Maesel, A., Ulmstein, V., Avstrom, K. & Maršál, K. (1991). Comparison of umbilical artery velocimetry and cardiotocography for surveillance of small for gestational age fetuses (Abstract). *Journal of Maternal and Fetal Investigation, * **1**, 127.

Arbeille, Ph., Roncin, A., Berson, M., Patat, F. & Pourcelot, L. (1987). Exploration of the fetal cerebral blood flow by duplex Doppler-linear array system in normal and pathological pregnancies. *Ultrasound in Medicine and Biology, * **13**, 329–37.

Berkowitz, G. S., Chitkara, U., Rosenberg, J., Cogswell, C., Walker, B., Lahman, E. A., Mehalek, K. E. & Berkowitz, R. L. (1988). Sonographic estimation of fetal weight and Doppler analysis of umbilical artery velocimetry in the prediction of intrauterine growth retardation: A prospective study. *American Journal of Obstetrics and Gynecology,* **158**, 1149–53.

Bilardo, C. M., Nicolaides, K. H. & Campbell, S. (1990). Doppler measurements of fetal and uteroplacental circulations: Relationship with umbilical venous blood gases measured at cordocentesis. *American Journal of Obstetrics and Gynecology,* **162**, 115–20.

Campbell, S., Diaz-Recasens, J., Griffin, D. R., Pearce, J., et al. (1983). New Doppler technique for assessing uteroplacental blood flow. *Lancet,* **i**, 675–7.

Campbell, S., Pearce, K. M. F., Hackett, G., Cohen-Overbeek, T. & Hernandex, C. (1986). Qualitative assessment of uteroplacental blood flow: early screening test for high risk pregnancies. *Obstetrics and Gynecology,* **69**, 649–53.

Chambers, S. E., Hoskins, P. R., Haddad, N. G., Johnstone, F. D., McDicken, W. N. & Muir, B. B. (1989). A comparison of fetal abdominal circumference measurements and Doppler ultrasound in the prediction of small-for-dates babies and fetal compromise. *British Journal of Obstetrics and Gynaecology,* **96**, 803–8.

Chambers, S. E., Johnstone, F. D., Muir, B. B., Hoskins, P., Haddad, N. G. & McDicken, W. N. (1988). The effects of placental site on the arcuate artery flow velocity waveform. *Journal of Ultrasound in Medicine,* **7**, 671–3.

Dawes, G. S. (1968). *Fetal and Neonatal Physiology.* Yearbook Medical Publishers, Chicago.

Eik-Nes, S. H., Brubakk, A. O. & Ulstein, M. K. (1980). Measurement of human fetal blood flow. *British Medical Journal,* **280**, 283–4.

Erskine, R. L. A. & Ritchie, J. W. L. (1985). Umbilical artery blood flow characteristics in normal growth retarded fetuses. *British Journal of Obstetrics and Gynecology,* **92**, 605–10.

Farmakides, G., Schulman, H., Saldana, L. R., et al. (1985). Surveillance of twin pregnancy with umbilical arterial velocimetry. *American Journal of Obstetrics and Gynecology,* **153**, 789–92.

Farmakides, G., Schulman, H., Winter, D., et al. (1988). Prenatal surveillance using non-stress testing and Doppler velocimetry. *Obstetrics and Gynecology,* **71**, 184–7.

Fitzgerald, D. E. & Drumm, J. E. (1977). Non-invasive measurement of human fetal circulation using ultrasound, a new method. *British Medical Journal,* **2**, 1450–1.

Giles, W. B., Trudinger, B. J. & Cook, C. M. (1982). Umbilical artery velocity time waveforms in pregnancy. *Ultrasound in Medicine,* **1**, 98.

Giles, W. B., Trudinger, B. J. & Baird, P. (1985*a*). Fetal umbilical artery flow velocity waveforms and placental resistance: pathological correlation. *British Journal of Obstetrics and Gynaecology,* **92**, 31–8.

Giles, W. B., Trudinger, B. J. & Cook, C. M. (1985*b*). Fetal umbilical artery flow velocity time waveforms in twin pregnancies. *British Journal of Obstetrics and Gynaecology,* **92**, 490–7.

Giles, W. B., Trudinger, B. J., Cook, C-M. & Connelly, A. (1988). Umbilical artery flow velocity waveforms and twin pregnancy outcome. *Obstetrics and Gynecology,* **72**, 894–7.

Giles W. B., Trudinger B. J., Cook C. M. & Connelly A. J. (1990). Umbilical artery waveforms in triplet pregnancy. *Obstetrics and Gynecology,* **75**, 813–16.

Gill, R. W. (1979). Pulsed Doppler with B-mode imaging for quantitative blood flow measurement. *Ultrasound in Medicine and Biology,* **5**, 223–35.

Griffin, D., Bilardo, K., Masini, L., Diaz-Racasens, J., Pearce, M., Willson, K. & Campbells, S. (1984). Doppler blood flow waveforms in the descending thoracic aorta of the human fetus. *British Journal of Obstetrics and Gynaecology,* **91**, 997–1006.

Gudmundsson, S. & Maršál, K. (1988). Umbilical and uteroplacental blood flow velocity waveforms in pregnancies with fetal growth retardation. *European Journal of Obstetrics, Gynecology and Reproductive Biology,* **27**, 187–96.

Hanretty, K. P., Whittle, M. & Rubin, P. C. (1988). Doppler uteroplacental waveforms in pregnancy induced hypertension: a reappraisal. *Lancet,* **i**, 850–2.

Jacobson, S-L., Imhof, R., Manning, N., Mannion, V., Little, D., Rey, E. & Redman, C. (1990). The value of Doppler assessment of the uteroplacental circulation in predicting preeclampsia or intrauterine growth retardation. *American Journal of Obstetrics and Gynecology,* **62**, 110–14.

Jouppila, P. & Kirkinen, P. (1984). Increased vascular resistance in the descending aorta of the human fetus in hypoxia. *British Journal of Obstetrics and Gynaecology,* **91**, 853–6.

McCallum, W. D., Williams, C. S., Napel, S. & Daigle, R. E. (1978). Fetal blood velocity waveforms. *American Journal of Obstetrics and Gynecology,* **132**, 425–9.

McParland P., Pearce J. M. & Chamberlain G. V. P. (1990). Doppler ultrasound and aspirin in recognition and prevention of pregnancy-induced hypertension. *Lancet,* **335**, 1552–5.

Mari, G. (1991). Arterial blood flow velocity waveforms of the pelvis and lower extremities in normal and growth retarded fetuses. *American Journal of Obstetrics and Gynecology,* **165**, 143–51.

Maršál, K., Eik-Nes, S. H., Lindblad, A. & Lingman, G. (1984). Blood flow in the fetal descending aorta. Intrinsic factors affecting fetal blood flow in fetal breathing movements and cardiac arrhythmia. *Ultrasound in Medicine and Biology,* **10**, 339–48.

Maršál, K. & Persson, P. (1988). Ultrasonic measurement of fetal blood velocity waveform as a secondary diagnostic test in screening for intrauterine growth retardation. *Journal of Clinical Ultrasound,* **16**, 239–44.

Newnham, J. P., Patterson, L. L., James, I. R., Diepeveen, D. A. & Reid, S. E. (1990). An evaluation of the efficacy of Doppler flow velocity waveform analysis as a screening test in pregnancy. *American Journal of Obstetrics and Gynecology,* **162**, 403–10.

Newnham, J. P., O'Dea, M., Reid, K., Diepeveen, D. A. & James, I. (1991). Doppler waveform analysis in high risk obstetric cases: a randomized controlled trial. *British Journal of Obstetrics and Gynaecology* (in press).

Nicolaides, K. H., Bilardo, C. M., Soothill, P. W. & Campbell, S. (1988).

Absence of end diastolic frequencies in umbilical artery: a sign of fetal hypoxia and acidosis. *British Medical Journal,* **297**, 1026–7.

Omtzigt, A. W. J. (1990). Clinical value of umbilical Doppler velocimetry. PhD Thesis, University of Utrecht.

Reuwer, P. J. H. M., Bruinse, H. W., Stoutenbeek, P. & Haspels, A. A. (1984). Doppler assessment of the feto-placental circulation in normal and growth retaded fetuses. *European Journal of Obstetrics, Gynecology and Reproductive Biology,* **18**, 199–205.

Schulman, H., Fleischer, A., Stern, W., Farmakides, G., Jagani, N. & Blottner, P. (1984). Umbilical velocity wave ratios in human pregnancy. *American Journal of Obstetrics and Gynecology,* **148**, 986–90.

Schulman, H., Fleischer, A., Farmakides, G., et al. (1986). Development of uterine artery compliance in pregnancy detected by Doppler ultrasound. *American Journal of Obstetrics and Gynecology,* **155**, 1031–6.

Soothill, P. W., Nicolaides, K. H., Bilardo, C. M. & Campbell, S. (1986). Relation of fetal hypoxia in growth retardation to mean blood velocity in the fetal aorta. *Lancet,* **ii**, 1118–19.

Spencer, J. A. D., Davies, J. A. & Gallivan, S. (1991). Randomised trial of routine Doppler screening during pregnancy (Abstract). *Journal of Maternal-Fetal Investigation,* **1**, 126.

Steel, S. A., Pearce, J. M., McParland, P. & Chamberlain, G. V. P. (1990). Early Doppler ultrasound screening in prediction of hypertensive disorders of pregnancy. *Lancet,* **225**, 1548–51.

Thompson, R. S. & Stevens, R. J. (1989). A mathematical model for interpretation of Doppler velocity waveform indices. *Medical and Biological Engineering and Computing,* **27**, 269–76.

Thompson, R. S. & Trudinger, B. J. (1990). Doppler waveform pulsatility index and resistance, pressure and flow in the umbilical placental circulation: An investigation using a mathematical mode. *Ultrasound in Medicine and Biology,* **16**, 449–58.

Trudinger, B. J. & Cook, C. M. (1982). Fetal umbilical artery velocity waveforms. *Ultrasound in Medicine,* **1**, 97.

Trudinger, B. J., Giles, W. B., Cook, C. M., Bombardieri, J. & Collins, L. (1985*a*). Fetal umbilical artery flow velocity waveforms and placental resistance: Clinical significance. *British Journal of Obstetrics and Gynaecology,* **92**, 23–30.

Trudinger, B. J., Giles, W. B. & Cook, C. M. (1985*b*). Uteroplacental blood flow velocity time waveforms in normal and complicated pregnancy. *British Journal of Obstetrics and Gynaecology,* **92**, 39–45.

Trudinger, B. J., Cook, C. M., Jones, L. & Giles, W. B. (1986). A comparison of fetal heart rate monitoring and umbilical artery waveforms in the recognition of fetal compromise. *British Journal of Obstetrics and Gynaecology,* **93**, 171–5.

Trudinger, B. J., Stevens, D., Connelly, A., Hales, J. R. S., Alexander, G., Bradley, L., Fawcett, A. & Thompson, R. S. (1987*a*). Umbilical artery flow velocity waveforms and placental resistance: The effects of embolization on the umbilical circulation. *American Journal of Obstetrics and Gynecology,* **157**, 1443–9.

Trudinger, B. J. Cook, C. M., Giles, W. B., Connelly, A. & Thompson, R. S. (1987*b*). Umbilical artery flow velocity waveforms in high-risk pregnancy. *Lancet,* **i**, 188–90.

Trudinger, B. J., Stewart, G., Cook, C-M., Connelly, A. & Exner, T. (1988*a*). Monitoring lupus anticoagulant positive pregnancies with umbilical artery flow velocity waveforms. *Obstetrics and Gynecology,* **72**, 215–18.

Trudinger, B. J., Cook, C-M., Thompson, R. S., Giles, W. B. & Connelly, A. (1988*b*). Low dose aspirin therapy improves fetal weight in umbilical placental insufficiency. *American Journal of Obstetrics and Gynecology* **159**, 681–5.

Trudinger, B. J. & Cook, C. M. (1990). Doppler umbilical and uterine flow waveforms in severe pregnancy hypertension. *British Journal of Obstetrics and Gynaecology,* **92**, 142–8.

Trudinger, B. J., Cook, C. M., Giles, W. B., Ng, S., Fong, E., Connelly, A. J. & Wilcox, W. (1991). Fetal umbilical artery velocity waveforms and subsequent neonatal outcome. *British Journal of Obstetrics and Gynaecology,* **98**, 378–84.

Tyrrell, S., Obaid, A. H. & Lilford, R. J. (1989). Umbilical artery Doppler velocimetry as a predictor of feta hypoxia and acidosis at birth. *Obstetrics and Gynecology,* **74**, 332–7.

van den Winjngaard, J. A. G. W., Groenenberg, I. A. L., Wladimiroff, J. W. & Hop, W. C. J. (1989). Cerebral Doppler ultrasound of the human fetus. *British Journal of Obstetrics and Gynaecology,* **96**, 845–9.

Vyas, S., Nicolaides, K. H. & Campbell, S. (1989). Renal artery flow velocity waveforms in normal and hypoxemic fetuses. *American Journal of Obstetrics and Gynecology* **161**, 168–72.

Vyas, S., Nicolaides, K. H., Bower, S. & Campbell, S. (1990). Middle cerebral artery flow velocity waveforms in fetal hypoxaemia. *British Journal of Obstetrics and Gynaecology,* **91**, 797–803.

Wilcox, G. R., Trudinger, B. J., Cook, C. M., Wilcox, W. R. & Connelly, A. J. (1989). Reduced fetal platelet counts in pregnancies with abnormal Doppler umbilical flow waveforms. *Obstetrics and Gynecology,* **75**, 639–43.

Wilcox, G. R. & Trudinger, B. J. (1990). Fetal platelet consumption: A feature of placental insufficiency. *Obstetrics and Gynecology,* **77**, 616–20.

16

Assessment of cerebral haemodynamics and oxygenation in the newborn human infant

JOHN S. WYATT, A. DAVID EDWARDS AND
E. OSMUND R. REYNOLDS

Introduction

Abnormalities of cerebral perfusion have been implicated in the patho-genesis of both the major causes of cerebral injury occurring in the perinatal period: hypoxia-ischaemia and periventricular haemorrhage (Pape & Wigglesworth, 1979). If the mechanisms of injury are to be investigated and therapeutic interventions tested, objective measure-ments of the newborn infant's cerebral circulation are required. A number of techniques have been employed although none has proved entirely satisfactory. This chapter aims to provide a critical review of these techniques, emphasising those which are novel or promising, and underlining problems of interpretation.

Measurement of cerebral blood flow (i) the Fick principle

The Fick principle is a restatement of the law of conservation of matter. Fick noted that if a substance (i) is not consumed or produced in an organ, the amount that accumulates during time t, ($Q(t)$) is equal to the difference between the amount supplied by the arteries and that removed by the veins (Siesjo, 1978a). The amount supplied (or removed) is the product of the concentration in the arteries (C_a) (or veins (C_v)), the flow rate (F) and the time period (t). Thus:

$$Q(t) = (F \cdot C_a \cdot t) - (F \cdot C_v \cdot t) \tag{1}$$

If arterial and venous flow are equal and constant, but C_a and C_v vary, then:

$$F = \frac{Q(t)}{\int_0^t (C_a - C_v)\, dt} \tag{2}$$

339

The substance (*i*) can be any metabolically inert molecule measurable in the vascular supply and brain, and is usually referred to as a 'tracer'; different formulations of the Fick principle are required depending on whether the tracer diffuses freely into cells or remains within the vasculature. Several methods for measuring cerebral blood flow (CBF) use this principle, including the Kety–Schmidt technique, the ^{133}Xe clearance method, positron emission tomography (PET) and near infrared spectroscopy (NIRS), all of which have provided useful data in newborn infants.

The Kety–Schmidt technique

Kety and Schmidt employed the Fick principle to make the first quantitative measurements of global CBF using nitrous oxide (N_2O) as a tracer (Kety & Schmidt, 1945). They determined C_a and C_v directly by placing catheters in the arterial and cerebral venous systems, and ingeniously overcame the problem of determining $Q(t)$ after realizing that because N_2O diffused easily across membranes, at equilibrium the venous concentration would have a direct relationship with the cerebral tissue concentration. This relationship could be expressed as the 'blood/brain partition coefficient' (ρ) which could be measured in vitro. Thus, providing equilibrium between blood and brain tracer concentrations was achieved at time (*t*), $Q(t)$ could be calculated from the product of ρ and $C(v)$. This enabled them to reformulate the Fick equation in terms of measured quantities:

$$F = \frac{\rho C(v)}{\int_0^t (C_a - C_v)\,dt} \tag{3}$$

This equation holds true for all fully diffusible tracers, both when increasing and decreasing in concentration. N_2O is administered by inhalation, and a period of at least 10 min is required for equilibrium to be established. A value for C_v is then obtained from which $Q(t)$ can be derived. C_v and C_a can be measured either during this accumulation phase or during desaturation of the brain when inhalation is discontinued.

There are several important requirements for the method to be valid. CBF must be constant throughout the measurement; if it is not, Equation 3 cannot be integrated. CBF must also be reasonably uniformly distributed as major inhomogeneities of flow or arteriovenous anastomoses will prevent equilibration between brain and venous blood. Critically, the blood sampled for C_v measurement must not be contaminated by extra-cerebral blood. Unfortunately none of these requirements can be strictly ensured in clinical practice, limiting the accuracy of the technique.

The Kety–Schmidt method has been used extensively in studies of adults (Siesjo, 1978*b*). However it is invasive, requiring catheterization of the cerebral venous and the arterial circulation, and this has limited its use in the newborn. A recent study of term infants who had suffered from severe birth asphyxia concluded that CBF was raised, and particularly so in infants with a worse outcome (Frewen et al., 1991). In view of the practical difficulties it seems unlikely that the technique will be applicable to small preterm infants.

^{133}*Xenon clearance technique*

The substitution of a γ emitting diffusible radiopharmaceutical tracer for N_2O has provided a practical method of CBF measurement in the newborn. γ emissions can be detected through the skull by scintillation counting allowing the cerebral concentration of tracer (Q) to be determined directly. The radiopharmaceuticals are fully diffusible so that the cerebral concentration is directly related to the venous concentration by the partition coefficient (ρ); thus C_v can be derived from $Q(t)$. In most studies the tracer is administered at a constant rate so as to saturate the brain. The administration is then stopped and the rate at which tracer is removed from the brain is measured. This rate of desaturation is used to determine CBF.

The mathematical analysis of desaturation curves is somewhat controversial, but the most commonly used method is an application of the Fick principle, not in the integrated form used by Kety and Schmidt but in an instantaneous formulation of Equation 2 which allows the derivation of exponential rate constants from the desaturation curve. From Equation 1, at any instant:

$$dQ = F(C_a - C_v)\, dt \qquad (4)$$

and Kety (1960) has shown that when C_a is negligible an exponential rate constant describing the rate of disappearance of tracer from the brain in terms of CBF can be derived from Equation 4.

In practice, experimental desaturation curves (see Fig. 16.1) require several exponential rate constants to fit the data, and therefore produce several measures of CBF, demonstrating the heterogeneity of CBF. This heterogeneity is often said to relate to grey and white matter in the brain,

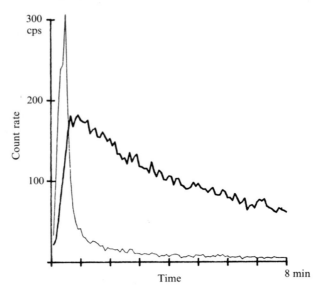

Fig. 16.1. Cranial (bold line) and chest (thin line) clearance curves after intra-venous injection of [133]Xenon (from Griesen, G. et al, *Pediatric Research* (1985), **19**, 1156–9, with permission).

but such claims have not been substantiated in the newborn. Most workers prefer to present an averaged blood flow with an explicit weighting of the different rate constants (Greisen & Pryds, 1988; Jaggi, Lipp & Duc, 1989).

It has been argued that to assume that the desaturation curve can be fitted by exponential terms is invalid, and a method has been proposed which calculates CBF by relating the maximum cerebral concentration of tracer to the concentration remaining at a given time interval (Zierler, 1965). This, the stochastic or 'height over area' method, involves other assumptions and has not been used extensively in newborn infants. It will not be discussed further here.

The most commonly used technique calculates a weighted average of the exponential rate constants describing the desaturation that follows intravenous injection of [133]Xenon dissolved in saline (Younkin et al., 1982). $Q(t)$ is determined by scintillation counters placed over the skull and C_v calculated from $Q(t)$ and the partition coefficient. C_a is assumed to be zero except for recirculation of tracer. This is thought to be small because 80% of the [133]Xenon is cleared at first pass through the lungs. However a small amount of recirculation does occur and this can be monitored by a detector placed over the chest with the assumption that alveolar gas is in equilibrium with pulmonary venous blood. The desaturation curve can then be corrected for the effects of recirculation, and Equation 4 applied.

The [133]Xenon clearance technique, however, is not without problems. First, it involves exposure to ionizing radiation. Thus, repeated measurements are restricted by the dose of radiation administered and ethical considerations preclude its use in normal subjects. Secondly, the procedure is technically exacting and requires continuous measurements over 12–15 min. The infant must be in a stable condition and must lie still for this often impractically lengthy period. The method then gives a value for the average flow over the whole measurement period; rapid changes in CBF will not only be missed but theoretically invalidate the calculation. It is not certain that the partition coefficient remains unchanged when brain tissue is injured, although this problem may have been exaggerated (Tomita & Gotoh, 1981). High flow rates, extreme heterogeneity of flow or arterio-venous anastomoses may prevent complete equilibrium between blood and brain, and low flow rates may allow diffusion of [133]Xenon from vein to artery violating the underlying assumptions of the method; it is possible that cerebral lesions may increase non-homogeneity of flow. Compton scattering of γ radiation from [133]Xenon in the airways may be detected by the cerebral scintillation counters, and right to left shunting at pulmonary and cardiac level will affect the measurement of C_a.

[133]Xenon has also been administered by intra-arterial injection (Lou, Lassen & Friis-Hansen, 1977) and inhalation (Ment et al., 1981). Unfortunately the results of different studies are not always directly comparable because global CBF is an average of the multiplicity of different regional flow rates, and technical factors may affect the proportion of high and low flow rates that are detected. There are additional problems of comparison because early studies used an adult value for ρ which caused flow to be overestimated by a factor of approximately 1/3 (Greisen, 1986).

[133]Xenon clearance measurements have been validated against other techniques in adult volunteers and experimental animals (Costeloe & Rolfe, 1988a), but in the newborn no studies have been published comparing the [133]Xenon technique against older quantitative methods for CBF determination. Internal validations have been performed however, and the intrasubject coefficient of variation has been estimated as between 8 and 17% (Greisen & Trojaborg, 1987).

Table 16.1. *Some values for cerebral blood flow in newborn infants*

Authors	Method	n	Gestation (weeks)	Age (days)	Mean CBF (range) (ml 100 g^{-1} min^{-1})
Cross et al. (1979)	JOP	16	Full term	2–8	40 (22–59)
Lou et al. (1979)	^{133}XE (IA)	5	29–39	1	40 (30–55)
Ment et al. (1981)	^{133}Xe (Inh)	15	26–32	1–2	37 (12–70)
Younkin et al. (1982)	^{133}Xe (IV)	15	31	3–57	28 (20–36)[a]
Greisen (1986)	^{133}Xe (IV)	11	21	0–5	20 (15–25)
Volpe et al. (1983)	PET	3	27–30	5–6	13 (9–20)[b]
Edwards et al. (1988b)	NIRS	9	25–44	1–10	18 (16–33)

Note: IV: intravenous; IA: intra-arterial; Inh: inhaled; JOP: jugular venous occlusion plethysmography; PET: positron emission tomography; NIRS: near infrared spectroscopy.
[a] Recalculated using a value for the neonatal blood–brain partition coefficient. The originally published value using the adult coefficient was 42 ml 100 g^{-1} min^{-1}
[b] In infants suffering from major intracerebral haemorrhage.

Despite these problems, the intravenous [133]Xenon technique has gained acceptance as a standard against which other methods have been tested, and has produced valuable information about CBF in sick new-born infants (see Table 16.1). Greisen and his colleagues obtained values for CBF in very preterm infants which are much lower than those in older children and adults (Greisen, 1986), but despite this most infants had a normal response of CBF to changes in arterial PCO_2; visual evoked responses were also intact despite low CBF (Greisen & Trojaborg, 1987). However, very low CBF values in the neonatal period have been associated with cerebral lesions detected by [133]Xenon single photon computerized tomography and poor performance on psychological testing at the age of 9 to 10 years (Lou, Skov & Henrikson, 1989). Unfortunately, but perhaps characteristically, the numerical values for CBF in these studies cannot be compared directly because different types of [133]Xenon clearance techniques were used.

Positron emission tomography

Positron emission tomography (PET) has considerable potential for studying cerebral haemodynamics and metabolism. A short half-life positron emitting diffusible tracer is injected into the blood stream. When the nucleus of the radioactive isotope decays the emitted positron collides with an electron within a few millimetres, and an annihilation event occurs which results in the emission of a pair of γ-ray photons which leave at an angle of 180^0 to each other. The photons are detected by an array of particle detectors arranged to detect photons which arrive in pairs. Using suitable computer algorithms it is possible to localize the annihilation event within a two-dimensional slice and thus detect both the position and the concentration of the positron emitting tracer (see Fig. 16.2). With suitable tracers, such as $H_2^{15}O$, CBF can be quantified, and PET has the great advantage therefore of providing information on the regional distribution of blood flow within a two-dimensional slice. Cerebral blood volume (CBV) can be obtained by using a haemoglobin-bound tracer such as ^{11}C labelled carboxyhaemoglobin. Other important variables including regional oxygen and glucose consumption and intracerebral haematocrit can also be measured with appropriate tracers (Volpe, 1987).

Practical difficulties, however, limit the widespread application of this technique to newborn infants. The PET scanner must be physically situated close to the cyclotron which produces the short-lived positron

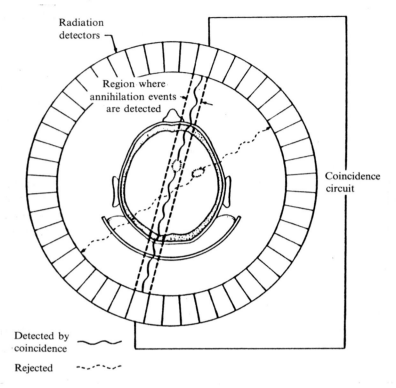

Radiation detectors

Region where annihilation events are detected

Coincidence circuit

Detected by coincidence

Rejected

Fig. 16.2. Schematic representation of arrangement of radiation detectors for positron emission tomography. The circumferential array of detectors is linked in coincidence circuits in order to detect simultaneously arriving x-rays, generated by an annihilation event between a positron and an electron. (From Volpe, J., 1987, *Neurology of the Newborn,* 2nd edn, p. 120, with permission.)

emitting isotopes. This implies that the infant to be studied must be transported away from the intensive care nursery to the detector site which precludes study of very sick or unstable infants. The exposure of the subject to ionising radiation limits the number of measurements that may be obtained and ethical considerations prohibit the use of the technique in normal infants. For absolute quantification of flow data, an arterial catheter must be inserted. Consequently, the amount of data from newborn infants that has been generated is small, although of great interest. In one study infants with intraparenchymal cerebral haemorrhage had marked reductions in regional CBF in parts of the brain quite distant from the anatomical site of the lesion (Volpe et al., 1983). Limited data on cerebral oxygen consumption rate in sick newborn infants have also been obtained (Altman et al., 1989).

Near infrared spectroscopy

Near infrared spectroscopy (NIRS), first described by Jobsis in 1977, is a novel technique which depends on the relative transparency of tissue to light in the near infrared spectrum (700–1000 nm). Light at several different wavelengths is transmitted from a fibreoptic bundle through the infant head where some photons are absorbed by pigmented compounds (chromophores) present in the tissue. Within the brain the three principal chromophores are oxyhaemoglobin (HbO_2), deoxyhaemoglobin (Hb), and oxidized cytochrome aa_3 (cyt aa_3), the terminal member of the mitochondrial respiratory chain. Changes in the concentration of these chromophores can be measured from changes in light absorption at the different wavelengths employed (Wray et al., 1988). Figure 16.3 shows a simplified diagram of the apparatus.

CBF is measured using a modification of the Fick principle. In contrast to previously discussed methods, the technique employs a purely intra-vascular and non-diffusible tracer. This is introduced rapidly into the

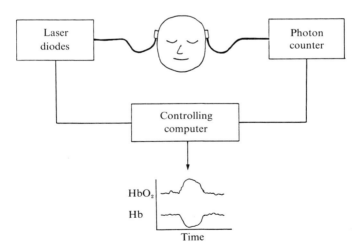

Fig. 16.3. Schematic representation of near infrared spectroscopy. A computer controls laser diodes which emit near infrared light which is transmitted to the infants head by optical fibres. After traversing the cranium, unabsorbed photons are transmitted by similar fibres to a photon counter. Changes in light absorption allow changes in the concentrations of chromophores to be calculated. (From Wyatt, J. S. et al., 1990, *Journal of Applied Physiology*, **68**, 1086–91, with permission.)

arterial supply of the brain, and the amount that has accumulated in the brain at time t (Qt) is measured. If it is less than the venous appearance time no tracer will have appeared in the venous system and C_v (referring to Equation 2) is zero. Thus:

$$F = \frac{Q(t)}{\displaystyle\int_0^t (C_a)\, dt} \qquad (2)$$

CBF can be determined from the ratio of the tracer accumulated at time t to the quantity of tracer introduced. Although exogenous infrared absorbing tracers (such as indocyanin green) can be used, and have been employed in animal studies (Colacino, Grubb & Jobsis, 1981), it is possible to make use of the presence of intravascular oxyhaemoglobin as an endogenous tracer. This method has been used for several studies in newborn infants (Edwards et al., 1988b).

A sudden increase in arterial saturation (SaO_2) over a few s is induced by a sharp but transient increase in inspired oxygen concentration. This causes an additional bolus of the tracer HbO_2 to enter the arterial supply. C_a is estimated from the change in SaO_2 measured by a pulse oximeter on the face or upper limb. The increase from baseline in $[HbO_2]$ is measured by NIRS (see Fig. 16.4). The cerebral haemoglobin flow (CHF) in mmol/l per min can then be calculated from the expression:

$$CHF = \frac{\Delta[HbO_2](t)}{\displaystyle\int_0^t (\Delta SaO_2)\, dt} \qquad (5)$$

CBF is obtained from the relationship:

$$CBF = K_{cbf} \cdot CHF/H \qquad (6)$$

where K_{cbf} is a constant reflecting the brain density and H is the large vessel haemoglobin concentration (in mol/l) measured from an arterial blood sample. In this calculation, the effects of dissolved oxygen have been ignored since it represents less than 1.5% of the total carried in the arterial blood.

The technique involves several assumptions. During the measurement, CBF, CBV and cerebral oxygen extraction must remain constant. Studies in animals and adult human subjects have shown that CBF and oxygen extraction do not alter significantly with changes in oxygen tension between 6 kPa and 13 kPa (Siesjo, 1978c) and any changes in CBV can be observed continuously by NIRS during the measurements. The period of

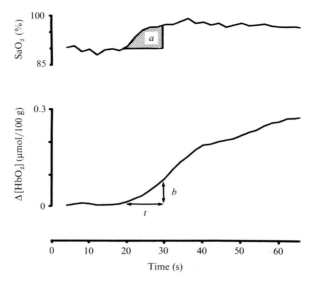

Fig. 16.4. Experimental record showing the calculation of cerebral blood flow by near infrared spectroscopy. Shaded area $a = \int_0^t (\Delta SaO_2)$, and $b = \Delta[HbO_2]$ over time t. Terms a and b are used to derive cerebral blood flow as described in the text. (From Wyatt, J. S. et al., 1989, *Archives of Disease in Childhood*, **64**, 953–63.)

measurement must be less than the venous appearance time. Studies in rats have shown that the venous appearance time is in excess of 10 s at flow rates below 100 ml/100 g per min; measurements made over a period of 8 s can thus be expected to be accurate (Jones, Korfali & Marshall, 1991). The head is assumed to be optically homogeneous with uniform and isotropic scattering. Large regional or compartmental fluctuations in haemoglobin concentration and CBF may cause significant errors on theoretical grounds.

The technique has been validated by comparison with two established methods of blood flow measurement. A study of blood flow in the adult forearm comparing flow measurements by NIRS with venous occlusion plethysmography (Edwards et al., 1988a) and two studies of CBF in sick newborn infants comparing NIRS measurements with [133]Xenon have all shown a close correspondence (Bucher et al., 1992). The average intra-subject coefficient of variation for NIRS measurements of CBF has been estimated to be 18% (Edwards et al., 1989).

NIRS has obvious advantages as a practical tool for CBF measurement in newborn infants. No ionizing radiation is employed and measurements can be obtained rapidly at the cotside. Provided that an appropriately rapid change in SaO_2 can be induced, estimations of CBF can be performed repeatedly without risk and with minimum interference to the infant. Cerebral oxygen delivery (COD) in ml/100 g per min may be obtained directly from the measured cerebral haemoglobin flow from the relationship:

$$COD = K_{cod} \cdot SaO_2 \cdot CHF \qquad (7)$$

where K_{cod} is a constant reflecting the quantity of oxygen in ml carried by each mmol of haemoglobin.

With existing apparatus a change in SaO_2 of about 4% over about 6 s is required for a satisfactory measurement. Although this is both feasible and safe in many infants undergoing intensive care, it may not be possible in infants with severe lung disease. In infants with normal lungs, whose baseline SaO_2 may be greater than 98%, an appropriate rise in SaO_2 may also not be obtained and the use of an hypoxic gas mixture may be necessary. With future improvements in NIRS and pulse oximetry technology it may become feasible to obtain satisfactory CBF measurements with smaller fluctuations in SaO_2.

NIRS has been used to study the effect on the brain of indomethacin administered for treatment of a patent ductus arteriosus (Edwards et al., 1990). In all 13 infants studied, CBF fell following indomethacin by about 45%. A similar study of the effect of administering exogenous surfactant to treat hyaline membrane disease showed no evidence of an effect on CBF except that caused by changes in arterial PCO_2 due to changes in alveolar ventilation (Edwards et al., 1992).

Because of the highly scattering nature of cerebral tissue no information on the regional distribution of CBF can be currently obtained with NIRS. However attempts are being made to develop apparatus which will provide spectroscopic imaging of the brain from an array of optical fibres, allowing localized quantification of haemodynamic variables (Jarry et al., 1984; Arridge et al., 1991). In future it may therefore be possible to quantify regional cerebral blood flow at the bedside.

Measurement of cerebral blood flow (ii) other techniques

Jugular venous occlusion plethysmography

Venous occlusion plethysmography has been employed for many years to measure blood flow in limbs by recording the change in limb volume that occurs following temporary occlusion of the venous drainage. Cross et al.

(1976) recognized that the neonatal skull was a compliant structure which changed in volume with changes in intracranial blood content. This characteristic of the infant head allowed the development of the technique of jugular venous occlusion plethysmography. Electrical impedance strain gauges are employed to measure minute changes in skull circumference, and gentle pressure is applied to the infant's neck to occlude the jugular venous flow temporarily. A considerable amount of data has been accumulated in the newborn using this technique, but it has recently fallen out of favour for several reasons. First the technique has never been properly validated by comparison against other available techniques for CBF measurement in the newborn. Secondly, anxiety has been expressed about the possible harmful consequences of a transient rise in cerebral venous pressure, especially in the preterm infant at high risk of periventricular haemorrhage. Thirdly, manual compression of the jugular vessels in the neck is often associated with some inadvertent compression of the carotid arteries thus contributing a major source of error (Cowan, Erikson & Thoresen, 1983). Finally, the compliance of the skull appears to be highly variable and unpredictable, and skull expansion is not isotropic, thus invalidating the underlying assumptions of the technique (Cooke, Rolfe & Howat, 1977).

Magnetic resonance imaging (MRI)

Several techniques have been devised for the manipulation of MRI data to provide information on cerebral perfusion, although this field is still at an early stage of development (Smith, 1990). Methods under investigation fall loosely into three main categories. First, motion sensitizing gradient pulses may be employed. These cause attenuation and/or detectable phase shifts in the signals from moving material dependent on the characteristics of the motion concerned. Secondly 'time of flight effects' which utilize the paradoxical enhancement or attenuation of an image caused by flow during an imaging sequence are used. Thirdly, a paramagnetic contrast agent such as Gadolinium–DTPA is used as a tracer for measurements employing the Fick principle. At the time of writing there have been no published studies in newborn infants, but it is likely that some will be reported in the near future. MRI has considerable potential for clinical studies of cerebral perfusion in vivo, but there are obvious disadvantages including the cost and complexity of the scanning equipment, and the need to transport the sick newborn infant away from the intensive care environment.

Other measurements of cerebral haemodynamics

Doppler ultrasound velocimetry

The widespread availability of Doppler ultrasound equipment has led to an explosion of interest in the measurement of cerebral arterial blood velocity as an indirect guide to fluctuations in CBF. By detecting the shift in frequency caused when ultrasound is reflected through moving red blood cells the velocity of the cells can be measured using the Doppler equation:

$$V = \frac{\Delta F \cdot c}{2F \cdot \cos \Omega} \tag{8}$$

where V = blood cell velocity; F = frequency; c = speed of sound in tissue; Ω = angle between direction of flow and ultrasound beam.

It can be seen from the equation that the angle Ω between the insonating beam and the direction of red cell flow is of crucial significance. As Ω increases from zero, the error in the measurement of blood flow velocity increases. Similarly, changes in Ω during insonation will lead to significant inaccuracies. Modern duplex ultrasound scanners allow two-dimensional imaging of the vessel at the same time that Doppler measurements are being made. This makes it possible to measure Ω directly and improves the accuracy and reproducibility of the measurements. Measurements are generally taken from the anterior or middle cerebral arteries (Archer & Evans, 1988).

Attempts have been made to produce quantitative data on CBF from Doppler measurements (Drayton & Skidmore, 1987), but the methods have not gained wide acceptance. Instead, most clinical studies have used the mean, peak systolic or diastolic velocities. In addition, the 'pulsatility index' (PI) may be calculated:

PI = (systolic velocity − diastolic velocity)/mean velocity

(Alternatively, systolic velocity may be substituted in the denominator.) It has been suggested that increases in these indices reflect increases in cerebral vascular resistance (Pourcelot, 1974), although this has been disputed (Costeloe & Rolfe, 1988*b*).

Although modern ultrasound equipment allows blood flow velocity to be measured easily and accurately, neither absolute velocity nor a calculated velocity index is any more than an indirect guide to trends in CBF. Blood velocity is related to blood flow by a function which includes the diameter of the insonated vessel. This diameter is too small to be measured directly from ultrasound imaging, and therefore it is not possible to convert velocity measurements directly into CBF. To infer changes in CBF from blood flow velocity it is necessary to assume that the diameter of the vessel is constant. However, even if the effects of transient vessel pulsations are disregarded, the mean diameter of large cerebral vessels may vary significantly under both physiological and pathological conditions. For example, in rabbits, it has been demonstrated that large arteries change diameter in response to noradrenaline, and that this effect is modulated by CO_2 (Flaim & Krol, 1983). Changes in sympathetic tone and arterial PCO_2 may therefore complicate the interpretation of velocity data considerably. In addition, flow in an individual cerebral artery may have a complex relationship to global or regional CBF, so that measurements in a single vessel may not be informative. Several studies have assessed the validity of Doppler velocity measurements in the newborn. Hancock et al. investigated interobserver variability and found considerable errors (Hancock et al., 1983). Studies in newborn animals have failed to demonstrate a correlation between PI and CBF (Batton et al., 1983). However, studies in newborn infants comparing Doppler velocity measurements and CBF measured by the intravenous [133]Xenon clearance method (Greisen et al., 1984) or PET (Perlman et al., 1985) have found a weak relation between CBF and both PI and absolute velocities.

Despite the difficulties in interpreting Doppler velocity measurements, the great ease with which they can be made has recommended the technique to many investigators. PI has been found to be significantly altered after birth asphyxia (Archer, Levene & Evans, 1986; den Ouden et al., 1987) but other studies give conflicting evidence. Thus early studies suggested that intracranial haemorrhage was associated with a high resistance index (Bada et al., 1979) but this has not been a general finding (Perlman & Volpe, 1982). The role of Doppler velocimetry in the investigation of the newborn cerebral circulation remains uncertain, although more sophisticated data analysis may hold promise for the future.

Cerebral blood volume measurement by NIRS

Global CBV can be quantified with NIRS by observing the effect of a small gradual change of 5–10% in SaO_2 on cerebral oxyhaemoglobin concentration over about 5 min. If it is assumed that CBF, CBV and cerebral oxygen extraction remain constant during this change then the total cerebral haemoglobin concentration [TCHb] in mmol/l can be calculated (Wyatt et al., 1990). If:

$$[HbO_2] = [TCHb] \cdot SaO_2$$

then:

$$\Delta[HbO_2] = [TCHb] \cdot \Delta SaO_2$$

and:

$$[TCHb] = \frac{\Delta[HbO_2]}{\Delta SaO_2} \tag{9}$$

and as CBV is assumed to be constant, changes in HbO_2 and deoxyhaemoglobin ([Hb]) are equal and opposite, thus:

$$\Delta[Hb] = -[TCHb] \cdot \Delta SaO_2$$

thus:

$$[TCHB] = (\Delta[HbO_2] - \Delta[Hb])/(2 \cdot \Delta SaO_2) \tag{10}$$

CBV in ml/100 g can be calculated from [TCHb] from the formula:

$$CBV = K_{cbv} \cdot [TCHb]/H \tag{11}$$

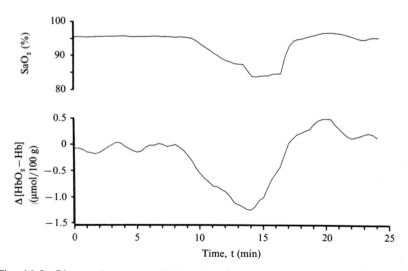

Fig. 16.5. Observations on an infant showing the effect of a small transient alteration in SaO_2, starting at 9 minutes. *Top trace*, SaO_2. *Bottom trace*, $[HbO_2 - Hb]$ determined by near infrared spectroscopy. (From Wyatt, J. S. et al., 1990, *Journal of Applied Physiology*, **68**, 1086–91, with permission.)

where K_{cbv} is a constant reflecting the cerebral:large vessel haematocrit ratio and the brain density in gm/ml. H is the large vessel haemoglobin concentration in mmol/l measured from an arterial or venous sample. Figures 16.5 and 16.6 show typical data obtained from a slow induced change in SaO_2 in a preterm infant undergoing intensive care. Although intraventricular haemorrhage is common in preterm infants, only blood participating in oxygen transport will be detected, so the presence of blood clot within the ventricles would not be expected to affect the results. This is because intraventricular blood is not involved in oxygen exchange with cerebral tissue and it would therefore be effectively 'invisible' during a small induced change in SaO_2.

No study has yet been undertaken to validate this technique in the newborn, not least because of a paucity of suitable methods with which to compare it. During the measurement of CBV, CBF and cerebral oxygen extraction are assumed to remain constant. CBV has been measured in 12 infants who were undergoing intensive care but were thought to have normal brains. Mean CBV was lower than values obtained by other techniques in adults and there was no evidence of a systematic change in CBV with increasing gestational age (Wyatt et al., 1990).

NIRS also allows the change in CBV in response to a small induced change in arterial PCO_2 to be quantified. Observations in 14 preterm and

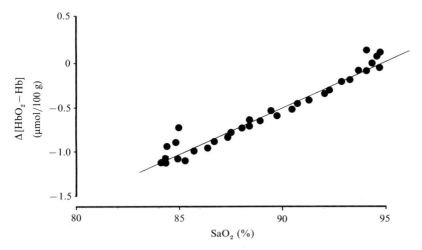

Fig. 16.6. Data from Figure 16.5 showing alterations in [HbO_2 − Hb] plotted against SaO_2, demonstrating the calculation of cerebral haemoglobin concentration. (From Wyatt, J. S. et al., 1990, *Journal of Applied Physiology*, **68**, 1086–91, with permission.)

term infants undergoing intensive care but with apparently normal brains gave values for this CBV response that ranged from 0.1 to 0.7 ml/100 g per kPa. A close linear correlation between CBV response and gestational age was observed with a marked increase in the cerebrovascular response to changing arterial PCO_2 with increasing maturity. The values obtained for CBV response in term infants were similar to those obtained previously in adult volunteers using radiolabelled erythrocytes (Wyatt et al., 1991). Preliminary studies employing NIRS in newborn infants who had suffered birth asphyxia demonstrated that CBV and CBF were both raised compared to control values. The magnitude of the derangement was related to the severity of adverse outcome. The response of CBV to changes in arterial PCO_2 was significantly attenuated in asphyxiated infants (McCormick et al., 1991), indicating the presence of both vasodilatation and vasoparalysis.

Cerebral impedance measurements

Small changes in transcephalic impedance recorded from surface electrodes on the scalp can be observed during the cardiac cycle. This signal is thought to derive from transient changes in the intracranial blood volume during systole. Using an array of four scalp electrodes it is possible to detect and measure the pulsatile impedance signal in the newborn (Costeloe et al., 1984). This signal appears to provide a qualitative indicator of changes in cerebral perfusion but attempts at quantitative analysis have so far been disappointing. Comparison of transcephalic impedance measurements with the intravenous ^{133}Xe technique has been

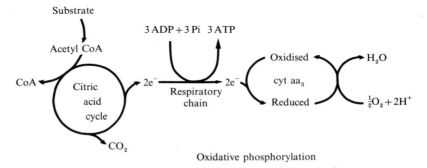

Fig. 16.7. Diagram showing oxidative phosphorylation. (From Wyatt, J. S. et al., 1989, *Archives of Disease in Childhood*, **64**, 953–63.)

undertaken (Colditz, Greisen & Pryds, 1988). This study showed that although there was a weak correlation between the two measurements, the accuracy of transcephalic impedance data was insufficient to draw firm conclusions about CBF.

Assessment of cerebral oxygenation

A very simplified representation of the relation between cellular energy metabolism and oxygenation is shown in Figs 16.7 and 16.8. Substrate (principally glucose) is metabolized by the glycolytic pathway leading to the production of electrons which are transferred to the respiratory chain in the mitochondrial membrane. Electrons flowing down an electrochemical gradient lead to the production of ATP from ADP and inorganic phosphate (Pi). The terminal enzyme complex cytochrome aa_3 passes electrons to molecular oxygen and free protons leading to the formation of water. Phosphocreatine (PCr) acts as a reserve source of intracellular high energy which allows ATP to be generated from ADP using the creatine kinase reaction. Two noninvasive techniques are available to investigate these metabolic processes directly: NIRS and magnetic resonance spectroscopy (MRS).

Near infrared spectroscopy

NIRS allows changes in the concentration of cerebral oxidized cytochrome aa_3 ($[cytO_2]$), to be quantified. This enzyme catalyses the reduction of molecular oxygen, and plays a crucial role in matching oxygen

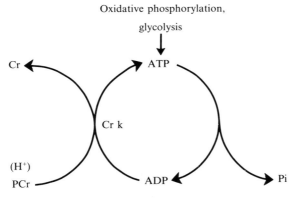

Fig. 16.8. Diagram showing the reaction of phosphocreatine, ADP and ATP.

availability to energy requirements. Variations in the enzyme redox state may reflect changes in the sufficiency of molecular oxygen at a mitochondrial level. In addition NIRS allows the global vascular supply of oxygen to be measured from the cerebral haemoglobin flow rate. Thus NIRS has the potential to assess both the vascular and the intracellular supply of oxygen to the brain. However measurements of $[cytO_2]$ demand scrupulous analysis of the optical data. Many early studies were significantly flawed because of contamination of the cytochrome optical signal by the much larger haemoglobin signal (Kariman & Scott Burkhart, 1985). Recent work has aimed to overcome this problem (Cope et al., 1991), and the results of studies on the newborn infant are becoming available. The effect of changes in SaO_2 and arterial PCO_2 on $[cytO_2]$ has been investigated (Edwards et al., 1991a). The results suggest that the brain of a preterm newborn infant may respond differently to falls in SaO_2 when compared to the brain of an adult. Whereas reductions in SaO_2 are reflected in the adult brain by a fall in $[cytO_2]$ (Hampson et al., 1990), in the newborn infant this was not observed. It was suggested that the low cerebral metabolic rate of the preterm infant retards the development of significant oxygen gradients between blood and mitochondria during hypoxia. Increasing arterial PCO_2 was associated with a rise in $[cytO_2]$, although whether this was due to a direct effect of CO_2 on the mitochondrion or the result of haemodynamic changes has yet to be ascertained.

The effect of indomethacin on $[cytO_2]$ in preterm infants has also been investigated by NIRS. In a group of infants where large changes in cerebral oxygen delivery were observed following administration of the drug, a proportion of infants demonstrated a fall in $[cytO_2]$, suggesting an imbalance between oxygen requirement and availability (McCormick et al., 1990).

Preliminary data on fetal cerebral oxygenation during labour have recently been obtained in a group of eight fetuses studied by NIRS. Optical fibres were passed through the cervix after rupture of the amniotic membranes and situated on the fetal scalp using a specially designed probe. During normal uterine contractions large changes in cerebral blood volume were observed without changes in cerebral oxygen saturation. However in contractions associated with fetal heart decelerations, the cerebral oxygen saturation fell suggesting a significant fall in cerebral oxygen delivery. Mean cerebral saturation calculated from the ratio of $[HbO_2]$ to $[Hb]$ was found to be 43 ± SD 10% during the first stage of labour, but was observed to fall to 1% just before delivery in an infant who was born with signs of intrapartum asphyxia (Peebles et al.,

1991). The effect of these changes on [cytO$_2$] have not yet been reported but NIRS has obvious potential as a clinically feasible technique for assessing fetal cerebral oxygenation.

Magnetic resonance spectroscopy (MRS)

[31]Phosphorus MRS allows quantification of the cerebral concentrations of ATP, PCr and Pi, as well as the intracellular pH; lactate concentrations can be measured by proton MRS (Cady, 1990). The PCr/Pi ratio is a sensitive index of the phosphorylation potential of the cell and the effect of substrate deprivation or of damage to the intracellular mechanisms for utilising oxygen can therefore be observed directly. Measurements have been obtained in normal term and preterm infants (Azzopardi et al., 1989a) allowing the effects of normal brain development to be assessed and the consequences of hypoxic–ischaemic brain injury have been observed (Azzopardi et al., 1989b). A late decline in phosphorylation potential has been seen at 24–72 h following severe birth asphyxia demonstrating a late or 'secondary' failure in energy metabolism (Hope et al., 1984) which has been attributed largely to damage in the mitochondrial electron transport chain. The severity of the derangement in energy metabolism measured after birth has been shown to correlate with the long-term neurodevelopmental outcome of the child (Azzopardi et al., 1989b). Advances in magnetic resonance techniques have allowed the regional concentrations of phosphorus metabolites to be measured, increasing the value of the investigation. Like MRI, MRS requires the transport of infants to a separate scanning facility which makes it a comparatively cumbersome and limited clinical tool. However, it is capable of supplying unique information about the state of important metabolic processes, and has great potential in the investigation of the neonatal brain.

Conclusion

Reliable measurements of cerebral haemodynamics and oxygenation are difficult to obtain in vivo. Methodological limitations and technical complexities abound, and data produced by the various methods require critical interpretation. No method for CBF measurement in the newborn is entirely satisfactory, although useful physiological and pathological data have been accumulated using a variety of different techniques. Table 16.1 gives a selection of representative values for CBF obtained using different methods. The intravenous ^{133}Xe technique has achieved some status as a standard for CBF measurement, but NIRS shows considerable promise as a practical non-invasive technique. Other indirect techniques for assessing cerebral perfusion, such as Doppler velocimetry, have also added useful information though their future role is uncertain. As technological and methodological advances are made, the newer techniques of MRS, MRI, NIRS and PET can be expected to make major contributions to our understanding of neonatal cerebral haemodynamics and oxygenation. In addition, it can be expected that some or all of these techniques will find a future role in studies of the fetus during labour.

References

Altman, D. I., Perlman, J. M., Volpe, J. J. & Powers, W. J. (1989). Cerebral oxygen metabolism in newborn infants measured by positron emission tomography. *Journal of Cerebral Blood Flow and Metabolism,* **9.1**, s25.
Archer, L. N. J. & Evans, D. H. (1988). Doppler assessment of the cerebral circulation. In *Fetal and Neonatal Neurology and Neurosurgery*, ed. M. I. Levene, M. J. Bennet & J. Punt. pp. 162–169. Churchill Livingstone, Edinburgh.
Archer, L. N. J., Levene, M. I. & Evans, D. H. (1986). Cerebral artery Doppler ultrasonography for prediction of outcome after perinatal asphyxia. *Lancet,* **ii**, 1116–18.
Arridge, S. R., van der Zee, P., Delpy, D. T. & Cope, M. (1991). Aspects of clinical infrared absorption imaging. In *The Formation, Handling and Evaluation of Medical Images*, ed. A. Todd-Pokropeck & M. A. Viergever. pp. 407–418. Springer-Verlag, Berlin.
Azzopardi, D., Wyatt, J. S., Hamilton, P. A., Cady, E. B., Delpy, D. T, Hope, P. L. & Reynolds, E. O. R. (1989a). Phosphorus metabolites and intracellular pH in the brains of normal and small for gestational age infants investigated by magnetic resonance spectroscopy. *Pediatric Research* **25(5)**, 440–4.
Azzopardi, D., Wyatt, J. S., Cady, E. B., Delpy, D. T., Baudin, J., Stewart, A. L., Hope, P. L., Hamilton, P. A. & Reynolds, E. O. R. (1989b). Prognosis of newborn infants with hypoxic-ischaemic brain injury assessed by magnetic resonance spectroscopy. *Pediatric Research,* **25(5)**, 445–51.
Bada, H. S., Hajjar, W., Chua, C. & Sumner, D. S. (1979). Non-invasive diagnosis of neonatal asphyxia and intraventricular haemorrhage by Doppler ultrasound. *Journal of Pediatrics,* **95**, 775–9.
Batton, D. G., Hellmann, J., Hernandez, M. J. & Maisels, M. J. (1983). Regional blood flow, cerebral blood velocity and pulsitility index in newborn dogs. *Pediatric Research,* **17**, 908–12.
Bucher, H. U., Lipp, A. E., Duc, G. & Edwards, A. D. (1992). Comparison between ^{133}Xe clearance and near infrared spectroscopy for estimation of cerebral blood flow in sick preterm infants. *Pediatric Research*, in press.
Cady, E. B. (1990). *Clinical Magnetic Resonance Spectroscopy*, pp 84–109, Pleunum Press, New York.

Colacino, J. M., Grubb, B. & Jobsis, F. F. (1981). Infrared technique for cerebral blood flow: comparison with [133]Xenon clearance. *Neurological Research,* **3** (1), 17–31.

Colditz, P., Greisen, G. & Pryds, O. (1988). Comparison of electrical impedance and [133]Xenon clearance for the assessment of cerebral blood flow in the newborn infant. *Pediatric Research,* **24**, 461–4.

Cooke, R. W. I., Rolfe, P. & Howat, P. (1977). A technique for the non-invasive investigation of cerebral blood flow in the newborn infant. *Journal of Medical Engineering and Technology,* **1**, 263–6.

Cope, M., van der Zee, P., Essenpreis, M., Arridge, S. R. & Delpy, D. T. (1991). Data analysis methods for near infrared spectroscopy of tissue: problems of determining the relative cytochrome aa_3 concentration. *Proc SPIE 1431*, in press.

Costeloe, K., Smyth, D. P. L., Murdoch, N., Rolfe, P. & Tizard, J. P. M. (1984). A comparison between electrical impedance and strain gauge plethysmography for the study of cerebral blood flow in the newborn. *Pediatric Research,* **18**, 290–5.

Costeloe, K. & Rolfe, P. (1988*a*). Techniques for studying cerebral perfusion in the newborn. In *Contemporary Issues in Fetal and Neonatal Medicine, vol 5*, ed. K. E. Pape & J. S. Wigglesworth. pp. 152–153. Blackwell Scientific Publications, USA.

Costeloe, K. & Rolfe, P. (1988*b*). Techniques for studying cerebral perfusion in the newborn. In *Perinatal Brain Lesions*, ed. K. E. Pape & J. S. Wigglesworth. Blackwell Scientific Publications, Boston.

Cowan, F., Erikson, M. & Thoresen, M. (1983). An evaluation of the plethysmographic method of measuring cranial blood flow in the newborn infant. *Journal of Physiology,* **335**, 41–50.

Cross, K. W., Dear, P. R. F., Warner, R. M. & Watling, G. B. (1976). An attempt to measure cerebral blood flow in the newborn infant. *Journal of Physiology,* **260**, 42–3P.

Cross, K. W., Dear, P. R. F., Hathorn, M. K. S., Hyams, A., Kerslake, D., Milligan, D. A. W., Rahilly, P. M. & Stothers, J. K. (1979). An estimation of intracranial blood flow in the newborn infant. *Journal of Physiology,* **289**, 329–45.

den Ouden, L., van Bel, F., van der Bor, M., Stijnem, T. & Ruys, J. (1987). Doppler flow velocity in anterior cerebral artery for prediction of outcome after perinatal asphyxia. *Lancet,* **i**, 562.

Drayton, M. R. & Skidmore, R. (1987). Vasoactivity in the major intracranial arteries in newborn infants. *Archives of Disease in Childhood,* **72**, 236–40.

Edwards, A. D., Reynolds, E. O. R., Richardson, C. & Wyatt, J. S. (1988*a*). Estimation of blood flow in man using near infrared spectroscopy. *Journal of Physiology,* **410**, 50P.

Edwards, A. D., Wyatt, J. S., Richardson, C., Delpy, D. T., Cope, M. & Reynolds, E. O. R. (1988*b*). Cotside measurement of cerebral blood flow in ill newborn infants by near infrared spectroscopy. *Lancet,* **ii**, 770–1.

Edwards, A. D., Wyatt, J. S., Richardson, C. E., Delpy, D. T., Cope, M. & Reynolds, E. O. R. (1989). Precision of cerebral blood flow measurement by near infrared spectroscopy. *Pediatric Research,* **26**, 520.

Edwards, A. D., Wyatt, J. S., Richardson, C., Potter, A., Cope, M. & Delpy, D. T. (1990). Effects of indomethacin on cerebral haemodynamics in very preterm infants. *Lancet,* **i**, 1491–5.

Edwards, A. D., Brown, G. C., Cope, M., Wyatt, J. S., McCormick, D. C., Roth, S. C., Delpy, D. T. & Reynolds, E. O. R. (1991*a*). Quantification of concentration changes in neonatal human cerebral oxidised cytochrone oxidase. *Journal of Applied Physiology*, **71**, 1907–13.

Edwards, A. D., McCormick, D. C., Roth, S. C., Wyatt, J. S., Cope, M., Delpy, D. T. & Reynolds, E. O. R. (1992). Effects of natural porcine surfactant (Curosurf) administration on cerebral oxygenation and haemodynamics investigated by near infrared spectroscopy. *Pediatric Research*, in press.

Flaim, S. F. & Krol, R. C. (1983). Effects of CO_2 to modulate the norepinephrine constrictor response in isolated perfused rabbit artery. *Pharmacology*, **26**, 150–6.

Frewen, T. C., Kissoon, N., Kronick, J., Fox, M., Lee, R., Bradwin, N. & Chance, G. (1991). Cerebral blood flow, cross-brain oxygen extraction, and fontanelle pressure after hypoxic-ischaemic injury in newborn infants. *Journal of Pediatrics*, **118**, 265–71.

Greisen, G. (1986). Cerebral blood flow in preterm infants during the first week of life. *Acta Paediatrica Scandinavica*, **75**, 43–71.

Greisen, G., Johansen, K., Ellison, P. H., Fredericksen, P. S., Mali, J. & Friis-Hansen, B. (1984). Cerebral blood flow in the newborn infant: comparison of Doppler ultrasound and ^{133}Xenon clearance. *Journal of Pediatrics*, **104**, 411.

Greisen, G. & Pryds, O. (1988). Intravenous ^{133}Xe clearance in preterm neonates with respiratory distress. Internal validation of CBF_{00} as a measure of global cerebral blood flow. *Scandinavian Journal of Clinical Laboratory Investigation*, **48**, 673–8.

Greisen, G. & Trojaborg, W. (1987). Cerebral blood flow, $PaCO_2$ changes and visual evoked potentials in mechanically ventilated preterm infants. *Acta Paediatrica Scandinavica*, **76**, 394–400.

Hampson, N. B., Camporesi, E. M., Stolp, B. W., Moon, R. E., Shook, J. E., Griebel, J. A. & Piantodosi, C. A. (1990). Cerebral oxygen availability by NIR during transient hypoxia in humans. *Journal of Applied Physiology*, **69(3)**, 907–13.

Hancock, P. J., Goldberg, R. N., Bancalarin, E., Hill, M. C. & Castillo, T. (1983). Limitation of pulsatility index as a diagnostic tool in the newborn. *Critical Care Medicine*, **11**, 186–8.

Hope, P. L., Costello, A. M. de L, Cady, E. B., Delpy, D. T., Tofts, P. S., Chu, A., Hamilton, P. A., Reynolds, E. O. R. & Wilkie, D. R. (1984). Cerebral energy metabolism studied with phosphorus NMR spectroscopy in normal and birth asphyxiated newborn infants. *Lancet*, **2**, 366–70.

Jaggi, J. L., Lipp, A. E. & Duc, G. (1989). Measurement of cerebral blood flow with a noninvasive Xenon–133 meethod in preterm infants in *Physiological Foundations of Perinatal Care*, ed. L. Stern, M. Orzalesi & B. Friis-Hansen. vol 3, Elsevier, New York.

Jarry, G., Ghesquiere, S., Maarek, J. M., Debrya, S., Bui-Mong-Hung & Laurent, D. (1984). Imaging mammalian tissues and organs using laser collimated transillumination. *Journal of Biomedical Engineering*, **6**, 70–4.

Jobsis, F. F. (1977). Noninvasive infrared monitoring of cerebral and myocardial oxygen sufficiency and circulatory parameters. *Science*, **198**, 1264–7.

Jones, S. C., Korfali, E. & Marshall, S. A. (1991). Cerebral blood flow with the indicator fractionation of [^{14}C]Iodoantipyrine: Effect of $PaCO_2$ on the cerebral venous appearance time. *Journal of Cerebral Blood Flow and Metabolism*, **11**, 236–41.

Kariman, K. & Scott Burkhart, D. (1985). Non-invasive in vivo spectrophotometric monitoring of brain cytochrone aa$_3$ revisited. *Brain Research*, **360**, 203–13.

Kety, S. S. (1960). Blood-tissue exchange methods. Theory of blood-tissue exchange and its application to measurement of blood flow. In *Methods of Medical Research, vol 8*, ed. H. D. Bruner. pp. 223–227. The Year Book Publishers Inc., Chicago.

Kety, S. S. & Schmidt, C. F. (1945). The determination of cerebral blood flow in man by the use of nitrous oxide in low concentrations. *American Journal of Physiology*, **143**, 53–66.

Lou, H., Lassen, N. A. & Friis-Hansen, B. (1977). Low cerebral blood flow in hypotensive perinatal distress. *Acta Neurologica Scandinavica*, **56**, 343–52.

Lou, H., Lassen, N. A. & Friis-Hansen, B. (1979). Impaired autoregulation of cerebral blood flow in the distressed newborn infant. *Journal of Pediatrics*, **94**, 118–21.

Lou, H., Skov, H. & Henrikson, L. (1989). Intellectual impairment with cerebral dysfunction after low neonatal cerebral blood flow. *Acta Paediatrica Scandinavica*, **360**, 72–82.

McCormick, D. C., Edwards, A. D., Wyatt, J. S., Potter, A., Cope, M., Delpy, D. T. & Reynolds, E. O. R. (1990). Effect of indomethacin on cerebral oxidised cytochrome aa$_3$ concentration in preterm infants. *Pediatric Research*, **28(3)**, 290.

McCormick, D. C., Edwards, A. D, Roth, S. C., Wyatt, J. S., Elwell, C. E., Cope, M., Delpy, D. T. & Reynolds, E. O. R. (1991). Relation between cerebral haemodynamics and outcome in birth asphyxiated newborn infants studied by near infrared spectroscopy (NIRS) *Pediatric Research* (in press).

Ment, L., Ehrenkrantz, R. A., Lange, R. C., Rothstein, P. T. & Duncan, C. C. (1981). Alterations in cerebral blood flow in preterm infants with intraventricular haemorrhage. *Pediatrics*, **68**, 763–9.

Pape, K. E. & Wigglesworth, J. S. (1979). Haemorrhage, ischaemia and the perinatal brain. Spastics International Medical Publications, London.

Peebles, D. M., Edwards, A. D., Wyatt, J. S., Bishop, A. P., Cope, M., Delpy, D. T. & Reynolds, E. O. R. (1992). Effect of uterine contraction during labour on human fetal cerebral haemoglobin concentration and oxygenation measured by near infrared spectroscopy. *American Journal of Obstetrics and Gynecology*, **166**, 1369–73.

Perlman, J. M., Herscovitch, P., Corriveau, S., Raichle, M. & Volpe, J. J. (1985). The relationship of cerebral blood flow velocity, determined by Doppler ultrasound, to regional blood flow determined by positron emission tomography. *Pediatric Research*, **19**, 357.

Perlman, J. M. & Volpe, J. J. (1982). Cerebral blood flow velocity in relation to intraventricular haemorrhage in the premature newborn infant. *Journal of Pediatrics*, **95**, 956–8.

Pourcelot, L. (1974). Applications cliniques de l'examen Doppler transcutane. In *Velocimetres ultrasonore Doppler, Vol 34*, ed. P. Perroneau. pp. 213–240. INSERM, Paris.

Siesjo, B. K. (1978a). *Brain Energy Metabolism*, pp. 56–58, Wiley, New York.

Siesjo, B. K. (1978b). *Brain Energy Metabolism*, p. 74, Wiley, New York.

Siesjo, B. K. (1978c). *Brain Energy Metabolism*, pp. 422–426, Wiley, New York.

Smith, M. A. (1990). The measurement and visualisation of vessel blood flow by magnetic resonance imaging. *Clinical Physics and Physiological Measurement,* **11**, 101–23.

Tomita, M. & Gotoh, F. (1981). Local cerebral blood flow values as estimated with diffusible tracers: validity of assumption in normal or ischaemic tissue. *Journal of Cerebral Blood Flow and Metabolism,* **4**, 403–11.

Volpe, J. J. (1987). *Neonatal Neurology* 2nd ed. pp. 119–123. WB Saunders, Philadelphia.

Volpe, J. J., Herscovitch, P., Perlman, J. M. & Raichle, M. E. (1983). Positron emission tomography in the newborn: extensive involvement of regional cerebral blood flow with intraventricular haemorrhage and haemorrhagic intracerebral involvement. *Pediatrics,* **72**, 589–601.

Wray, S. C., Cope, M., Delpy, D. T., Wyatt, J. S. & Reynolds, E. O. R. (1988). Characterisation of the near infrared absorption spectra of cytochrome aa$_3$ and haemoglobin for the non-invasive monitoring of cerebral oxygenation. *Biochimica et Biophysica Acta,* **933**, 184–92.

Wyatt, J. S., Cope, M., Delpy, D. T., Richardson, C. E., Wray, S. C. & Reynolds, S. C. (1990). Quantitation of cerebral blood volume in human infants by near infrared spectroscopy. *Journal of Applied Physiology,* **68(3)**, 1086–91.

Wyatt, J. S., Edwards, A. D., Cope, M., Delpy, D. T., McCormick, D. C., Potter, A. & Reynolds, E. O. R. (1991). Response of cerebral blood volume to changes in arterial carbon dioxide tension in preterm and term infants. *Pediatric Research* (in press).

Younkin, D. P., Reivitch, M., Jaggi, J., Obrist, W. & Delivoria-Papudopulos, M. (1982). Noninvasive method of estimating human newborn regional cerebral blood flow. *Journal of Cerebral Blood Flow and Metabolism,* **2**, 415–20.

Zierler, K. L. (1965). Equations for measuring blood flow by external monitoring of radioisotopes. *Circulation Research,* **16**, 309–21.

17

Structural and functional anomalies of the heart

LINDSEY D. ALLAN

Introduction

The cross-sectional appearance of the normal fetal heart was described by several authors almost simultaneously in 1980 (Lange et al., 1980; Kleinman, Hobbins & Jaffe, 1980; Allan et al., 1980). Since then, cardiac abnormalities, in all the forms recognized in childhood, have been detected during pregnancy from the mid-trimester onwards (Allan, 1986). Pulsed and colour flow Doppler adds further information to the cross-sectional images in terms of assessment of cardiac function and accuracy in the diagnosis of abnormalities.

Congenital heart disease is now the most common congenital anomaly in children, affecting about eight in 1000 live-births of which about three are severe malformations. Despite advances in paediatric cardiac surgery over the last 20 years, the outlook for children with many forms of heart disease remains poor. In addition, although the short-term results of cardiac surgery in children are improving, long-term results are still very uncertain. There is little information concerning late complications, quality of life, and lifespan in adults whose congenital heart disease was corrected in childhood. Table 17.1 gives a classification of congenital anomalies.

Fetal screening

Over 90% of pregnancies in the UK have a routine scan, the timing and intensity of which varies. Where a thorough detailed scan takes place at 18 weeks gestation or after, major cardiac anomalies of the fetus can be detected by obtaining an image of the four-chamber view. This examination will allow many major defects to be excluded and detects abnormality in about two in 1000 pregnancies. Thus it is possible to screen the

Table 17.1. *Classification of congenital heart disease abnormalities of connection*

(*a*) Abnormalities of connection	
Right heart	Left heart
At the venous–atrial junction	
Interrupted inferior vena cava	Total anomalous pulmonary venous drainage*
At the atrioventricular junction	
Tricuspid atresia*	Mitral atresia*
Atrioventricular septal defect*	
Double inlet ventricle*	
At the ventriculo–arterial junction	
Pulmonary atresia*	Aortic atresia*
Tetralogy of Fallot	
Common arterial trunk	
Transposition of the great arteries	
Double outlet ventricle	

(*b*) Additional abnormalities	
Right heart	Left heart
Pulmonary stenosis (*if severe)	Aortic stenosis (*if severe)
Tricuspid dysplasia*	Interrupted aortic arch*
Ebstein's anomaly*	Coarctation of the aorta*
Tumour*	
Ventricular septal defect (*if large)	
Ectopia cordis*	
Conjoint twins*	

* Indicates anomalies in which the four-chamber view would be abnormal.

whole pregnant population for major forms of congenital heart disease (Allan et al., 1986). The four-chamber view of the total heart should be identified in every pregnancy from 18 weeks gestation onwards with standard real-time equipment. Failure to obtain the normal appearance of four chambers is an indication for referral to a specialized centre for further investigation.

The four chambers of the fetal heart are seen in a horizontal section of the fetal thorax just above the level of the diaphragm (Fig. 17.1). The appearance of the four-chamber view will vary according to the orien-

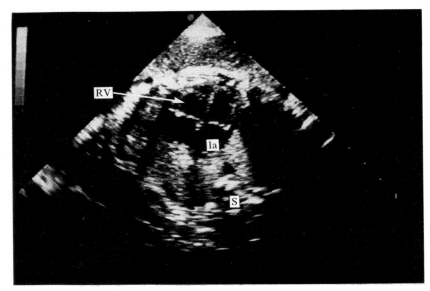

Fig. 17.1. The four-chamber view of the fetal heart is obtained in a horizontal section of the thorax, just above the diaphragm. Here the fetus lies in an ideal position with the apex of the heart closest to the transducer. RV = right ventricle, la = left atrium, S = spine.

tation of the fetus to the ultrasound beam but, whatever the fetal lie, the following important points can always be seen in the normal heart.

1. The heart occupies about one-third of the thorax.
2. There are two atria of approximately equal size.
3. There are two ventricles of approximately equal size and thickness, both showing equal contraction in the moving image.
4. The atrial and ventricular septa meet the two atrio-ventricular valves in the centre of the heart.
5. Two opening atrio-ventricular valves are seen in the moving image.

However, after about 32 weeks gestation, the right ventricle may look slightly larger than the left in the normal fetus.

The complete fetal echocardiogram

At the present time, a more detailed cardiac scan which examines all the cardiac structures is limited to pregnancies at increased risk of congenital heart disease and is only available at some specialized centres. Pregnancies at increased risk of congenital heart disease (CHD) include:

1. A family history of CHD. If one previous child has had CHD, the recurrence risk is 1 in 50. Where there have been two affected children, the risk increases to 1 in 10. When a parent is affected, the risk in the next generation is of the order of 1 in 10.
2. Maternal diabetes. This condition is associated with a statistical risk of cardiac malformation of about 1 in 50. Good diabetic control in early pregnancy probably diminishes this risk.
3. Teratogens. Exposure to teratogens in early pregnancy such as lithium, phenytoin or steroids is reported to be associated with a 1 in 50 risk of heart malformation.
4. Other structural abnormality. The detection of an extracardiac fetal anomaly on ultrasound should lead to a complete examination of the fetal heart as many types of abnormality are often linked with heart disease. Abnormalities in more than one system in the fetus should arouse suspicion of a chromosome defect.
5. Fetal arrhythmia. Some fetal arrhythmias are associated with structural heart disease, especially complete heart block, which produces a sustained bradycardia of less than 100/min.
6. Fetal hydrops. Non-immune fetal hydrops can be due to congenital heart disease and a fetal echocardiogram should be an essential part of the work-up of these patients. Fetal hydrops will have a cardiac cause in up to 25% of cases.
7. Abnormal four-chamber view. By far the most important high-risk group now seen are those pregnancies where the ultrasonographer or obstetrician notices an abnormality of the four-chamber view on a routine scan. Over 80% of the last 100 anomalies seen in our department have been referred for this reason.

High risk patients are booked for elective scans at 18 and 24–28 weeks gestation. At 18 weeks all the connections are seen. Later, more minor defects are sought. On the right side of the heart, the inferior and superior vena cavae can be seen to drain to the right atrium, which connects through the tricuspid valve to the right ventricle. The pulmonary artery then arises from the right ventricle. On the left side of the heart, the left atrium receives the pulmonary veins. The left atrium connects via the mitral valve to the left ventricle which then gives rise to the aorta. Once the method of imaging all these connections is learned, major forms of heart disease can be excluded.

The great arteries can be imaged in a variety of projections but there are several important features to note:

1. Two arterial valves can always be seen.
2. The aorta arises wholly from the left ventricle.
3. The pulmonary artery at the valve ring is slightly bigger than the aorta.
4. The pulmonary valve is anterior and cranial to the aortic valve.
5. At their origins, the great arteries lie at right angles to, and cross over, each other.
6. The arch of the aorta is of similar size to the pulmonary artery and duct and is complete.

If all these normal features are seen, major anomalies of the great arteries can be excluded.

Over 8000 patients have been examined in our unit since early 1980. Over 600 anomalies have been accurately detected. In no patient has it proved impossible to visualise the atrio-ventricular connections and the two great arteries. Heart defects which do not involve a connection abnormality are usually relatively minor defects with a good chance of successful correction, although many can be recognized prenatally. However, it is mainly the more severe forms of heart disease which are important to diagnose in fetal life. Some minor defects, such as small ventricular septal defect, secundum atrial septal defects, and valve stenosis have been overlooked but no major false positive predictions have been made.

Cardiac malformations

Abnormalities of connection can occur at the venous-atrial, the atrioventricular or the ventricular-arterial connection. Any of the connections may be absent (or atretic), displaced (or inappropriate). Examples of absent connections include total anomalous pulmonary venous drainage, tricuspid, mitral, pulmonary or aortic atresia. Two of these conditions are illustrated in Figs. 17.2 and 17.3. Infants with total anomalous pulmonary venous drainage have a good prognosis if they survive early surgery but the outlook for most conditions where there is an absent connection is poor. Mitral and aortic atresia usually occur together in the setting of the hypoplastic left heart which is a fatal defect. The most recent results of staged palliative surgery are still poor (<24% surviving the final stage) and the scarcity of organs for neonatal heart transplantation does not make this a viable alternative (Stuart et al., 1991). Right-sided lesions are

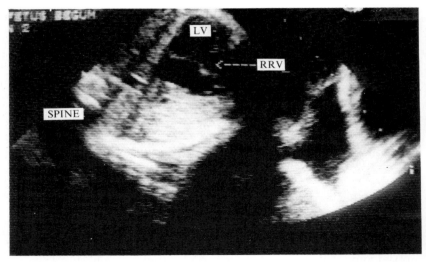

Fig. 17.2. The right ventricle is much smaller than the left and there was no opening valve in the position of the tricuspid valve. This is tricuspid atresia. LV = left ventricle, RRV = rudimentary right ventricle.

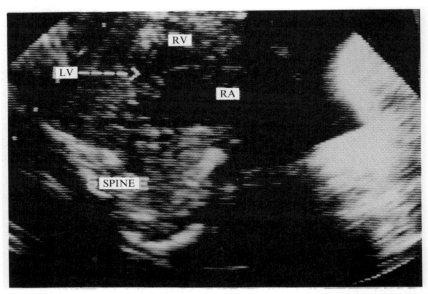

Fig. 17.3. In this fetus the left atrioventricular valve is atretic. There is a small left atrium and a small discernible left ventricle. RA = right atrium.

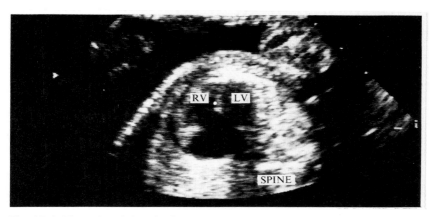

Fig. 17.4. There is a defect in the atrial and ventricular septum with a common atrioventricular valve seen open in diastole in this frame. The normal 'cross' at the crux of the heart is lost.

usually successfully palliated in the short term but the prognosis for corrective surgery in later childhood is poor.

Another defect recognizable on the four chamber view is seen in Fig. 17.4. This is a common atrioventricular valve in the context of an atrioventricular septal defect. This is one of the most frequent diagnoses made in prenatal life and its presence will indicate Down's syndrome in 50% of cases (Machado et al., 1988).

Examples of inappropriate connections include transposition of the great arteries, aortic override and double outlet right ventricle. The normal position of the aortic origin is seen in Fig. 17.5 for comparison with aortic override in Fig. 17.6. As many of these conditions can be successfully treated surgically, it is important to make accurate diagnosis. An example of a displaced connection is Ebstein's anomaly of the tricuspid valve, where the septal leaflet of this valve is positioned further down into the right ventricle than normal. This can be of varying severity but, if associated with severe incompetence (on Doppler examination) and right atrial dilatation, the outlook is poor.

One of the difficulties in predicting prognosis has been the observation that some defects progress or change as pregnancy advances. For example, when critical aortic stenosis occurs in the mid-trimester fetus, the lack of forward flow through the left ventricle and aorta leads to underdevelopment of these structures. Relief of aortic stenosis after birth

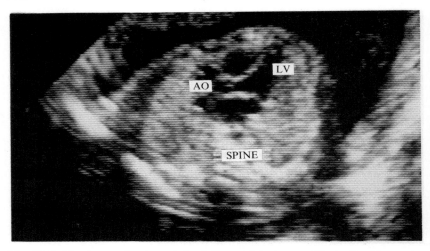

Fig. 17.5. The long-axis view of the left ventricle is seen illustrating the aorta arising from the left ventricle, with the anterior wall of the aorta (AO) continuous with the ventricular septum.

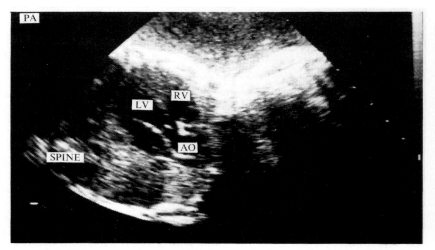

Fig. 17.6. The aorta arises astride the ventricular septum. There is a large ventricular septal defect positioned below the aorta. Examination of the pulmonary outflow tract will differentiate the three possible underlying diagnoses in this condition.

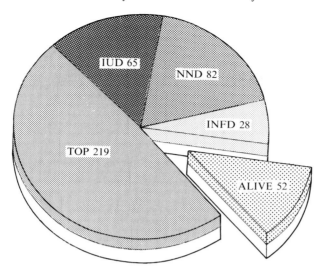

Fig. 17.7. The outcome of 446 cases of congenital heart disease detected prenatally up to the end of 1989. TOP = termination of pregnancy, IUD = intrauterine death, NND = neonatal death, INFD = infant death, ALIVE = alive.

is then of no avail as the left ventricle is by this time too small and damaged to support the circulation. These observations of the natural history of heart disease in prenatal life have led us to consider intrauterine valvoplasty which has been achieved with technical success by inflating a balloon catheter within the aortic valve ring (Maxwell, Tynan & Allan, 1991).

It is apparent from a consideration of the forms of CHD seen prenatally that it is a different spectrum of disease than that which presents in infancy. This is reflected in the outcome of the pregnancies where fetal heart disease has been detected (Fig. 17.7). Malformations detected tend to be the most severe forms of heart disease or defects such as tricuspid dysplasia & cardiac tumours which are not commonly seen postnatally. Many of these fetuses do not survive intrauterine life which accounts partly for the discrepancy between prenatal and postnatal life. Up to 25% of continuing pregnancies with CHD resulted in spontaneous fetal loss. Four-chamber view scanning selects the more severe defects. Referral of fetuses with extracardiac anomalies leads to the preferential detection of defects such as atrioventricular septal defects and tetralogy of Fallot, which are commonly associated with trisomies. Fetal hydrops is a common presenting finding in cases of cystic hygroma, coarctation and Turner's syndrome. Of 467 cases of structural heart disease seen in the series, 77 (16.5%) were found to have chromosome defects. The expected figure would be about 12% of live-births (Allan et al., 1991). For all these reasons, the epidemiology of congenital heart disease in prenatal life is proportionally quite different to that found in infants or children.

Heart rate abnormalities

The normal fetal heart rate is around 140 beats/min and the rhythm is regular. The heart rhythm can, however, be disturbed in one of three ways. Tachycardias, particularly rates over 200 beats/min; bradycardias, rates less than 100 beats/min; or irregular rhythms may occur. Rhythm disturbances are evaluated by M-mode echocardiography or Doppler and should be assessed and treated by the paediatric cardiologist.

Tachycardias

It is important that atrial and ventricular tachycardias are distinguished from each other as the therapy for one would not be appropriate for the other. Anti-arrhythmic therapy therefore should not be prescribed until the rhythm disturbance has been defined on M-mode echocardiography. Atrial tachycardias are much more common. A supraventricular tachycardia can be distinguished from atrial flutter by examining the relationship of atrial to ventricular contraction on the M-mode echocardiogram. As a tachycardia can result in intrauterine cardiac failure, all sustained tachycardias should be treated. The drug of choice for an atrial tachycardia in the non-hydropic patient is digoxin. A dose of 0.75mg per day is often necessary as the maternal serum digoxin level should be maintained at 2.0 μg/l. If the rhythm fails to convert after two weeks of adequate serum levels, verapamil may have to be added.

Conversion of the arrhythmia is usually achieved in non-hydropic cases and there should be no morbidity or mortality if these fetuses are delivered at term.

Fetuses in cardiac failure with an atrial tachycardia are more difficult to treat as digoxin is not adequately transferred across the hydropic placenta. The drug of choice remains controversial. Flecanide or a combination of digoxin and verapamil has been used with success (Maxwell et al., 1988) but there have been reports of the successful use of procainamide and quinide. If conversion occurs and delivery is delayed until close to term, hydrops can resolve and the outcome will be good. Premature delivery should be avoided as this is the major cause of morbidity and mortality.

Bradycardias

Short episodes of sinus bradycardia are normal in the midtrimester fetus. A bradycardia is important only if it is sustained. A prolonged sinus bradycardia can occur as a sign of fetal distress. It may indicate the need for urgent obstetric intervention and must be distinguished from complete heart block which is not an emergency situation. Complete heart block occurs in two sets of circumstances. It may occur in association with complex structural congenital heart disease, or it may be the result of damage to the developing conduction tissue by circulating anti-SSA antibodies associated with subclinical maternal connective tissue disease. The prognosis, when there is associated heart disease, is very poor whereas the prognosis in isolated complete heart block is usually good if antenatal care and delivery are carefully managed. However, both types of complete heart block can be associated with the development of intrauterine heart failure which has poor survival.

Irregular rhythms

Irregular rhythms are due to ectopic beats of atrial or ventricular origin. They can be as frequent as every second beat, occur with regular or irregular frequency or alternatively may be very occasional. Dropped beats are almost invariably found in every fetus between 30 weeks gestation and term, although the frequency will vary. They are not associated with morbidity or mortality and the mother and the obstetrician can be reassured if the structure of the fetal heart is normal. No treatment or intervention is necessary.

References

Allan, L. D. (1986). *Manual of Fetal Echocardiography*. MTP Press, Lancaster, England.

Allan, L. D., Crawford, D. C., Chita, S. K. & Tynan, M. J. (1986). Prenatal screening for congenital heart disease. *British Medical Journal,* **292**, 1717.

Allan, L. D., Sharland, G. K., Chita, S. K., Lockhart, S. & Maxwell, D. J.

(1991). Chromosomal anomalies in fetal congenital heart disease. *Ultrasound in Obstetrics and Gynecology,* **1**, 8–11.

Allan, L. D., Tynan, M. J., Campbell, S., Wilkinson, J. & Anderson, R. H. (1980). Echocardiographic and anatomical correlates in the fetus. *British Heart Journal,* **44**, 444.

Kleinman, C. S., Hobbins, J. C. & Jaffe, C. C. (1980). Echocardiographic studies of the human fetus: prenatal diagnosis of congenital heart disease and cardiac dysrhythmias. *Pediatrics,* **65**, 1059.

Lange, L. W., Sahn, D. J., Allen, H. D., Goldberg, S. J., Anderson, C. & Giles, H. (1980). Qualitative real-time cross-sectional echocardiographic imaging of the human fetus during the second half of pregnancy. *Circulation,* **62**, 799.

Machado, M. V. L., Crawford, D. C., Anderson, R. H. & Allan, L. D. (1988). Atrioventricular septal defect in prenatal life. *British Heart Journal,* **59**, 352.

Maxwell, D. J., Crawford, D. C., Curry, P. V. M., Tynan, M. J. & Allan, L. D. (1988). Obstetric significance, diagnosis and management of fetal tachycardias. *British Medical Journal,* **297**, 107–110.

Maxwell, D. J., Tynan, M. J. & Allan, L. D. (1991). Balloon valvoplasty in prenatal life. *British Heart Journal* (in press).

Stuart, A. G., Wren, C., Hunter, S., Sharples, P. M. & Hey, E. N. (1991). Neonatal transplantation for hypoplastic left heart syndrome: the shortage of suitable donors. *Lancet,* **337**, 956.

18

Management of fetal cardiac anomalies

JEFFREY M. DUNN, SHARON R. WEIL AND
PIERANTONIO RUSSO

The rationale for fetal cardiac intervention

With the increasing accuracy of fetal cardiac diagnosis, an understanding of the fetal development of congenital abnormalities, and a growing frustration with the long-term clinical results of many cardiac lesions treated conventionally after birth, it is inevitable that we consider the role of fetal cardiac intervention. In addition, non-cardiac fetal surgery has demonstrated the feasibility of fetal surgery with minimal maternal morbidity and acceptable fetal morbidity and mortality in selected cases.

Fetal ultrasonography, amniocentesis for chromosome and chemical analysis, and percutaneous umbilical blood sampling has allowed the perinatologist and pediatric cardiologist the ability to diagnose significant cardiac lesions, evaluate the fetus's well-being, and document the presence of other non-cardiac lesions. At present, this information can be used primarily for counselling the family, allowing timely termination of the pregnancy, and preparing for the birth of an infant requiring surgical or medical intervention. Human fetal intervention has been limited to the pharmacological management of tachydysrhythmias (Allan et al., 1983; Maxwell et al., 1988) and preliminary attempts at percutaneous balloon valvuloplasty of left sided lesions (Maxwell, Allan & Tynan, 1991).

The congenital cardiac lesions presenting after birth are often complex and represent not only a primary lesion, which most likely occurs early in fetal life, but also secondary lesions of maldevelopment produced over time in response to the haemodynamic effects of the primary lesion. It is often these secondary lesions that are the limiting factors preventing an adequate postnatal repair and acceptable clinical outcome. It is in these settings that fetal cardiac intervention for structural abnormalities becomes an attractive proposition. Fetal cardiac surgery would appear to be an attractive approach for the following reasons:

377

1. Primary cardiac lesions may be relatively easy to repair.
2. Secondary lesions may be prevented, halted, or even reversed.
3. The fetus is usually haemodynamically and physiologically stable despite congenital cardiac lesions.
4. Fetal circulation may prevent haemodynamic derangements while the left or right circulations are temporarily recovering following fetal surgery.
5. Competent pulmonary function will not be required following fetal surgery.

Fetal diagnosis

The progress of fetal intervention will be largely dependent on advances in diagnostic imaging. The development of real-time two-dimensional echocardiography as well as pulsed wave, continuous wave, and colour Doppler have contributed enormously to our now quite sophisticated ability to diagnose most significant heart disease prenatally as early as 18 weeks (Allan, 1986; de Araujo et al., 1987; Allan et al., 1988; Machado et al., 1988*a*; Schmidt & Silverman, 1988; Groenenberg, Wladimiroff & Hop, 1989; Reed, 1989). A population of pregnancies that will benefit most from fetal echocardiographic evaluation can be identified. These include pregnancies in which:

1. there is a family history of congenital heart disease or history of a genetic disease known to be associated with congenital heart disease (such as Noonan Syndrome);
2. there is maternal disease or drug ingestion predisposing to congenital heart disease (such as the presence of diabetes mellitus or systemic lupus erythematosus or the ingestion of lithium, alcohol, indomethacin or progesterones);
3. chromosomal defects such as trisomies 21, 13, or 18 are identified in the fetus;
4. cardiac structural, functional or rhythm abnormality are suspected by the obstetrician;
5. other organ systems abnormalities of the fetus are identified.

The fetal circulation

In most cases the fetus with congenital heart disease remains haemodynamically stable despite lesions that are life-threatening after birth. The fetal circulation affords this protection (Fig. 18.1). While the mature

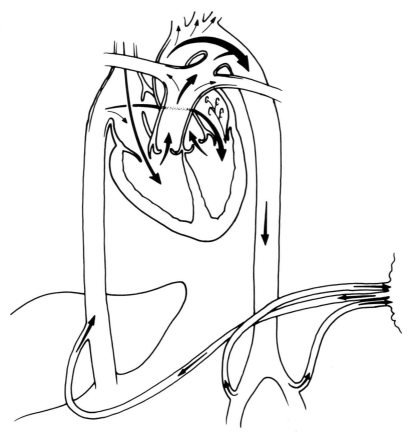

Fig. 18.1. Normal fetal circulation. A large patent foramen ovale and the ductus arteriosus afford free shunting of blood from the right to left atrium and from the pulmonary artery to the aorta respectively. The two ventricles function in parallel in contrast to the series circuit in the mature heart.

heart requires competent lungs for gas exchange and two separate series circulations (systemic and pulmonary), the fetal circulation is essentially a single circulation (Rudolph, 1974). The patent foramen ovale at the atrial level and the patent ductus arteriosus at the level of the great vessels allows the two ventricles to work in parallel rather than in series (Fig. 18.2) as in the mature heart. In addition, pulmonary blood flow is not essential for fetal survival, gas exchange being provided by the umbilical circulation, part of the single systemic circulation. This parallel circuitry of the left and right hearts militates against detrimental haemodynamic sequelae secondary to either structural or functional abnormalities of the

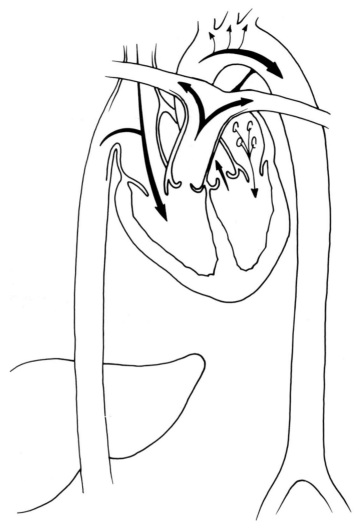

Fig. 18.2. Normal adult (mature) heart. The foramen ovale and patent ductus
arteriosus have closed. The right and left hearts function in series.

heart. For example, a hypoplastic left ventricle can be tolerated by the
fetus, since blood normally pumped by the left ventricle is directed
instead from the obstructed left ventricle to the right heart via the
foramen ovale. It is then pumped by the right ventricle to be delivered
ultimately to the aorta through the ductus arteriosus (Fig. 18.3). After

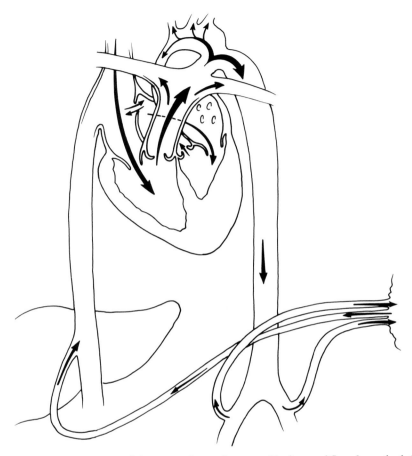

Fig. 18.3. Hypoplastic left heart syndrome in utero. No forward flow from the left ventricle to the aorta is possible. Systemic flow is maintained by the parallel right heart. Left atrial blood is diverted to the right atrium through the patent foramen. Systemic flow is maintained through the ductus arteriosus.

birth, closure of the patent ductus is incompatable with life since systemic circulation cannot be maintained (Fig. 18.4). It appears that either the left or right circulation can function as the dominant, or even the single circulation in the face of an obstructive, functional, or mixing lesion affecting the other side (Fig. 18.5). In addition to the complementary nature of the right and left ventricular outputs, other mechanisms contribute to the compensatory mechanisms of the fetal circulatory system in the face of structural or functional cardiac disease. For

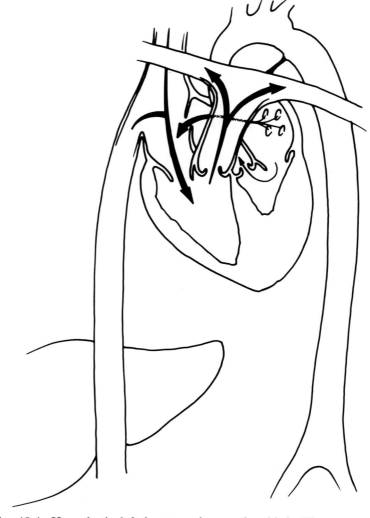

Fig. 18.4. Hypoplastic left heart syndrome after birth. The patent ductus arteriosus has closed. Systemic flow is thus not maintained. This is incompatible with life.

example, the low afterload of the placental circuit affords the fetus great compensation for myocardial dysfunction. In addition, the fetus has relatively low oxygen requirements due to the neutral thermal environment of the uterus and the use of the placenta for respiration and nutrition.

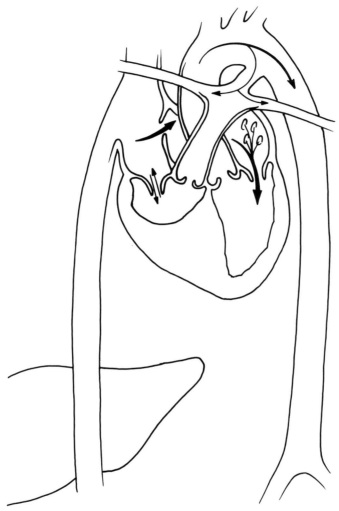

Fig. 18.5. Right-sided obstruction in utero. The tricuspid valve is stenotic or atretic. Flow is decompressed through the patent foramen to the left atrium and left-sided circulation.

In contrast, on transition to extrauterine life, the neonate requires pulmonary blood flow for adequate gas exchange. In addition, closure of the patent foramen ovale and the ductus arteriosus necessitate separate and competent left and right circulations. Thus, the fetus with congenital heart disease may only demonstrate difficulties on transition from fetal to neonatal circulation, particularly once fetal bypass pathways close. Medical management with prostaglandins after birth to preserve ductal patency are only temporizing measures, providing stabilization until surgical intervention can be performed.

Non-cardiac fetal intervention

In 1963, Liley first reported the performance of in utero peritoneal transfusion of a fetus for Rh incompatibility (Liley, 1963). Others, including Freda and Adamson in 1964, later developed open transfusion techniques involving exteriorization of a fetal part for venous or arterial cannulation (Freda & Adamson, 1964; Pringle, 1986). The advent of ultrasonography allowed this procedure to be performed without a hysterotomy (Pringle, 1986). In 1970, Nadler and Gerbie reported extensive use of amniocentesis for prenatal genetic diagnosis. More recently invasion of the uterus for diagnosis and treatment has become increasingly commonplace. Percutaneous umbilical blood sampling is routinely performed for fetal diagnosis and treatment (Ludomirski & Weiner, 1988; Ludomirski et al., 1987). Studies of fetoplacental pharmacology and visualization by two-dimensional and M-mode echocardiography have allowed effective diagnosis and treatment of fetal dysrhythmia by maternal medication (Hamamoto et al., 1990).

Surgical procedures developed in the fetal lamb and primate model have been extended to the clinical arena by Harrison et al. (Abrams, 1972; Harrison et al., 1982; Redwin & Petres, 1983; Nakayama et al., 1984; Adzick et al., 1986; Crombleholme et al., 1988; Evans et al., 1989; Harrison et al., 1990; Harrison, personal communication). They have performed over 23 human procedures of surgical fetal exteriorization and repair. Although they have not attempted cardiac repairs, they have experience with decompression of renal obstruction (seven open procedures and more than 500 closed bladder catheterizations), resection of cystic adenomatoid malformation of the lung (two cases, one survivor), resection of a sacrococcygeal teratoma (one case with successful surgery, but fetal demise due to maternal mirror syndrome), and repair of diaphragmatic hernias (13 cases total with 6 deaths in the early cases but three of seven survivors in the most recent cases). Their experience with in utero surgery offers insight into the potential for fetal cardiac repairs. Other surgeons have performed decompressions of hydrocephalus, but with disappointing results with regard to recovery of brain function (Pringle, 1986). These pioneers in fetal surgery have demonstrated both maternal and fetal safety in selected cases. The lesions they have chosen to repair in utero have demonstrated a common rationale that can equally be applied to fetal cardiac intervention. These fetal lesions all consist of a primary lesion that is easily amenable to surgical intervention, and severe secondary lesions not amenable to postnatal repair or reversal. The common rationale that Harrison et al. have applied is that the secondary lesions can be reversed, arrested, or prevented simply by managing the primary lesion in utero. For example, renal obstruction can be easily treated, the decompression allowing more normal development of renal parenchyma. This rationale can be used to select cardiac lesions that are likely to be helped by fetal intervention.

Appropriate cardiac lesions for fetal repair

As in non-cardiac lesions, fetal intervention for cardiac lesions will only be successful with proper selection. The following criteria seem appropriate.

1. The lesion must be readily diagnosable by ultrasound.
2. The natural history and progression of the fetal lesion must be understood.
3. The lesion must be life-threatening either in utero or
4. The results of postnatal repair are unacceptable.
5. The lesion will have two components: a primary lesion easily amenable to fetal repair and severe secondary lesions that are not amenable to postnatal repair but are reversible with fetal repair.

Any attempt at fetal cardiac intervention must be preceded by a firm understanding of the cause of these defects. A basis for this understanding is offered by a number of animal models of congenital heart disease which have been created in which primary surgical lesions have resulted in a constellation of secondary abnormalities which resemble recognized forms of human congenital heart disease (Gessner, 1966; Harh et al., 1973; Fishman et al., 1978). Similar spontaneously occurring human models have been proposed (Lev et al., 1963). Clearly, fetal surgical intervention is based on the assumption that these secondary abnormalities can be reversed or arrested. Unfortunately, this assumption has not yet been proven.

The many chromosomal abnormalities known to be associated with congenital heart lesions (Jones, 1988) will give the molecular biologists a basis to identify the gene sequences necessary for normal (and abnormal) cardiac development. In addition, as we get closer to identifying gene defects associated with specific cardiac syndromes (such as Williams & Noonan Syndromes), we will get closer to the responsible gene aberrations. Cell cycle genes, or oncogenes, have been found to contribute to hypertrophy and hyperplasia, and, we suspect, hypoplasia (Claycomb & Lanson, 1987; Simpson, 1989). Although studies are now demonstrating the role of oncogenes in pathologic states of the mature or adult heart, little is understood about the contribution of these oncogenes to pathologic fetal development of the heart. Studies of neural crest cell derivatives, including selective neural crest cell ablations, have demonstrated association of these predetermined cells with development (and maldevelopment) of cardiac truncal septation as well as components of the pharyngeal pouches known to be abnormal in DiGeorge Syndrome (Kirby & Waldo, 1990). The multitude of cardiac abnormalities is overshadowed by the even greater multitude of gene abnormalities responsible for them. Thus, the deciphering task will take time.

Certain lesions seem most amenable to fetal cardiac intervention.

Semilunar valve obstruction

Severe obstruction of the aortic or pulmonary valves rarely presents as a completely isolated lesion. Secondary lesions often include maldevelopment of the aorta or pulmonary arteries respectively. These secondary changes often preclude complete repair after birth, and indeed may necessitate only unattractive palliation even though the valve obstruction itself may be amenable to surgical repair. This group is by far the most likely group to be aided by fetal surgery. Realistically, fetal intervention will not become appropriate until we demonstrate that surgical repair of the abnormal valve will indeed result in more normal development of the aorta or pulmonary artery. In addition, skills will have to be developed for predicting which prenatally diagnosed cases of valvular stenosis will progress to include hypoplastic vessels not amenable to postnatal repair.

Stenotic foramen ovale

The stenotic foramen ovale has been implicated in the development of the hypoplastic left heart syndrome (Fishman et al., 1978; Lev et al., 1963). With our recently acquired capabilities of measuring fetal cardiac blood flows with echo-Doppler, the role of the stenotic foramen ovale in maldevelopment of the left heart and great vessels may be confirmed.

After birth, surgical results for the hypoplastic left heart syndromes, whether by Norwood palliation and modified Fontan (Pigott et al., 1988), or by transplantation (Bailey et al., 1988) are improving but are not optimal. Thus, surgical creation of an adequate intra-atrial communication in order to foster left ventricular growth will be very attractive.

Congenital heart block

In most cases, isolated congenital heart block is well tolerated by the fetus. In association with other fetal cardiac abnormalities, fetal heart block can be lethal. Prenatal diagnosis of fetal distress associated with heart block and medical management are discussed in Chapter 17 (see also Kleinman, Copel & Hobbins, 1987; Machado et al., 1988*b*). Epicardial pacing is technically feasible, but, to our knowledge, fetal pacemaker placement has only been clinically attempted using a closed technique without exteriorization of the fetus. Neither has transvenous pacing via umbilical vein catheterization been attempted although this approach should also be feasible. The risk of lead displacement or strangulation of a fetal part entangled in a chronic transuterine wire are major concerns. Interest in this area has thus been minimal especially since intervention is usually not required for isolated block.

Patent ductus arteriosus

The patent ductus arteriosus is essential for normal fetal circulation and inappropriate persistent patency postnatally cannot be predicted. Premature closure of the patent ductus has been associated with the development of pulmonary vascular disease (Huhta, Cohen & Wood, 1990). Of interest, management of premature labour or polyhydramnios with maternally administered indomethacin is associated with constriction of the ductus arteriosus (Huhta et al., 1990; Kirshon et al., 1990). Cardiac sequelae include dilatation of the right ventricle and tricuspid valve insufficiency. The ductal constriction and cardiac changes are reversible with cessation of the drug.

Therefore, fetal ligation of the ductus arteriosus will almost always be contra-indicated. However, normal ductal patency has been implicated in contributing to fetal demise in cases of absent pulmonary valve syndrome, in which severe pulmonary regurgitation leads to profound right ventricular dilatation and consequent compression of intrathoracic structures. It has been suggested that fetal ductal ligation in these cases might improve fetal survival (Ettedgui et al., 1990). Conversely, maintaining ductal patency may be indicated in prenatally diagnosed ductal-dependent cardiac lesions. In addition, creation of a systemic to pulmonary shunt mimicking the ductus will be feasible and may be indicated in documented cases of premature spontaneous ductal closure.

Certain lesions will not be amenable to fetal repair, or repair in utero will carry little or no advantage to repair after birth.

Ventricular septal defect

A small ventricular septal defect may evade prenatal diagnosis since the equal right and left ventricular pressures in the fetus preclude visualization of shunting. Due to the haemodynamic insignificance of these lesions, they would not appropriately be treated, even if diagnosed, in utero. Likewise, even large ventricular septal defects are more easily and safely addressed postnatally. An exception to this is when a ventricular septal defect, because of its size, location, or configuration, leads to underdevelopment of the left ventricular outflow tract and/or ascending or transverse aorta. While this meets criteria for causing maldevelopment, it might be very difficult to address surgically in the fetus.

Atrial septal defect

As discussed above, the intra-atrial communication by the patent foramen ovale or other intra-atrial shunt is essential for normal fetal circulation. After birth, isolated atrial septal defects are rarely life-threatening and are virtually always amenable to surgical repair. Therefore, fetal closure of atrial septal defects is not indicated.

Other lesions

A number of lesions are likely to be more appropriately treated postnatally. These lesions, which generally are not associated with irreversible secondary lesions, include transposition of the great arteries, total anomalous pulmonary venous return, and truncus arteriosus.

Experimental fetal cardiac surgery

Carpenter et al. (1986) reported a case of fetal complete atrioventricular block and hydrops. After conventional medical management failed, they attempted pacing of the right ventricle using a pacing catheter passed directly across the maternal abdomen and fetal thorax into the right ventricular cavity. The fetus was successfully paced for over 4 h before fetal asystole ensued. Crombleholme et al. (1990) recently reported epicardial pacing in fetal lambs with experimentally produced complete heart block.

Anderson, Askin & Pupkin (1983) used cryosurgical treatment of the ductus arteriosus in the fetal sheep, which successfully maintained ductal patency after birth. Although this therapy would have applications in a vast number of ductal dependent lesions, to our knowledge, it has not yet been attempted in humans.

Turley et al. (1982) created simulated congenital cardiac lesions in a group of fetal sheep by placing bands around either the main pulmonary artery or the ascending aorta. They subsequently performed in utero repair of two simulated semilunar valve obstructions by performing open balloon dilatation.

Bical et al. (1987) also created simulated pulmonary stenosis in a large number of fetal sheep. They subsequently performed in utero repair by clamping and patching the pulmonary artery without cardiopulmonary bypass.

Allan et al. (1983) have performed transuterine valvuloplasty to dilate critically stenotic aortic valves in two fetuses. In one fetus, attempts to position the balloon across the aortic valve were unsuccessful. In the other fetus, obstruction was successfully relieved and the fetus remained in utero for 1 week prior to preterm delivery. A repeat valvuloplasty was performed on the first day of postnatal life, but the infant died 5 weeks later of complex problems including renal failure. Marked endocardial fibroelastosis was present, and no significant changes in left ventricular morphology were noted following the procedure, probably due to the short in utero postoperative period prior to delivery. The safety and efficacy of this treatment is unclear, but the technique is promising.

The cardiac surgeon has a large repertoire of techniques to allow intracardiac repair in the infant and adult. These same techniques will be applicable to fetal cardiac surgery. Pulmonary artery occlusion, hypothermic arrest, and cardiopulmonary bypass have all been performed in the fetal lamb model (Verrier, 1989). Each of these techniques holds promise. Stevens et al. (1988) studied in fetal lambs the circulatory effects of acute pulmonary artery occlusion, a technique that might allow in utero repair of the pulmonary valve (Adzick et al., 1984). Using microspheres, blood flow to various organs was measured prior to, during, and after 30 min of pulmonary artery occlusion. Their results demonstrated that brain and heart blood flows increased in response to pulmonary artery occlusion, and these flows increased further above baseline after occlusion was released. Conversely, combined ventricular output and flows to the lungs, kidney, and placenta all decreased in response to pulmonary artery occlusion, and all increased toward baseline after occlusion was released. Although these results suggest that this technique is feasible, the residual diminished blood flows after release of occlusion, particularly to the placenta (68% of baseline), are worrying. Adzick et al. (1984) performed surface cooling of six exteriorized fetal lambs to produce moderate hypothermia (22–25 °C), under the assumption that this might provide enough myocardial protection to allow for intracardiac repair (Stevens et al., 1988). After rewarming, some fetuses were electively sacrificed while the others were allowed to survive beyond term delivery, demonstrating that viability is possible following fetal hypothermic arrest. Richter et al. (1985) performed hypothermic cardiopulmonary bypass in nine fetal lambs (128 to 135 days gestation), using right atrial and ascending aortic cannulae, a roller pump, the placenta as the oxygenator, and microspheres to measure blood flows. They demonstrated that, during 10 min of bypass, all organ flows decreased, although flows to left ventricle and brain decreased relatively less than flows to other organs. During bypass, tissue oxygen requirements were probably met, as demonstrated by only a mild decrease in fetal arterial pH. Following bypass, organ blood flows increased, with flows to the left ventricle and brain increasing above baseline levels. However, kidney and, more importantly, placental blood flows remained below baseline (53% & 37% of baseline respectively), suggesting placental blood flow and, therefore, fetal viability, may remain significantly compromised following cardiopulmonary bypass using the placenta as the oxygenator. Fetal compromise was further suggested by the presence of postbypass acidemia. Seven of the nine fetuses survived bypass. Russo, Hanson & Dunn (1988) and Dunn et al. (1989) have utilized modified cardiopulmonary bypass with mild hypothermia (30 °C) in 21 fetal lambs between 90 and 140 days gestation. (Fig. 18.6). The technique is technically feasible even in the younger animals. Venous cannulation sites included the superior vena cava, inferior vena cava, right atrium or left atrium. Both single and double venous cannulae techniques were employed. In addition to right-sided cannulation, a left atrial cannula appeared necessary to accomplish complete cardiopulmonary bypass. Arterial cannulation sites included the ascending aorta, carotid artery (right, left or common), or ductus arteriosus. During bypass, PO_2 remained normal but PCO_2 was abnormally elevated. All fetuses survived replacement into the uterus, but hypercapnia without hypoxaemia persisted, resulting in eventual demise of all fetuses. The authors' results correlate with those of Richter et al. (1985), suggesting that circulatory changes, including severe umbilical–placental vasoconstriction, obviate against the use of the placenta for gas exchange during bypass. Thus an artificial oxygenator in the bypass circuit is necessary for fetal viability during bypass. Recently, Russo et al. (1988)

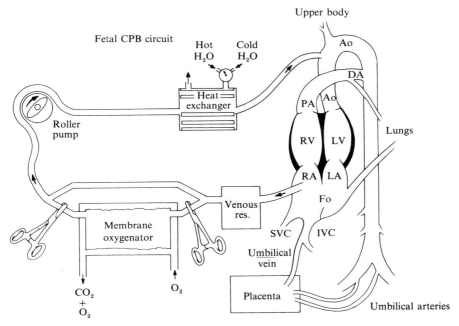

Fig. 18.6. Cardiopulmonary bypass circuitry for a fetal lamb. Although the placenta remains in the circuit, umbilical blood flow is reduced during bypass, and an artificial membrane oxygenator is essential for adequate gas exchange.

and Dunn et al. (1989) have been able to inhibit the umbilical vaso-constriction with aggressive pretreatment with α blockers and/or nitro-prusside and nitroglycerine. Improvement in fetal hypothermic cardiopulmonary bypass techniques will be crucial to the future develop-ment of fetal cardiac surgery.

Conclusion

The prenatal diagnosis of fetal cardiac lesions, the futility or inadequacy of conventional postnatal management of some cardiac lesions and early success following non-cardiac fetal surgery all suggest a role for fetal cardiac surgery in the future. Certainly, this mode of therapy will not replace traditional postnatal surgical repair. However, adding it to the surgical armament will greatly increase the surgical options, and salvage infants with lesions that today are only palliatable.

Before fetal cardiac surgery becomes a clinical reality, its safety to both

392   *Jeffrey M. Dunn* et al.

the mother and fetus must be demonstrated, the moral and ethical questions must be addressed, and belief that fetal surgical intervention can return the circulation to a more normal state must be confirmed, thus stimulating a more normal cardiac development. Simply stated, fetal cardiac surgery can only become practical if it is demonstrated to be clearly superior to traditional postnatal intervention.

References

Abrams, J. S. (1972). Fetal surgery in sheep: Technique and results of fifty-three intrauterine procedures. *Journal of Surgical Research,* **13**, 249–59.

Adzick, N. S., Harrison, M. R., Slate, R. K., Glick, P. L. & Villa, R. (1984). Surface cooling and rewarming the fetus: A technique for experimental fetal cardiac operation. *Surgery,* **35**, 314–16.

Adzick, N. S., Harrison, M. R., Glick, P. L., Anderson, J., Villa, R. L., Flake, A. W. & Laberge, J. M. (1986). Fetal surgery in the primate III. Maternal outcome after fetal surgery. *Journal of Pediatric Surgery,* **21**, 477–80.

Allan, L. D. (1986). Pulmonary atresia in prenatal life. *Journal of the American College of Cardiology,* **8**, 1131–6.

Allan, L. D., Anderson, R. H., Sullivan, I. D., Campbell, S., Holt, D. W. & Tynan, M. (1983). Evaluation of fetal arrhythmias by echocardiography. *British Heart Journal,* **50**, 240–5.

Allan, L. D., Chita, S. K., Anderson, R. H., Fagg, N., Crawford, D. & Tynan, M. J. (1988). Coarctation of the aorta in prenatal life: an echocardiographic, anatomical, and functional study. *British Heart Journal,* **59**, 356–60.

Anderson, P. A. W., Askin, F. B. & Pupkin, M. J. (1983). Cryosurgery of the fetal ductus arteriosus. *Journal of the American College of Cardiology,* **51**, 1446–50.

Bailey, L. L., Assaad, A. N., Tremm, R. F., Nehlsen-Cannarella, S. L., Kanakriyeh, M. S., Haas, G. S. & Jacobson, J. G. (1988). Orthotopic transplantation during early infancy as therapy for incurable congenital heart disease. *Annals of Surgery,* **45**, 279–86.

Bical, O., Gallix, P., Toussaint, M., Hero, M., Karam, J., Sidi, D. & Neveux, J. Y. (1987). Intrauterine creation and repair of pulmonary artery stenosis in the fetal lamb. *Thoracic and Cardiovascular Surgery,* **93**, 761–6.

Carpenter, R. J., Jr., Strasburger, J. F., Garson, A., Jr., Smith, R. T., Deter, R. L. & Engelhardt, H. T., Jr. (1986). Fetal ventricular pacing for hydrops secondary to complete atrioventricular block. *Journal of the American College of Cardiology,* **8**, 1434–6.

Claycomb, W. C. & Lanson, N. A., Jr. (1987). Proto-oncogene expression in proliferating and differentiating cardiac and skeletal muscle. *Biochemical Journal,* **247**, 701–6.

Crombleholme, T. M., Harrison, M. R., Langer, J. C., Longaker, M. T., Anderson, R. L., Slotnick, N. S., Filly, R. A., Callen, P. W., Goldstein, R. B. & Golbus, M. S. (1988). Early experience with open fetal surgery for congenital hydronephrosis. *Journal of Pediatric Surgery,* **23**, 1114–21.

Crombleholme, T. M., Harrison, M. R., Longaker, M. T., Langer, J. C.,

Adzick, N. S., Bradley, S., Duncan, B. & Verrier, E. D. (1990). Complete heart block in fetal lambs. I. Technique and acute physiological response. *Journal of Pediatric Surgery,* **25**, 587–93.

de Araujo, L. M. L., Schmidt, K., Silverman, N. H. & Finkbeiner, W. E. (1987). Prenatal detection of truncus arteriosus by ultrasound. *Pediatric Cardiology,* **8**, 261–3.

Dunn, J. M., Balsara, R. K., Heckman, J., Hanson, M. & Russo, P. (1989). Technical considerations of fetal cardiopulmonary bypass. Presented at the Society for the Study of Fetal Physiology, 16th Meeting, Reading, Pa.

Ettedgui, J. A., Sharland, G. K., Chita, S. K., Cook, A., Fagg, N. & Allan, L. D. (1990). Absent pulmonary valve syndrome with ventricular septal defect: Role of the arterial duct. *American Journal of Cardiology,* **66**, 233–4.

Evans, M. I., Drugan, A., Manning, F. A. & Harrison, M. R. (1989). Fetal surgery in the 1990's. *American Journal of Disease in Childhood,* **143**, 1431–6.

Fishman, N. H., Hof, R. B., Rudolph, A. M. & Heymann, M. A. (1978). Models of congenital heart disease in fetal lambs. *Circulation,* **58**, 354–64.

Freda, V. J. & Adamson, F. J. (1964). Exchange transfusion in utero: Report of a case. *American Journal of Obstetrics and Gynecology,* **89**, 817–21.

Gessner, I. H. (1966). Spectrum of congenital cardiac anomalies produced in chick embryos by mechanical interference with cardiogenesis. *Circulation Research,* **18**, 625–32.

Groenenberg, I. A. L., Wladimiroff, J. W. & Hop, W. C. J. (1989). Fetal cardiac and peripheral arterial flow velocity waveforms in intrauterine growth retardation. *Circulation,* **80**, 1711–17.

Hamamoto, K., Iwamoto, H. S., Roman, C. M., Benet, L. Z. & Rudolph, A. M. (1990). Fetal uptake of intraamniotic digoxin in sheep. *Pediatric Research,* **27**, 282–5.

Harh, J. Y., Paul, M. H., Gallen, W. J., Friedberg, D. Z. & Kaplan, S. (1973). Experimental production of hypoplastic left heart syndrome in the chick embryo. *American Journal of Cardiology,* **31**, 51–6.

Harrison, M. R., Anderson, J., Rosen, M. A., Ross, N. A. & Hendrick, A. G. (1982). Fetal surgery in the primate I. Anesthetic, surgical, and tocolytic management to maximize survival. *Journal of Pediatric Surgery,* **17**, 115–22.

Harrison, M. R., Langer, J. C., Adzick, N. S., Golbus, M. S., Filly, R. A., Anderson, R. L., Rosen, M. A., Callen, P. W., Goldstein, R. B. & deLorimier, A. A. (1990). Correction of congenital diaphragmatic hernia in utero, V. Initial clinical experience. *Journal of Pediatric Surgery,* **25**, 47–57.

Huhta, J. C., Cohen, A. W. & Wood, D. C. (1990). Premature constriction of the ductus arteriosus. *Journal of the American Society of Echocardiography,* **3**, 30–4.

Jones, K. L. (1988). *Smith's recognizable patterns of human malformation.* W. B. Saunders Co., Philadelphia.

Kirby, M. L. & Waldo, M. S. (1990). Role of neural crest in congenital heart disease. *Circulation,* **82**, 332–40.

Kirshon, B. Mari, G., Moise, K. J., Jr. & Wasserstrum, N. (1990). Effect of indomethacin on the fetal ductus arteriosus during treatment of symptomatic polyhydramnios. *Journal of Reproductive Medicine,* **35**, 529–32.

Kleinman, C. S., Copel, J. A. & Hobbins, J. C. (1987). Combined echocardiographic and Doppler assessment of fetal congenital atrioventricular block. *British Journal of Obstetrics and Gynaecology,* **94,** 967–74.

Lev, M., Arcella, R., Remolde, H. J. A., Licata, R. H. & Gasul, B. M. (1963). Premature narrowing or closure of the foramen ovale. *American Heart Journal,* **65,** 638–47.

Liley, A. W. (1963). Intrauterine transfusion of foetus in haemolytic disease. *British Medical Journal,* **2,** 1107–9.

Ludomirski, A., Nemiroff, R., Johnson, A., Ashmead, G. G., Weiner, S. & Bolognese, R. J. (1987). Percutaneous umbilical blood sampling: A new technique for prenatal diagnosis. *Journal of Reproductive Medicine,* **32,** 276–9.

Ludomirski, A. & Weiner, S. (1988). Percutaneous fetalumbilical blood sampling. *Clinical Obstetrics and Gynecology,* **31,** 19–26.

Machado, M. V. L., Crawford, D. C., Anderson, R. H. & Allan, L. D. Atrioventricular septal defect in prenatal life (1988*a*). *British Heart Journal,* **59,** 352–5.

Machado, M. V. I., Tynan, M. J., Curry, P. V. I. & Allan, L. D. (1988*b*). Fetal complete heart block. *British Heart Journal,* **60,** 512–15.

Maxwell, D. J., Allan, L. D. & Tynan, M. J. (1991). Balloon aortic valvotomy in the fetus: A report of two cases. *British Heart Journal,* in press.

Maxwell, D. J., Crawford, D. C., Curry, P. V. M., Tynan, M. J. & Allan, L. D. (1988). Obstetric importance, diagnosis, and management of fetal tachycardias. *British Medical Journal,* **297,** 107–10.

Nadler, H. L. & Gerbie, A. B. (1970). Role of amniocentesis in the intrauterine detection of genetic disorders. *New England Journal of Medicine,* **282,** 596–9.

Nakayama, D. K., Harrison, M. R., Seron-Ferre, M. & Villa, R. L. (1984). Fetal surgery in the primate II. Uterine electromyographic response to operative procedures and pharmacologic agents. *Journal of Pediatric Surgery,* **19,** 333–9.

Pigott, J. D., Murphy, J. D., Barber, G. & Norwood, W. I. (1988). Palliative reconstructive surgery for hypoplastic left heart syndrome. *Annals of Thoracic Surgery,* **45,** 122–8.

Pringle, K. C. (1986). In utero surgery. In *Advances in Surgery.* ed. J. A. Mannick. vol. 19, 101–38.

Redwin, F. & Petres, R. E. (1983). Fetal surgery – past, present and future. *Clinics in Perinatology,* **10,** 399–409.

Reed, K. L. (1989). Doppler ultrasound studies of human fetal blood flow. *Circulation,* **80,** 1914–17.

Richter, Slate, R. K., Rudolph, A. M. & Turley, K. (1985). Fetal blood flow during hypothermic cardiopulmonary bypass in utero. *Journal of Cardiovascular Surgery,* **26,** 86.

Rudolph, A. M. (1974). The Fetal Circulation. In *Congenital Heart Disease.* Year Book Medical Publishers, Inc. pp. 1–16.

Russo, P. A., Hanson, M. & Dunn, J. M. (1988). Fetal cardiopulmonary bypass without artificial oxygenator. *American Journal of Cardiology,* **62,** 503.

Schmidt, K. G. & Silverman, N. H. (1988). Evaluation of the fetal heart by ultrasound. In *Ultrasonography in Obstetrics and Gynecology,* ed. P.W. Callen. pp. 165–206. W.B.Saunders Co., Philadelphia.

Simpson, P. C. (1989). Proto-oncogenes and cardiac hypertrophy. *Annual Review of Physiology*, **51**, 189–202.

Stevens, M. B., Hill, A. C., Turley, K. & Hoffman, J. I. E. (1988). Circulatory responses to pulmonary artery occlusion in fetal lambs. *Circulation*, **71** (Supp.II), p. 1187.

Turley, K., Vlahakes, G. J., Harrison, M. R., Messina, L., Hanley, F., Uhlig, P. N. & Ebert, P. A. (1982). Intrauterine cardiothoracic surgery: the fetal lamb model. *Annals of Thoracic Surgery*, **34**, 422–6.

Verrier, E.D. (1989). Fetal cardiac surgery. *Annual of Cardiac Surgery*, 3–7.

19

Persistent fetal circulation: principles of diagnosis and management

SHEILA G. HAWORTH

Introduction

The term persistent fetal circulation implies a postnatal right to left shunt through the ductus arteriosus, foramen ovale or both. William Harvey first described the fetal circulation correctly (see p. 160) (Harvey, 1628). In 1628 he emphasized that Aristotle had been correct in saying that the fetal heart pulsates and went on to say that the heart 'propels the blood . . . from the vena cava to the aorta throught the cavities of both ventricles, the right one receiving blood from the auricle and propelling it by the vena arteriosa, or pulmonary artery, and its continuation named the ductus arteriosus, into the aorta; the left which has received its supply through the foramen ovale from the vena cava, contracting and project-ing the blood through the root of the aorta into the trunk of that vessel. In the embryo, whilst the lungs are yet in a state of inanition nature uses the two ventricles of the heart as if they form but one, for the trans mission of the blood'. Harvey then described persistence of the fetal circulation in 'the unripe births of mankind'.

In 1950 Novelo et al. described persistence of the fetal flow pattern in the presence of pulmonary hypertension (Novelo, Limon Lason & Bouchard, 1950). In 1952 Lind and Wegelius, injecting contrast material into the umbilical vein observed that the foramen ovale had either failed to close or had reopened in several asphyxiated babies (Lind & Wegelius, 1952). These investigators subsequently carried out venous angiography on 30 cyanosed infants during the first week of life and demonstrated a right to left atrial shunt in all and a reversed flow from the pulmonary artery to the aorta in three babies (Lind & Wegelius, 1954). James and Rowe (1957) studied normal newborns in whom the circulation had adapted to extra-uterine life and by exposing them to a short period of hypoxia were able to induce a return to the fetal flow pattern, emphasizing the lability of the newborn circulation. Studies carried out between 1959 and 1965 demonstrated right to left shunting in the presence of asphyxia (James, Burnard & Rowe, 1961), the respiratory distress syndrome and meconium aspiration (Rowe, 1959; Rudolph et al., 1961; Stahlman et al., 1966). Greater recognition of the clinical problem followed the presentation of a paper by Gersony, Duc and Sinclair (1969) in which persistence of the fetal circulation was described in two babies with pulmonary hypertension. The association between congenital heart disease and transitional right to left ductal and atrial shunting was described by Rowe (1959). Preservation of the fetal flow pattern is life-saving in many infants with congenital heart disease who first present to the cardiologist when the ductus arteriosus closes.

Thus persistence of the fetal circulation is caused either by pulmonary hypertension in the presence of an anatomically normal heart, or by pulmonary hypertension due to congenital heart disease, as in, for example, obstructed total anomalous pulmonary venous drainage. In addition, flow through the fetal channels persists after birth when either right or left heart output is obstructed or impaired. In such instances flow may be left to right through the ductus arteriosus or foramen ovale. *Persistence of the fetal circulation is therefore not a diagnosis but a manifestation of many abnormalities and diseases.* Accurate diagnosis of the underlying cause requires a logical approach to the problem. This is facilitated by understanding the physiology of the principal causes of persistent fetal circulation (Fig. 19.1) which can be summarized as follows:

1. Failure of the pulmonary circulation to adapt normally to extra-uterine life, either idiopathic or secondary to pulmonary disorders.
2. Persistent fetal circulation due to obstructed pulmonary venous drainage.
3. Persistence of an abnormal fetal circulation due to left ventricular outflow obstruction.
4. Persistence of an abnormal fetal circulation due to obstructed or impaired right ventricular outflow.
5. Persistence of the fetal circulation due to ventricular dysfunction.
6. Persistence of the fetal circulation due to 'obligatory' shunts.

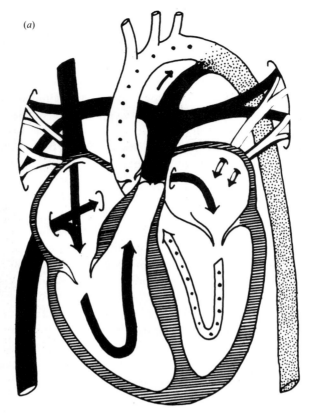

Fig. 19.1(*a*). Persistent pulmonary hypertension, indicating right to left shunts at ductal and atrial level.

Principal causes of persistent fetal circulation

Failure of the pulmonary circulation to adapt normally to extrauterine life: either idiopathic or secondary to pulmonary disorders (see Fig. 19.1(a))

Physiology

Failure of the pulmonary circulation to adapt normally to extrauterine life is usually caused by hypoxic lung disorders, congenital or acquired. Less than 20% of cases are idiopathic (Drummond, 1984). The peripheral pulmonary arteries retain their thick walled fetal appearance (Fig. 19.2) and pulmonary vascular resistance remains high (Haworth & Reid, 1976). Blood continues to shunt from right to left across the ductus arteriosus. Right ventricular and right atrial pressures are elevated, the

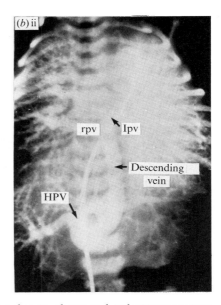

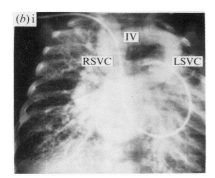

Fig. 19.1(*b*). Persistent fetal circulation due to obstructed pulmonary venous return. (i) Supradiaphragmatic total anomalous pulmonary venous return. Cineangiogram showing pulmonary venous blood draining into left superior vena cava (LSVC), thence into innominate vein (IV) to right superior vena cava (RSVC) and right atrium. Tortuous intrapulmonary arteries indicate pulmonary hypertension. (ii) Infradiaphragmatic total anomalous pulmonary venous return. Cineangiogram showing right and left pulmonary veins (RPV & LPV) draining to common pulmonary vein, which descends below the diaphragm to drain into hepatic sinusoids and thence to inferior vena cava. (Reproduced with permission from: Sullivan, I.D., & Gooch, V.M. (1991). Venous anomalies. In *Clinical Ultrasound,* ed. H. Meire, K.C. Dewbury, D.O. Cosgrove & P. Wilde. Churchill Livingstone, in press.)

flap valve of the fossa ovalis remains open and a right to left atrial shunt persists. Cross-sectional echocardiography reveals right-to-left bulging of the atrial septum.

Pulmonary hypoplasia causes persistent pulmonary hypertension because the pulmonary vasculature is underdeveloped. Such abnormalities include congenital diaphragmatic hernia, renal agenesis or dysplasia and rhesus isoimmunization (Fig. 19.3) (Hislop & Reid, 1981).

Differential diagnosis

Is the cyanosis primarily pulmonary or cardiac in origin? The distinction is made on the basis of the obstetric and postnatal history, the clinical

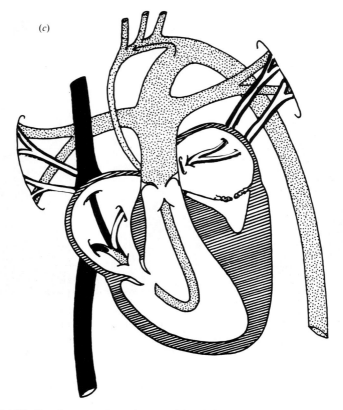

Fig. 19.1(*c*). Persistence of an abnormal fetal circulation due to obstructed left ventricular outflow, showing a right-to-left ductal shunt and a left-to-right atrial shunt.

findings and the response to hyperoxia. The presence of congenital heart disease is excluded or confirmed by cross-sectional echocardiography. Colour flow imaging and Doppler techniques demonstrate the direction and magnitude of ductal and interatrial shunting and permit non-invasive determination of the pulmonary arterial pressure. Thus cardiac catheterization is no longer required to confirm the diagnosis of persistent fetal circulation and is seldom required to define the nature of an intracardiac abnormality. In babies with pulmonary hypertension due to parenchymal lung disease the pulmonary vascular resistance falls on inhalation of 100% oxygen, right to left shunting decreases and the systemic arterial oxygen tension usually increases by more than 100 mm Hg (Lees & Sunderland, 1981). In cyanotic congenital heart disease inhalation of

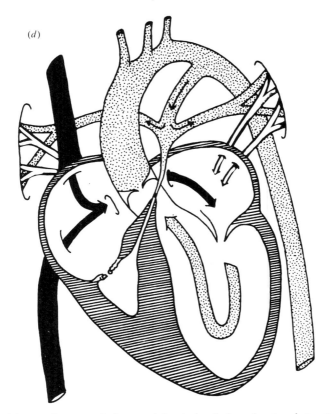

Fig. 19.1(*d*). Persistence of abnormal fetal circulation due to obstructed right ventricular outflow, showing a left to right ductal shunt and a right to left atrial shunt.

100% oxygen usually fails to increase the systemic arterial oxygen tension by more than 20 mm Hg. However, a more marked increase in arterial oxygen tension does occur occasionally in cyanotic congenital heart disease and, conversely, refractory hypoxaemia in persistent fetal circulation due to lung disease. The predictive value of the hyperoxia test is improved when 100% oxygen is given by face mask and continuous positive airway pressure (10 cm water) is applied (Shannon, Lusser & Goldblatt, 1972). The greatest discrimination is seen when newborn infants are manually ventilated through an endotracheal tube at a fast rate, to achieve a low PCO_2 and a pH greater than 7.55 (Fox & Duara, 1983). In babies with pulmonary hypertension due to parenchymal lung disease the systemic arterial PO_2 usually increases by 50–100 mm Hg.

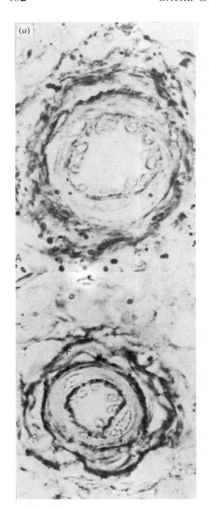

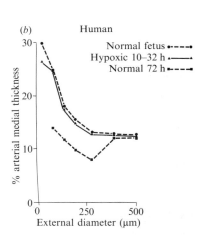

(b) Human

Normal fetus •----•
Hypoxic 10–32 h ▲———▲
Normal 72 h ■----■

% arterial medial thickness

External diameter (μm)

Fig. 19.2 (*a*). Photomicrographs of alveolar wall arteries from the lung of a baby who died 24 hours after an hypoxic delivery, showing an unadapted thick walled artery. m = media. (*b*). Pulmonary arterial medial thickness related to external diameter showing that the mean percentage arterial medial thickness of seven infants dying at between 10 and 32 hours of age was similar to the normal fetal level and greater than that in normals of similar age.

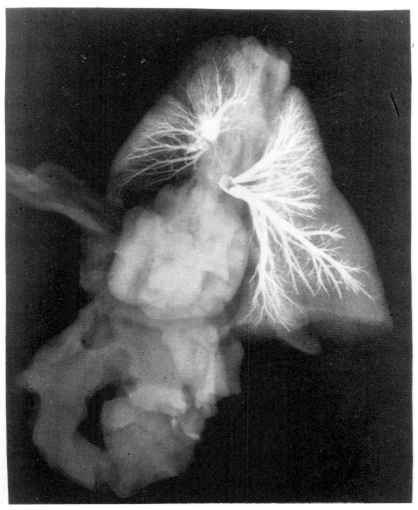

Fig. 19.3. Postmortem arteriogram of the lungs of a newborn infant with congenital diaphragmatic hernia showing hypoplasia of both lungs and their vasculature. (Reproduced with permission from Kitagawa, M., Hislop, A.A., Boyden, E.A. & Reid, L. (1971).)

Using this approach the hyperoxia test is not foolproof but it is helpful. However, it can be unnecessarily invasive and disturbing in babies who have been maintained satisfactorily without mechanical ventilation. The combination of clinical judgment, the chest X-ray and cross-sectional echocardiography and Doppler studies should suffice to make the diagnosis of persistent fetal circulation and its cause.

Persistent fetal circulation of pulmonary origin

The majority of babies with persistent fetal circulation due to pulmonary hypertension in the presence of an anatomically normal heart have lung disease (Table 19.1). Meconium aspiration is the commonest problem. Such babies and those who have developed hyaline membrane disease or have transient tachypnoea of the new born can be cyanosed and show signs of respiratory distress, tachypnoea, intercostal and subcostal recession, râles, bronchi and wheezing, as detailed in Chapter 10. Accentuation of the pulmonary component of the second heart sound can be difficult to confirm in distressed, tachypnoeic infants with tachycardia. A systolic murmur at the lower left sternal border can frequently be heard due to functional tricuspid regurgitation. The ECG usually shows nonspecific changes and is most helpful in identifying babies with congenital heart disease. On the chest radiograph, the appearance of the lung fields may be diagnostic. Patchy atelectasis and focal hyperaeration are seen following aspiration but the degree of lung involvement may be less than expected given the severity of the hypoxaemia, particularly in cases of meconium aspiration. In hyaline membrane disease with a dominantly right to left ductal shunt, the lung fields may have a ground glass

Table 19.1. *Pulmonary disorders causing PFC*

Aspiration of meconium, amniotic fluid, blood
Severe intrapartum hypoxia
Pulmonary infection
Pulmonary haemorrhage
Hyaline membrane disease
Transient tachypnoea of the newborn

Congenital diaphragmatic hernia
Pulmonary hypoplasia
Thrombo emboli
Congenital abnormalities of alveolar development

appearance and an air bronchogram. Small pneumothoraces or a pneumomediastinum can be overlooked. In transient tachypnoea of the newborn the clearance of intrapulmonary fluid is delayed and the chest radiograph usually shows fluffy opacified areas which disappear during the first 2–3 days of life.

In some babies with persistent pulmonary hypertension there is a history of prenatal or intrapartum asphyxia (Haworth, 1979). The lung fields are clear on the chest radiograph. Depending upon the duration and severity of the hypoxic insult, the pulmonary vascular resistance usually falls more rapidly than in babies who have aspirated.

Approximately 20% of cases of persistent pulmonary hypertension are idiopathic (Drummond, 1984). In these, there appears to be a primary failure of the pulmonary circulation to adapt normally to extrauterine life and pulmonary vascular resistance remains elevated. Typically, the pregnancy and labour have been normal and the baby is born at term (Haworth & Reid, 1976). Mild cyanosis is noticed during the first few hours of life, but the baby is not hypoxic or acidotic initially and the lung fields are clear on the chest radiograph. When treated with tolazoline and/or prostacyclin there may be an initial improvement but cyanosis usually increases and eventually there is no response to increasing doses of medication (Fig. 19.6). The baby becomes hypoxaemic and acidotic despite the administration of vasodilator drugs and mechanical ventilation and usually dies between one week and three months of age.

Natural history

Treatment is supportive, because the mechanisms underlying normal adaptation of the pulmonary circulation to extrauterine life are not understood. This means maintaining body temperature and correcting the hypoxaemia and acidosis which promote vasoconstriction. Tolazoline or prostacyclin are given to aid pulmonary vasodilatation but are not selective pulmonary vasodilators, and therefore careful monitoring of the systemic arterial pressure is essential. When appropriate, surfactant replacement therapy is given and in critically ill babies inotropic agents are required (Hallman & Kankaanpaa, 1980). Extra corporeal membrane oxygenation can allow time for the lungs to recover (Bartlett et al., 1985). Recent experience has shown that inhaled nitric oxide is an extremely effective pulmonary vasodilator in babies with persistent pulmonary hypertension, acting selectively on the pulmonary vasculature and improving ventilation : perfusion matching. In some babies its use can obviate the need for extracorporeal membrane oxygenation.

Pathological findings

In babies who die with idiopathic persistent pulmonary hypertension or as a result of intrauterine or intrapartum hypoxia without parenchymal lung damage, post mortem examination shows that the pulmonary arteries within the respiratory unit have the thick walled undilated appearance of fetal vessels (Haworth, 1979; McKenzie & Haworth, 1981; Raine et al., 1991). In those dying after the first few days of life the medial smooth muscle cells are differentiated prematurely into a more contractile phenotype than normal, connective tissue deposition in and around the media is excessive, and the vessel appears to have become fixed in an incompletely dilated state (Raine et al., 1991). The vessel wall is also surrounded by sympathetic-like vasoconstrictor nerves. The change in morphological appearance with time emphasizes the vital importance of achieving pulmonary vasodilatation as soon as possible after birth. Changes are uniform throughout the lung. Similar abnormalities in the pulmonary vasculature are seen in babies in whom pulmonary hypertension is a consequence of lung disease when the changes are most severe in the regions of lung showing the greatest parenchymal damage.

Persistent fetal circulation due to obstructed pulmonary venous drainage (see Fig. 19.1(b))

Physiology

During fetal life only 8–10% of the combined ventricular output perfuses the pulmonary vascular bed (Rudolph, 1974) and therefore anomalous drainage of all the pulmonary veins into the systemic circulation (total anomalous pulmonary venous drainage) is usually well tolerated during fetal life. However, obstruction to pulmonary venous return can develop in utero and the baby is then born with thick walled excessively muscularized intrapulmonary arteries and veins (Fig. 19.4) (Haworth, 1982).

Total anomalous pulmonary venous drainage is described according to the route by which pulmonary venous blood returns to the heart (Table 19.2, Figs. 19.1(b)). In all children with total anomalous pulmonary

---

Fig. 19.4. Infra-diaphragmatic total anomalous pulmonary venous return, obstructed in utero. Photomicrographs of a 3 day-old showing (a) thick-walled muscular alveolar wall arteries, (b) thick-walled small pulmonary veins, (c) descending vertical vein obstructed by fibrosis tissue just above the diaphragm.

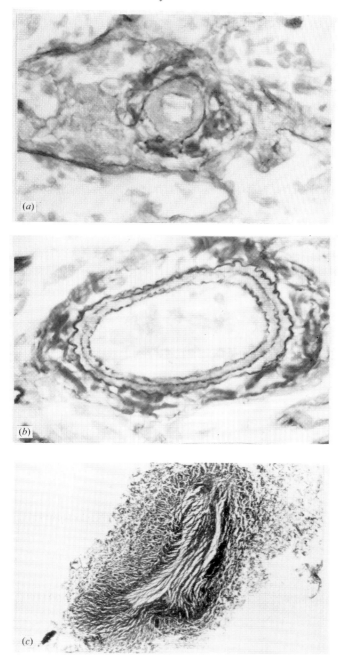

Fig. 19.4.

Table 19.2. *Classification of total
anomalous pulmonary venous
drainage*

	%
Supracardiac	50
Left superior vena cava	40
Right superior vena cava	10
Cardiac	25
Coronary sinus	20
Right atrium	5
Infradiaphragmatic	20
Mixed	5

Note: Adapted from Gersony, W. M.
(1979).

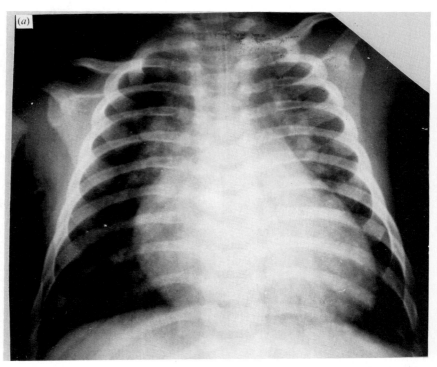

Fig. 19.5(*a*). Supracardiac total anomalous pulmonary venous return (TAPVR).
Chest radiograph showing cardiac enlargement and increased hilar vessel size.

venous drainage, after birth both pulmonary and systemic blood returns to the right atrium, the pressure in the right atrium exceeds that in the left, and the mixture of oxygenated and deoxygenated blood shunts from right to left atrium and is eventually ejected into the aorta. The physiological and therefore the clinical picture is determined by the presence or absence of obstruction to pulmonary venous return. In the absence of obstruction, pulmonary arterial pressure and vascular resistance fall after birth, right ventricular compliance decreases, the right ventricle becomes more thin walled relative to the left and pulmonary venous return to the right heart and then to the pulmonary artery increases (Fig. 19.5(*a*)). Pulmonary blood flow may be three times the systemic flow, which can remain normal. Such a high pulmonary blood flow ensures a relatively high systemic arterial oxygen saturation of 85% or more, and cyanosis will not be evident. By contrast, in the presence of obstruction to pulmonary venous drainage, right to left interatrial shunting will persist

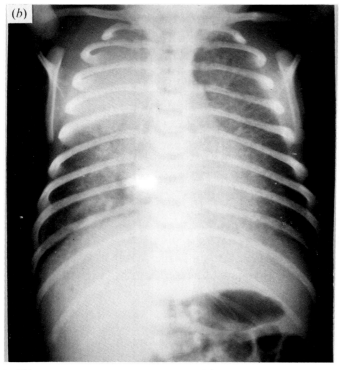

Fig. 19.5(*b*). Infradiaphragmatic TAPVR. Chest radiograph showing normal heart shadow and perihilar haze, fine nodular shadows and an opacification of right upper lobe due to pulmonary oedema.

Table 19.3. *Prevalence and site of obstruction*

Drainage site	Severe obstruction (%)	Site of obstruction
Left superior vena cava (LSVC)	40	LSVC compressed by L main bronchus ± stenosis at LSVC and innominate vein junction
Right superior vena cava (RSVC)	75	Common pulmonary venous channel and RSVC junction
Coronary sinus	10	Coronary sinus ostia
Right atrium	5	Pulmonary vein – right atrial junction
Infracardiac	nearly 100	At diaphragm, entrance to portal vein, hepatic capillaries, ductus venosus

All may have obstruction at foramen ovale

Note: Adapted from Gersony, W.M. (1979).

but less blood returns to the right atrium, the heart remains small, and the child is cyanosed (Fig. 19.5(*b*)). The pulmonary arterial pressure remains elevated and can become suprasystemic. A right to left shunt persists through the ductus arteriosus. Within the lung, the capillary hydrostatic pressure exceeds the plasma oncotic pressure and pulmonary oedema develops. Small pulmonary arteries and veins rapidly become as thick walled as those illustrated in Fig. 19.4.

Table 19.3 shows that severe obstruction develops commonly in all types of total anomalous pulmonary venous drainage save those in which blood returns to the coronary sinus or directly to the right atrium. Obstruction is almost inevitable in the presence of infradiaphragmatic total anomalous pulmonary venous return when closure of the ductus venosus forces the pulmonary venous blood through the hepatic venous bed.

The physiology of uncommon abnormalities such as cortriatriatum when obstructed, and pulmonary venous atresia or stenosis is akin to that of obstructed total anomalous pulmonary venous drainage. Left ventricular inflow obstruction, namely mitral atresia or critical stenosis or supramitral valve ring causes a high left atrial pressure and a left to right atrial shunt.

Clinical manifestations and principles of treatment

The clinical findings depend on the physiology. The magnitude of the pulmonary blood flow determines systemic arterial oxygen saturation and heart size (Fig. 19.5(*a*),(*b*)). In the presence of early pulmonary venous obstruction the baby is moderately cyanosed and shunts right to left across the ductus arteriosus, and the heart is small on X-ray (Fig. 19.5(*b*)). The differential diagnosis is between other conditions causing persistent pulmonary hypertension in the newborn. In the presence of severe obstruction, pulmonary oedema decreases lung compliance and the baby is dyspnoeic. Hepatic enlargement can result from a high pulmonary blood flow, a restricted foramen ovale or overinflated lungs.

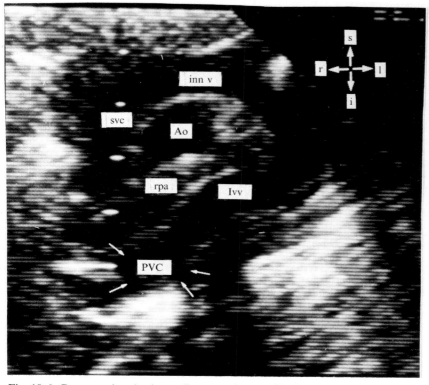

Fig. 19.6. Cross-sectional echocardiogram of supra-diaphragmatic TAPVR. Four pulmonary veins drain into the pulmonary venous confluence (PVC) which connects with a left vertical vein (LVV) to enter the innominate vein (Inn V), thence to the superior vena cava (SVC) to right atrium. RPA= right pulmonary artery. (Reproduced with permission from Sullivan, I.D. & Gooch, V.M. (1991).)

Tachycardia, poor peripheral pulses and peripheral cooling reflect a low systemic output. A systolic murmur is audible if the pulmonary vascular resistance is sufficiently low to permit a high flow through the pulmonary valve. The ECG is unhelpful, showing right ventricular dominance similar to that seen in healthy neonates. Cross-sectional echocardiography is usually diagnostic (Fig. 19.6) but it is probably more difficult to make a confident echocardiographic diagnosis in total anomalous pulmonary venous drainage than in any other condition. Since children with obstructed total anomalous pulmonary venous drainage deteriorate with alarming rapidity, even if the diagnosis is only suspected the baby should be transferred to a cardiac unit quickly for evaluation and, if necessary, immediate surgery. Before and during transfer the baby's condition can be immensely improved by treating acidosis and often by instituting mechanical ventilation to reduce pulmonary oedema and relieve the work of breathing. Infusing prostacyclin E_1 (0.01 μg/kg per min) dilates the ductus arteriosus to help perfuse the systemic circulation with oxygenated blood and may be helpful in dilating the ductus venosus in babies with infradiaphragmatic total anomalous pulmonary venous drainage.

In babies who survive neonatal surgery the long-term outlook is excellent.

Persistence of an abnormal fetal circulation due to left ventricular outflow obstruction (see Fig. 19.1(c))

Left ventricular outflow obstruction may be due to aortic atresia, critical aortic stenosis, an interrupted arch or severe coarctation of the aorta.

Physiology

In the presence of left ventricular outflow obstruction the systemic circulation is perfused by the right ventricle and pulmonary artery, before and after birth. Blood flows from left to right through the foramen ovale to increase right ventricular output and ductal flow. The aortic isthmus, brachiocephalic vessels and coronary arteries are perfused retrogradely across the ductus arteriosus. The abnormal fetal flow pattern does not usually embarass the fetus but the newborn is compromised as soon as the ductus begins to constrict. In each baby, the haemodynamic findings at cardiac catheterisation depend on the condition of the ductus arteriosus, foramen ovale and pulmonary vascular bed. If the ductus is at all constricted the right ventricular and pulmonary arterial pressure may exceed the systemic arterial pressure. Any restriction at the foramen ovale causes differences in the right and left atrial pressures. Severe foramenal restriction leads to pulmonary venous obstruction and pulmonary oedema. Oxygenated and deoxygenated blood mix in the right heart and the systemic arterial oxygen concentration correlates with the pulmonary blood flow. Babies become cyanosed when flow across the foramen ovale becomes restricted and pulmonary vascular resistance increases.

The abnormal fetal flow pattern and haemodynamics help explain the development of endocardial fibroelastosis, commonly seen in babies with aortic atresia or critical aortic stenosis particularly in the presence of a severely hypoplastic left ventricle. In critical aortic stenosis the degree of left ventricular hypoplasia and severity of endocardial fibroelastosis correlate with morbidity and mortality and severely affected infants do badly (Mocellin et al., 1983).

Clinical manifestations and principles of treatment

The clinical findings are determined by the site of obstruction, whether the left ventricular outflow or aortic arch, and its severity. The extreme example, aortic atresia, is usually associated with hypoplasia of the aortic arch and left ventricle and is known as the hypoplastic left heart syndrome. This syndrome is the commonest cardiac cause of death during the first week of life, in one study comprising 22% of deaths (Lambert, Canent & Hohn, 1966). The baby appears pink and well at birth but becomes acutely ill when the ductus closes. Respiratory symptoms predominate and the baby develops a shock-like state with tachypnoea, poor peripheral pulses, hepatomegaly and cold extremities. Auscultation reveals a loud single second sound, accompanied by a soft systolic murmur and possibly a tricuspid flow murmur. The ECG shows signs of right ventricular hypertrophy with ST and T wave changes and right atrial hypertrophy. Chest radiography shows a large globular heart with increased pulmonary vascular markings. The radiographic features of pulmonary venous obstruction indicate a restricted foramen ovale.

Infusion of prostaglandin E_1 maintains ductal patency to ensure perfusion before and during transfer to a cardiac unit (Fig. 19.7). Management is dictated by the type of abnormality. Urgent cardiac catheterization may be indicated to carry out atrial septostomy to relieve a restricted foramen ovale. The results of balloon angioplasty of critical aortic stenosis are similar to those achieved surgically. Results are poor using either approach.

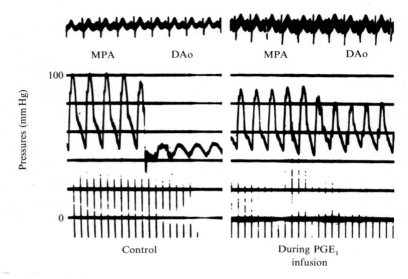

Fig. 19.7. Pressure tracing showing increase in systemic arterial pressure following infusion of PGE$_1$.

Persistence of an abnormal fetal circulation due to obstructed or impaired right ventricular outflow (see Fig. 19.1(d))

Physiology

Before and after birth, in the presence of tricuspid atresia, pulmonary atresia or critical pulmonary stenosis, a right to left atrial shunt persists and the pulmonary circulation is supported by the left ventricle and perfused through a left to right shunt across the ductus arteriosus (Fig. 19.8). Thus during fetal life both caval streams mix in the right atrium and there is no preferential streaming of oxygenated blood across the foramen ovale. The brain and upper part of the body is perfused with blood at an abnormally low PO_2. This does not appear to impair development. In the normal fetus, pulmonary blood flow is low. In the presence of obstructed right ventricular outflow the ductus is often small, arises at an acute angle from the descending thoracic aorta and closes soon after birth. The baby becomes deeply cyanosed rapidly and immediate survival depends upon maintaining ductal patency by infusion of prostaglandin E$_1$.

Right ventricular output can be severely reduced in Ebstein's anomaly. In Ebstein's anomaly the septal and posterior leaflets of the tricuspid

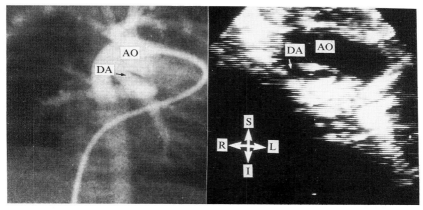

Fig. 19.8. Angiogram and cross-sectional echocardiogram showing ductus perfusing pulmonary artery in pulmonary atresia.

valve are displaced into the right ventricle and adhere to the inflow portion. Presentation in the newborn period is associated with severe right atrial dilatation and marked apical displacement of the tricuspid valve (Celermejer et al., 1991*a*). 80% of newborns present with cyanosis (Celermejer et al., 1991*b*). While the pulmonary vascular resistance is still elevated after birth, a considerable amount of blood is regurgitated into the right atrium with each right ventricular contraction. The pressure in the right atrium exceeds that in the left, and right to left shunting occurs. Systemic arterial desaturation can become marked when forward flow into the pulmonary circulation is low. Forward flow may be so low that the condition may mimic pulmonary stenosis or even atresia. In such babies the outlook is poor. One study reported a neonatal mortality of 18% (Calermajer et al., 1991*b*). Less severely affected infants improve as the pulmonary vascular resistance falls after birth.

Clinical manifestations and principles of treatment

In all these conditions, the clinical picture is determined by the magnitude of the pulmonary blood flow. In tricuspid atresia about half the patients present on the first day of life with cyanosis, tachypnoea, a prominent *a* wave in the jugular venous pulse when the foramen ovale is restrictive, and a single second heart sound (Dick, Fyler & Nadas, 1975). The lung fields are oligaemic on the chest X-ray. In the presence of an associated large ventricular septal defect pulmonary flow is high, cardiac failure develops during the first weeks of life and cyanosis is moderate. Chest radiography then shows a large heart with pulmonary plethora. In tricuspid atresia the ECG is characteristic, showing signs of right atrial hypertrophy, a reduction in right ventricular forces and a superior QRS axis. Pulmonary atresia and critical pulmonary stenosis present with severe cyanosis as the ductus closes. In all these conditions cross-sectional echocardiography defines the intracardiac anatomy. Cardiac catheterization is indicated to clarify the haemodynamic picture and to perform balloon atrial septostomy if a restrictive foramen ovale obstructs the flow of blood from right to left atrium. In the presence of a low pulmonary blood flow, medical management consists of giving prostaglandin E_1 to maintain ductal patency until a systemic–pulmonary shunt is carried out. Patients with a high pulmonary blood flow and pulmonary hypertension are at risk of developing pulmonary vascular disease which will preclude an intracardiac repair in late childhood. In such cases the pulmonary artery is banded.

Persistence of the fetal circulation due to ventricular dysfunction

In the presence of an anatomically normal heart myocardial disease can lead to impaired function of one or both ventricles. Asphyxia is the commonest cause of such a cardiomyopathy and may effect either ventricle causing a ductal shunt in either direction. Riemenschneider et al. (1976) and Fiddler et al. (1980) reported a total of 40 newborn infants with persistent pulmonary hypertension who improved with diuretic and inotropic therapy. Transient tricuspid regurgitation in newborn infants has also been attributed to intrauterine or intrapartum asphyxia (Boucek et al., 1976). The pathogenesis of asphyxia-induced cardiomyopathy is uncertain but coronary arterial thrombosis or embolism has been incriminated in some patients and rarely can lead to myocardial infarction. Other congenital cardiomyopathies include endocardial fibroelastosis and Pompe disease, both of which primarily affect the left ventricle.

Persistence of the fetal circulation due to 'obligatory' shunts
Physiology

The magnitude of many left to right shunts, such as those due to a ventricular septal defect or persistent ductus arteriosus is determined by the relative resistances of the pulmonary and systemic circulations. Others are not, and are therefore said to be obligatory (Rudolph, 1974).

Examples of these include a complete atrioventricular septal defect with a left ventricular to right atrial communication, a sinus of Valsalva fistula from aortic root to right atrium and a cerebral or hepatic arteriovenous malformation. All these malformations cause persistent pulmonary hypertension. A right to left shunt is usually present across the ductus, and also across the foramen ovale in babies with a cerebral arteriovenous malformation.

Babies with a cerebral arteriovenous malformation present in severe heart failure, with signs of a left to right shunt. They may have severe pulmonary hypertension and the pressure may be suprasystemic. Cranial bruits are not always heard. Cranial ultrasonography is indicated in newborns with unexplained congestive heart failure or persistent pulmonary hypertension.

Anticipation and recognition of persistent fetal circulation and its cause

The speed with which persistent fetal circulation is recognized and the underlying cause is diagnosed depends upon close liaison between obstetrician, neonatologist and, when appropriate, the paediatric cardiologist.

Obstetrician

The obstetrician can anticipate the development of persistent fetal circulation in a fetus compromised by diseases which reduce placental blood flow, maternal oxygen or blood pressure. Maternal ingestion of cyclo-oxygenase inhibitors such as aspirin, indomethacin and naproxin are thought to cause persistent fetal circulation by inducing intrauterine closure of the ductus arteriosus (Levin et al., 1978; Csaba, Sulyok & Ertle, 1978; Wilkinson, Aynsley-Green & Mitchell, 1979; Rudolph, 1981). Pulmonary blood flow is then excessive before birth and congestive cardiac failure develops after birth in fetuses who survive. Risk is related to gestational age at the time of drug administration, and presumably to the dose and duration of medication. In any patient unknown factors include the extent of placental drug transfer and metabolism. Inhibition of premature labour with cyclo-oxygenase inhibitors has not been associated with persistent pulmonary hypertension of the premature newborn. This is possibly because indomethacin causes reversable cyclo-oxygenase inhibition and does not cross the placenta until late gestation (Dudley & Hardie, 1985). The level of prostaglandin E increases towards term and the lower level in the preterm fetus may help maintain ductal patency when indomethacin is given.

Rarely, the obstetrician may be aware of a family history of persistent pulmonary hypertension in the newborn or of so-called primary pulmonary hypertension in childhood. The Eisenmenger syndrome in the mother is associated with a high fetal mortality. Babies who survive may be at risk of developing persistent fetal circulation.

Congenital heart disease may be diagnosed on routine four-chamber fetal echocardiography although the 'pick-up' rate is not yet satisfactory (Cullen et al., 1990). Extra-cardiac malformations such as congenital diaphragmatic hernia can also be detected. Certain chromosomal abnormalities are associated with congenital heart disease, the commonest being trisomy 21 in which between a third and a half of patients have congenital heart disease, usually an atrioventricular septal defect or a ventricular septal defect (VSD). Approximately 90% of infants with trisomy 18 and nearly all those with trisomy 13 have congenital heart disease, usually a VSD.

At delivery, intrapartum hypoxia and acidosis prejudice the fetus. Late cord clamping can lead to polycythaemia which increases pulmonary vascular resistance in the newborn. Elective Caesarian section may disturb the optimum balance of pulmonary vasodilator and vasoconstrictor prostanoids and so promote persistent pulmonary hypertension.

Neonatologist

The neonatologist first must distinguish between a pulmonary and cardiac cause of persistent fetal circulation and idiopathic persistent pulmonary hypertension. Recently, group B streptococcal infection has been associated with persistent pulmonary hypertension, as has Haemophilus influenzae, *Escherichia coli* and Listeria monocytogene (Shankaran, Farooki & Desai, 1982; Skidmore, Shennan & Hoslans, 1985).

If the advice of a paediatric cardiologist is sought, the telephone conversation between neonatologist and cardiologist can be structured in such a way that the likelihood of making a correct diagnosis is significantly increased (Franklin et al., 1991). A diagnostic algorithm has been designed which relies only on clinical examination, the hyperoxia test, a chest X-ray and ECG and does not require specialist knowledge (Fig. 19.9) (Franklin et al., 1991). The paediatrician and cardiologist can then

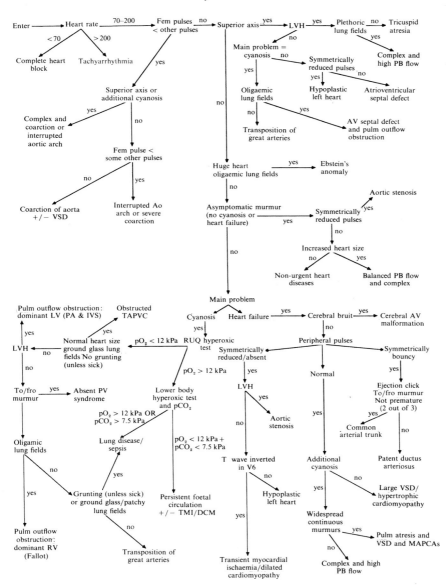

Fig. 19.9. Algorithm for use as an aid in the diagnosis of possible cardiovascular anomalies in the newborn. (Modified from Franklin et al. (1991).)

discuss the most appropriate form of treatment to be instituted in the neonatal nursery. They can discuss if, when and how best the baby should be transferred to a cardiac unit and the supportive treatment to be given during the journey. The outcome of newborn infants with severe congenital heart disease is mainly determined by the condition in which they arrive at a cardiac unit.

Cardiologist

A very sick baby requires supportive treatment while making a diagnosis as non-invasively as possible. Cross-sectional echocardiography and continuous wave Doppler studies are carried out immediately to diagnose the principal abnormality, ensure that this is the only abnormality and, if possible, ensure that all the information needed for immediate management is obtained. If a systemic pulmonary shunt is required, for example, then one needs to be sure that there is a central pulmonary artery present into which the shunt can be inserted. Cardiac catheterization is avoided in sick babies except when an intervention is indicated, such as balloon angioplasty of a critically stenosed valve, or when atrial septostomy is required.

When a sick baby is transferred to a cardiac unit, close liaison between obstetrician, paediatrician and cardiologist is essential in order to ensure the support of shocked and distressed parents.

Acknowledgement

The author wishes to thank Dr P Rees for helpful advice and encouragement.

References

Bartlett, R. H., Roloff, D. W., Cornell, R. G., Andrews, A. F., Dillon, P. W. & Zwischenberger, J. B. (1985). Extra corporeal circulation in neonatal respiratory failure: a prospective randomized study. *Pediatrics,* **76**, 479–87.

Boucek, R. J. Jr., Graham, T. P. Jr., Morgan, J. P., Atwood, G. F. & Boeth, R. E. (1976). Spontaneous resolution of massive congenital tricuspid insufficiency. *Circulation,* **54**, 795–800.

Celermejer, D. S., Cullen, S., Sullivan, I. D., Wyse, R. K. & Deanfield, J. E. (1991*a*). What happens to neonates with Ebstein's anomaly? *British Heart Journal,* **52** (abst).

Celermejer, D., Dodd, S. M., Greenwald, S. E., Wyse, R. K. H. & Deanfield, J. E. (1991*b*). Morbid anatomy in neonates with Ebstein's anomaly of the tricuspid valve: pathophysiological and clinical implications, in press.

Csaba, I. P., Sulyok, E. & Ertle, T. (1978). Relationship of maternal treatment with indomethacin to persistent fetal circulation syndrome. *Journal of Pediatrics*, **92**, 484.

Cullen, S., Franklin, R., Sharland, G., Allan, L. & Sullivan, I. (1990). Potential impact of population screening for prenatal diagnosis of congenital heart disease. *British Heart Journal*, **64** (1), 90.

Dick, M., Fyler, D. C. & Nadas, A. S. (1975) Tricuspid atresia: clinical course 101 patients. *American Journal of Cardiology*, **36**, 327–37.

Drummond, W. H. (1984). Persistent pulmonary hypertension of the newborn (persistent fetal circulation syndrome). *Advances in Pediatrics*, **30**, 61–91.

Dudley, D. K. & Hardie, M. J. (1985). Fetal and neonatal effects of indomethacin used as a tocolytic agent. *American Journal of Obstetrics and Gynecology*, **51**, 181–4.

Fiddler, G. I., Chatrath, R., Williams, G. J., Walker, O. R., & Scott, O. (1980). Dopamine infusion for the treatment of myocardial dysfunction associated with persistent transitional circulation. *Archives of Diseases in Childhood*, **55**, 194–8.

Fox, W. W. & Duara, S. (1983). Persistent pulmonary hypertension in the neonate: diagnosis and management. *Journal of Pediatrics*, **103**, 505–14.

Franklin, R. C. G., Spiegelhalter, D. J., Macartney, F. J. & Bull, K. (1991). Evaluation of a diagnostic algorithm for heart disease in neonates. *British Medical Journal*, **302**, 935–9.

Gersony, W. M. (1979). Presentation, diagnosis and natural history of TAPVD. In *Paediatric Cardiology*, ed. M.J. Godman & R. Marquis, vol. 2, Churchill Livingstone, London.

Gersony, W. M., Duc, G. V. & Sinclair, J. C. (1969). 'PFC' syndrome (persistence of the fetal circulation). (abstract). *Circulation*, **40** (suppl III), 87.

Hallman, M. & Kankaanpaa, K. (1980). Evidence of surfactant deficiency in persistence of the fetal circulation. *European Journal of Pediatrics*, **134**, 129–34.

Harvey, W. H. (1628). K. Exercitatio anatomica de motu cordiset sanguinis in animalibus. Francofurti: Fitzeri; quoted from the works of William Harvey MD, translated by R. Willis. Printed for the Sydenham Society, London 1847.

Haworth, S. G. (1979). Pulmonary vascular structure in persistent fetal circulation. In *Paediatric Cardiology and Heart Disease in the Newborn*, ed. M.J. Godman & R.M. Marquis. pp. 67–68. Churchill Livingstone, Edinburgh.

Haworth, S. G. (1982). Total anomalous pulmonary venous return. Prenatal damage to pulmonary vascular bed and extrapulmonary veins. *British Heart Journal*, **48**, 513–24.

Haworth, S. G. & Reid, L. (1976). Persistent fetal circulation: newly recognised structural features. *Journal of Pediatrics*, **88**, 614–20.

Hislop, A. & Reid, L. (1981). Growth and development of the respiratory system-anatomical development. *Scientific Foundations of Paediatrics*, 2nd edn. Heineman, London.

James, L. S., Burnard, E. D. & Rowe, R. D. (1961). Abnormal shunting through the foramen ovale after birth. *American Journal of Diseases in Childhood*, **102**, 550.

James, L. S. & Rowe, R. D. (1957). The pattern of response of pulmonary and systemic arterial pressures in newborn and older infants to short periods of hypoxia. *Journal of Pediatrics,* **51**, 5–11.

Kitagawa, M., Hislop, A. A., Boyden, E. A. & Reid, L. (1971). Lung hypoplasia in congenital diaphragmatic hernia. *British Journal of Surgerty,* **58**, 342–6.

Lambert, E. C., Canent, R. V. & Hohn, A. R. (1966). Congenital cardiac anomalies in the newborn. A review of conditions causing death or severe distress in the first month of life. *Pediatrics,* **37**, 343–51.

Lees, M. H. & Sunderland, C. O. (1981). Diseases of the cardiovascular system. In *Neonatal Perinatal Medicine: Diseases of the Fetus and Infant,* ed. J. B. Behrman. p. 572. Lippincott, Philadelphia.

Levin, D. L., Fixler, D. E., Morriss, F. C. & Tyson, J. (1978). Morphologic analysis of the pulmonary vascular bed in infants exposed in utero to prostaglandin synthetase inhibitors. *Journal of Pediatrics,* **92**, 478–83.

Lind, J. & Wegelius, E. (1952). Changes in the circulation at birth. *Acta Pediatrica,* **42**, 495–6.

Lind, J. & Wegelius, C. (1954). Human fetal circulation: changes in the cardiovascular system at birth and disturbances in the postnatal closure of the foramen ovale and ductus arteriosus. *Cold Spring Harbor Symposia on Quantitative Biology,* **19**, 109–25.

McKenzie, S. & Haworth, S. G. (1981). Occlusion of peripheral pulmonary vascular bed in a baby with idiopathic fetal circulation. *British Heart Journal,* **46**, 675–8.

Mocellin, R., Sauer, U., Simon, B., Comazzi, M., Sebening, F. & Buhlmeyer, K. (1983). Reduced left ventricular size and endocardial fibrolastosis as correlates of mortality in newborns and young infants with severe aortic valve stenosis. *Pediatric Cardiology,* **4**, 265–72.

Novelo, S., Limon Lason, R. & Bouchard, F. (1950). Un nouveau syndrome avec cyanose congenitale: la persistence du canal arte rial avec hypertension pulmonaire. *Paris Les Congres Mondial de Cardiologie.*

Raine, J., Hislop, A. A., Redington, A. N., Haworth, S. G. & Shinebourne, E. A. (1991). Persistent pulmonary hypertension of the newborn. *Archives of Diseases in Childhood,* **66**, 398–402.

Riemenschneider, T. A., Nielsen, H. C., Ruttenberg, H. D. & Jaffe, R. B. (1976). Disturbances of the transitional circulation: spectrum of pulmonary hypertension and myocardial dysfunction. *Journal of Pediatrics,* **89**, 622–25.

Rowe, R. D. (1959). Clinical observation of transitional circulations. In *Adaptation to Extra-uterine Life.* Report of Thirty-First Ross Conference on Pediatric Research, ed. T.K. Oliver, p. 339, Ross Laboratories, Ohio.

Rudolph, A. M. (1974). Congenital diseases of the heart. Clinical-physiologic considerations in diagnosis and management. Year Book Medical Publishers Inc., 35, East Wacker Drive, Chicago.

Rudolph, A. M. (1981). Effects of aspirin and acetaminopher in pregnancy and in the newborn. *Archives of Internal Medicine,* **141**, 358–63.

Rudolph, A. M., Drorbaugh, J. E., Auld, P. A. M., Rudolph, A. J., Nadas, A. S., Smith, C. A. & Hubbell, J. P. (1961). Studies on the circulation in the neonatal period: the circulation in the respiratory distress syndrome. *Pediatrics,* **27**, 551–66.

Shankaran, S., Farooki, Z. Q. & Desai, R. (1982). B-haemolytic streptococcal infection appearing as persistent fetal circulation. *American Journal of Disease in Childhood,* **136**, 725–7.

Shannon, D. C., Lusser, M. & Goldblatt, A. (1972). The cyanotic infant-heart disease or lung disease? *New England Journal of Medicine,* **287**, 951–53.

Skidmore, M. B., Shennan, A. R. & Hoslans, E. M. (1985). Tolazoline in the treatment of persistent fetal circulation. In *Persistent Fetal Circulation: Etiology, Clinical, Manifestations and Therapy,* ed. G. S. Sandor, A. J. McNab & R. B. Ratogi, pp. 189–93, Ratogi Futura Medical Services, Mt Kisco.

Stahlman, M., Shepard, F. M., Young, W. C., Gray, J. & Blankenship, W. (1966). Assessment of the cardiovascular status of infants with hyaline membrane disease. In *The Heart and Circulation in the Newborn and Infant,* ed. D. E. Cassels. pp. 121–140. Grune & Stratton, New York & London.

Sullivan, I. D. & Gooch, V. M. (1991). Venous anomalies. In *Clinical Ultrasound,* ed. H. Meire, K. C. Dewbury, D. O. Cosgrove & P. Wilde, Churchill Livingstone, in press.

Wilkinson, A. R., Aynsley-Green, A. & Mitchell, M. D. (1979). Persistent pulmonary hypertension and abnormal prostaglandin E levels in preterm infants after maternal treatment with naproxen. *Archives of Diseases in Childhood,* **54**, 942–5.

Index

myocardial blood flow, fetal
  acute hypoxaemia 28–9, 57, 108, 109,
    206–7
  asphyxia 28–9, 35, 37, 38
  changes at birth 177–9
  chronic hypoxaemia 43, 219, 221
  factors controlling 107–8
  immature fetuses 45, 47
  normoxaemia 25, 26
myocardial contractility
  early postnatal 176
  fetal 144, 153–5
myocardial depression, fetal hypoxaemia
  51
myocytes, cardiac
  contractility 153, 154–5
  development 139–41
myofibrils 139–40, 141
myosin 139–40

naproxin 417
near infrared spectroscopy (NIRS)
  CBF 344, 347–50
  cerebral blood volume 353–6
  cerebral oxygenation 357–9
necrotizing enterocolitis 62
neonatal circulation 162, 180–9
  autonomic nervous system 183–5
  baroreceptor and chemoreceptor control
    182–3
  perinatal transitions 160, 166–80
  postnatal changes 180–1
  responses to stress 181–2
  sleep states and 187–9
  vasoactive agents 185–7
neonatal intensive care, umbilical artery
  FVWs and 327, 329, 331
neonates
  cerebral haemodynamics and
    oxygenation 339–60
  persistent fetal circulation, *see* persistent
    fetal circulation
  persistent pulmonary hypertension, *see*
    persistent pulmonary hypertension
    of newborn
neurodevelopmental outcome
  FHR monitoring and 291
  neonatal CBF and 345
neuronal death, hypoxaemia/asphyxia 56
neuropeptide Y (NPY) 54
nitroprusside 241
nitrous oxide (N_2O) 340
noradrenaline (norepinephrine)
  asphyxiated immature fetuses 46, 47
  cerebral artery diameter and 353
  fetal blood volume and 83, 86
  fetal heart 142

fetal hypoxaemia 61, 220
  neonates 184–5
  umbilical–placental blood flow and 105,
    205–6
nutrition, maternal
  adult/childhood blood pressure and
    260–2
  fetal arterial pressure and 17
Nyquist limit 299

oesophagus, fetal, ligation 92
Ohm's law, hydraulic equivalent 233
oncogenes, heart development and 386
opioids, endogenous 54, 208
organ blood flow
  changes at birth 177–80
  fetal 25, 26–7, 54–65, 166
    acute hypoxaemia 28–9, 30–4, 40–1,
     204, 205–9
    asphyxia 28–9, 34–40, 47, 54–65
    cardiac surgery 389–90
    chronic hypoxaemia 43, 219–22
    immature asphyxiated fetuses 45, 47
    mechanisms of redistribution 51–2
    tissue metabolism and 50
  neonatal hypoxaemia 181
  see also specific organs
osmolality
  intravascular infusions, fetal blood
    volume and 90
  maternal, fetal blood volume and 93–4
oxidative phosphorylation 356
oximetry, pulse 242
oxygen consumption (VO_2), fetal
  acute hypoxaemia/asphyxia 48–50, 124,
    125
  cerebral 55–6, 103
  chronic hypoxaemia 42, 220
  fetal carcass 62–3
  fetal placental blood flow and 120,
    124–6
  hepatic 58
  myocardial 57, 107–8
  placental 48, 49, 59
  renal 60
oxygen delivery (DO_2)
  cerebral, *see* cerebral oxygen delivery
  oxygen consumption and 48–50, 124,
    125
  reduced fetal, *see* fetal hypoxaemia/
    hypoxia
oxygen radicals, neuronal death and 56
oxygen saturation, arterial (SaO_2)
  cerebral oxygenation and 358
  near infrared spectroscopy 348, 349,
    350, 353–5